FallProof!

A Comprehensive Balance and Mobility Training Program

Debra J. Rose

California State University, Fullerton

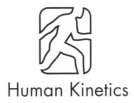

Human Kinetics

Library of Congress Cataloging-In-Publication Data

Rose, Debra J.
    FallProof! : a comprehensive balance and mobility training pro-
    gram / Debra J. Rose.
        p. ; cm.
    Includes bibliographical references and index.
    ISBN 0-7360-4088-9 (soft cover)
    1. Falls (Accidents) in old age--Prevention.   I. Title.
    [DNLM: 1. Accidental Falls--prevention & control--Aged. 2.
    Equilibrium--Aged. 3. Motor Skills--Aged. 4. Movement--Aged.
    5. Safety Management--Aged.   WT 104 R7953f 2003]
    RC952.5.R6657 2003
    617.1'0084'6--dc21   2003002621

ISBN: 0-7360-4088-9

Notice: Permission to reproduce the following material is granted to instructors and agencies who have purchased *FallProof! A Comprehensive Balance and Mobility Training Program*: pp. 18-20, 22-24, 51-54, 60, 64, 69-70, 73-76, 80, 82, 83-85, 245, 258, 266-268, 270. The reproduction of other parts of this book is expressly forbidden by the above copyright notice. Persons or agencies who have not purchased *FallProof! A Comprehensive Balance and Mobility Training Program* may not reproduce any material.

Permission notices for material reprinted in this book from other sources can be found on page x.

The Web addresses cited in this text were current as of February 21, 2003, unless otherwise noted.

Acquisitions Editor: Judy Patterson Wright, PhD; **Developmental Editor:** Rebecca Crist; **Assistant Editor:** Sandria M. Washington; **Copyeditor:** Barb Field; **Proofreader:** Sarah Wiseman; **Indexer:** Bobbi Swanson; **Permission Manager:** Dalene Reeder; **Graphic Designer:** Nancy Rasmus; **Graphic Artist:** Kim McFarland; **Photo Manager:** Kareema McLendon; **Cover Designer:** Robert Reuther; **Photographer (cover):** Titan Communications; **Photographer (interior):** Titan Communications, except where otherwise noted; **Art Manager:** Kelly Hendren; **Illustrator:** Accurate Art, Inc.; **Printer:** Custom Color Graphics

Printed in the United States of America   10   9   8   7   6   5   4   3   2   1

Human Kinetics
Web site: www.HumanKinetics.com

United States: Human Kinetics
P.O. Box 5076
Champaign, IL 61825-5076
800-747-4457
e-mail: humank@hkusa.com

Canada: Human Kinetics
475 Devonshire Road Unit 100
Windsor, ON N8Y 2L5
800-465-7301 (in Canada only)
e-mail: orders@hkcanada.com

Europe: Human Kinetics
107 Bradford Road
Stanningley
Leeds LS28 6AT, United Kingdom
+44 (0) 113 255 5665
e-mail: hk@hkeurope.com

Australia: Human Kinetics
57A Price Avenue
Lower Mitcham, South Australia
5062
08 8277 1555
e-mail: liahka@senet.com.au

New Zealand: Human Kinetics
P.O. Box 105-231
Auckland Central
09-523-3462
e-mail: hkp@ihug.co.nz

In memory of Liam,
a young man who possessed the wisdom
of an older adult

CONTENTS

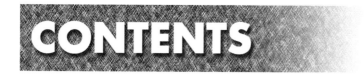

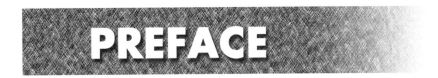

PREFACE

Maintaining a high level of balance and mobility is essential to aging successfully. In addition to making it possible to perform basic activities of daily living easily, such as rising from a chair or climbing a flight of stairs, good balance is the foundation on which a healthy and active lifestyle is built. Impairments in any of the multiple systems that contribute to postural stability will not only limit the extent and type of physical activities pursued as we grow older, but ultimately may result in falls, leading to further restrictions in activity and profound psychological consequences. This strong association between impairments in balance and mobility and increased falls suggests the need for activity-based programs that specifically *and* systematically focus on improving the multiple dimensions of the balance system, particularly among older adults.

FallProof! A Comprehensive Balance and Mobility Training Program is the first structured balance and mobility program to be published that not only provides the reader with the fundamental theoretical concepts and practical skills needed to assess and design effective activity programs for older adults with balance and mobility disorders, but also describes a comprehensive set of progressive balance activities that specifically address the important dimensions of balance and mobility. The program content in this instructor guide is based on sound, theoretical research, and a group-based version of the program has been extensively field-tested by many physical activity instructors and rehabilitation specialists working with older adults across a broad continuum of functional levels. The innovative balance and mobility program described in this book was developed at the Center for Successful Aging at California State University at Fullerton and is currently being implemented in numerous community-based and residential care settings with considerable success. Physical activity professionals who embrace this unique multidimensional programming approach to treating balance and mobility disorders can expect to achieve the same level of success.

FallProof! A Comprehensive Balance and Mobility Training Program is divided into three parts. Part I, The Theory Behind the Program, provides the reader with in-depth knowledge about the various body systems that contribute to balance and mobility and the common age-related changes occurring in each of these systems. The external and internal risk factors known to be strongly associated with the increased incidence of falls in the older adult population are also discussed, as well as the common medical conditions and medications known to adversely affect balance and mobility.

Part II of the instructor guide begins by describing a comprehensive set of balance and mobility assessments used to evaluate every client prior to entering the FallProof™ program and at regular intervals throughout the program. This assessment is designed to measure the multiple dimensions of balance and mobility and provide the instructor with the information needed to determine the starting level for each participant in each of the six major program components. These components, described in the remainder of part II, include (1) center-of-gravity control training, (2) multisensory training, (3) postural strategy training, (4) gait pattern enhancement and variation training, (5) strength and endurance training, and (6) flexibility training. In addition to a set of progressive exercises for each component of the program, ideas for increasing the challenge associated with each balance activity are included in each chapter. Advanced progressions are based on manipulating the demands of the task and the environment to progressively challenge the individual's capabilities. At-a-glance summary tables are also provided at the end of each chapter to further guide the less experienced instructor.

Part III of the book describes how to implement the FallProof program. The first chapter in this part describes contemporary motor learning principles that will enable instructors to foster optimal learning, develop effective lesson plans, organize the classroom environment for optimal safety and efficiency, and provide meaningful feedback to program participants. The second and final chapter describes the leadership and class management skills needed to be a successful FallProof instructor. It covers the important activities that must be completed (a) following the initial assessment of program participants and prior to the start of the program, (b) prior to the start of each class, (c) during each class session, (d) between class sessions, and (e) after each follow-up assessment. It also describes how to communicate effectively with program participants.

This instructor guide will be an invaluable resource for experienced health care professionals and physical activity instructors who want to acquire the specialized knowledge and practical skills needed to develop and implement programs directed at improving the balance and mobility of older adults. The wide range of exercise progressions described and the ideas for further increasing the challenge associated with the exercises following each set of progressions makes *FallProof! A Comprehensive Balance and Mobility Training Program* a versatile instructional guide in programming for older adults representing a broad range of functional levels. Although physical activity instructors who have not yet completed the academic and practical skills training needed to work with at-risk older adults can also use this instructor guide to learn how to incorporate more balance and mobility exercises into their senior fitness programs, they should not consider developing specialty balance and mobility programs for at-risk older adults until they have completed additional training in the area.

FallProof! A Comprehensive Balance and Mobility Training Program represents the first systematic effort to develop a structured and progressive program of activities specifically designed to address the multiple dimensions that contribute to balance and mobility. Heartfelt thanks are extended to the Archstone Foundation of California for providing the generous funding necessary to test the efficacy of this program in a large number of community-based centers serving the needs of older adults. Thanks also to the Retirement Research Foundation for providing additional funding to examine the long-term efficacy of the program in residential care facilities throughout southern California.

The Archstone Foundation has also provided the Center for Successful Aging at Cal State Fullerton with additional funding for implementation of an instructor certification program designed to provide health care professionals with the specialized knowledge needed to implement this program in their immediate communities. This instructor guide serves as the core text for the balance and mobility instructor specialist certification program that began operating at Cal State Fullerton in 2001. Readers interested in developing their knowledge and practical skills in the area of balance and mobility so they can successfully implement the FallProof program should consider enrolling in this certification program. The program is staffed by an outstanding group of experienced kinesiologists and physical therapists with expertise in the area of geriatric assessment and rehabilitation. Information about the certification program and an on-line application can be obtained by logging onto the Center for Successful Aging Web site at http://hdcs.fullerton.edu/csa.

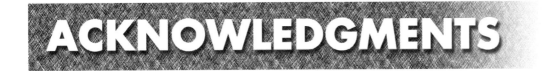

ACKNOWLEDGMENTS

I could not have completed this book without the help and support of many wonderful colleagues within the kinesiology and physical therapy profession. Special thanks are extended to Leslie Allison, PT; Janene Burton, PT; Dr. Courtney Hall, PhD, PT; Laura Morris, PT; and Dr. Peggy Trueblood, PhD, PT, whom I have had the pleasure of teaching with and learning from over the past 10 years. I would also like to thank the many instructors who have been certified to teach the FallProof program over the past two years for providing me with invaluable feedback on the early versions of this book and the program itself as they implemented it in their communities. Special thanks also to two outside reviewers, Judy Aprile and Leslie Kranz, who critically reviewed the book from the perspective of the instructor, and to the editorial staff at Human Kinetics, who waited patiently for me to send the final manuscript. Thanks also to the wonderful group of older adults who served as models for the book: Rodolfo Amaya, Lou Arnwine, Myrt and John Brothers, Fritz von Coelln, Ann Gardner, Connie Haddad, Carlos Estrada, Mio Sakai, and Ann Siebert. Finally, I would like to thank Dr. Jessie Jones, PhD, a wonderful colleague and "best" friend, who has encouraged and supported me in every way since my arrival at California State University, Fullerton.

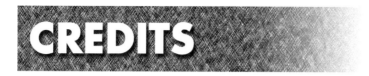

CREDITS

Figures

Figure 1.3 Dynamic Equilibrium Model reprinted, by permission, from NeuroCom International.

Figure 1.4 a-d Courtesy of the National Eye Institute, National Institutes of Health.

Figure 1.5 Reprinted from the Center for Successful Aging at California State University, Fullerton. Question 18 of this form is reprinted, by permission, from R. Rikli and J. Jones, 1999, "The reliability and validity of a 6-minute walk test as a measure of physical endurance in older adults," *Journal of Aging and Physical Activity,* 6: 367.

Figure 1.6 Reprinted from the Center for Successful Aging at California State University, Fullerton. Question 18 of this form is reprinted, by permission, from R. Rikli and J. Jones, 1999, "The reliability and validity of a 6-minute walk test as a measure of physical endurance in older adults," *Journal of Aging and Physical Activity,* 6: 367.

Figure 3.1 Reprinted, by permission, from R. Rikli and J. Jones, 1999, "Development and validation of a functional fitness test for community-residing older adults," *Journal of Aging and Physical Activity,* 7: 132.

Tables

Table 2.1 Reprinted from "Falls as risk factors for fractures," J.A. Grisso, E. Capezuti, and A. Schwartz, in *Osteoporosis,* R. Marcus, D. Feldman, and J. Kelsey (Eds.), pp. 599-611, Copyright 1996, with permission from Elsevier.

Table 2.2 Reprinted from "Falls as risk factors for fractures," J.A. Grisso, E. Capezuti, and A. Schwartz, in *Osteoporosis,* R. Marcus, D. Feldman, and J. Kelsey (Eds.), pp. 599-611, Copyright 1996, with permission from Elsevier.

Table 2.3 Reprinted, by permission, from *Assessment of Fracture Risk and Its Application to Screening for Postmenopausal Osteoporosis,* 1994, WHO Technical Report Series, No. 843 (Geneva, Switzerland: World Health Organization).

Table 3.1 Adapted, by permission, from R. Rikli and J. Jones, 2001, *Senior Fitness Test Manual* (Champaign, IL: Human Kinetics), 61-73.

Table 3.7 Reprinted from R. Bohannon, "Comfortable and maximum walking speed of adults aged 20-79 years: Reference values and determinants," *Age and Aging,* 1997, 26: 17, by permission of the Oxford University Press.

Boxes

Test Administration Procedures for the 50-ft Walk (p. 79) Reprinted by permission of the Center for Successful Aging at California State University, Fullerton.

Forms

Form 3.1 Reprinted by permission of the Center for Successful Aging at California State University, Fullerton. Question 18 of this form is reprinted, by permission, from R. Rikli and J. Jones, 1999, "The reliability and validity of a 6-minute walk test as a measure of physical endurance in older adults," *Journal of Aging and Physical Activity,* 6: 367.

Form 3.5 Reprinted, by permission, from K. Berg, 1992, *Measuring Balance in the Elderly: Development and Validation of an Instrument,* Dissertation. (Montreal, Canada: McGill University).

Form 3.8 Reprinted by permission of the Center for Successful Aging at California State University, Fullerton.

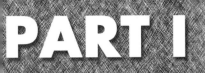

The Theory Behind the Program

Understanding Balance and Mobility

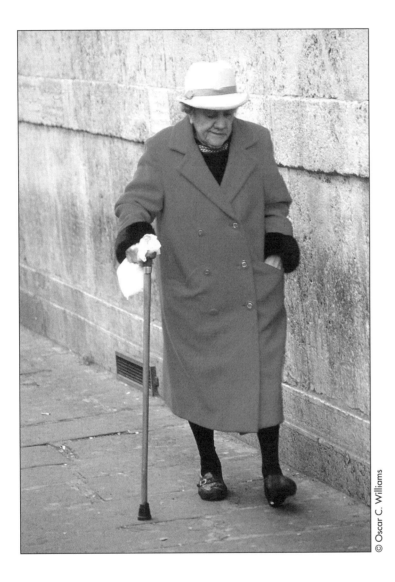

© Oscar C. Williams

Objectives

After completing this chapter, you will be able to

- describe important terminology used in the study of balance and mobility,
- identify the multiple systems that contribute to postural stability, and
- describe the major age-related changes in balance and mobility.

The successful control of balance depends on a series of complex processes that are triggered by either a conscious or unconscious decision to act. Our decision to act may be in response to an internal desire to perform a certain task, to sensory events occurring in the environment that require action, or a combination of the two. Although many of the decisions we make during the day are made at a conscious level, such as rising from a chair to answer the door or walk to the neighborhood store to purchase milk, others are made at a subconscious level. These more subconscious responses are most often associated with well-learned skills that require little or no conscious attention or with the need to respond rapidly to an unexpected event that threatens our stability. Whether the decision to act is a conscious or subconscious one, multiple systems within the body are involved.

What Is Balance?

center of mass (COM)—The point at which all the mass of a body may be considered to be concentrated in analyzing the forces that act on it and the body's motion. Also referred to as the center of gravity (COG) because the gravitational force due to the weight of the body also acts through this point.

Balance can be defined as the process by which we control the body's **center of mass (COM)** with respect to the base of support, whether it is stationary or moving. For example, when standing upright in space, our primary goal is to maintain the COM within the confines of the base of support, whereas when we are walking, we are continuously moving the COM beyond the base of support and reestablishing a new base of support with each step taken. Although we often consider standing upright in space to be a static balance task and leaning through space or walking as dynamic balance tasks, remember that maintaining a stable upright position also involves the active contraction of various muscle groups to control the position of the COM against the destabilizing force of gravity.

Important Terminology

balance—Process by which we control the body's center of mass with respect to the base of support, whether it is stationary or moving.

Inevitably, when we are first introduced to a new area of study, we are overwhelmed by the many new and unfamiliar terms presented. As you read each of the chapters in this instructor guide, you too will be confronted by many new terms that are specific to the study of balance and mobility. In addition to understanding what is meant by the term **balance,** which was defined at the outset of this chapter, other important terms you will need to be able to define include posture, anticipatory and reactive postural control, stability limits, the sway envelope, and mobility.

Good **posture** is critical to good balance and refers to the biomechanical alignment of each of our body parts as well as the orientation of the body to the environment (Shumway-Cook & Woollacott, 2001). When we are standing quietly in space, our goal is to align each of the body parts vertically and thereby expend the least amount of internal energy necessary to maintain an upright and stable position relative to gravity. To counteract the forces of gravity, a number of muscles are active during quiet standing (see figure 1.1). These include the soleus and gastrocnemius muscles, the tibialis anterior (when the body sways in a backward direction), the gluteus medius and tensor fasciae latae, the iliopsoas, the erector spinae muscles in the thoracic region of the trunk, and the abdominal muscles, somewhat more intermittently (Basmajian & De Luca, 1985).

posture—Refers to the biomechanical alignment of the individual body parts as well as the orientation of the body to the environment.

anticipatory postural control—Advance planning of actions.

Although many of the balance- and mobility-related activities we perform allow us to consciously plan our actions in advance, there will be times when an unexpected event forces us to respond more subconsciously or automatically. Anticipatory postural control is the term often used to describe those actions that can be planned in advance, whereas reactive postural control is a term used to describe those situations that cannot be planned in advance of action being required. **Antici-**

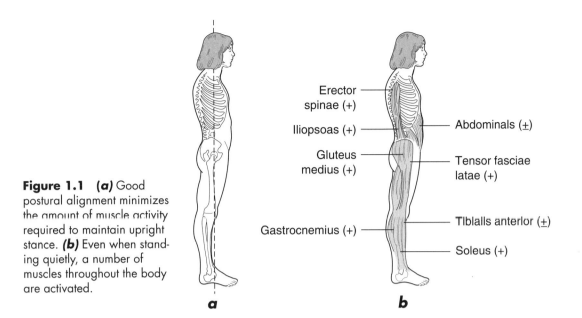

Figure 1.1 (*a*) Good postural alignment minimizes the amount of muscle activity required to maintain upright stance. (*b*) Even when standing quietly, a number of muscles throughout the body are activated.

patory postural control is used to avoid obstacles in our path as we walk to the store or run through the forest. It also assists us in adapting our gait pattern as we move between different types of surfaces (e.g., firm to compliant or moving surfaces, wide to narrow surfaces). In contrast, **reactive postural control** becomes necessary when we have to respond quickly to an event we did not expect (e.g., stepping in an unseen hole, being bumped in a crowd). Many exercises in chapters 4 and 5 are designed to help your older adult clients improve both of these abilities.

How far older adults are willing or able to lean in any direction without having to change their base of support constitutes their stability limits. Estimates are that people who are able to align their COM directly above their base of support during quiet standing can sway as much as 12° in a forward and backward direction and 16° laterally before it is necessary to take a step because their **stability limits** have been exceeded (Nashner, 1990). Of course, this **sway envelope,** as it is called, is often much smaller among older adults who are beginning to experience balance problems. Reduced or asymmetric limits of stability may be the result of such factors as musculoskeletal abnormalities caused by weakness in the muscles of the ankle joint or reduced range of motion about the ankles, neurological trauma that has resulted in muscle weakness that affects movement in a particular direction (i.e., stroke, Parkinson's disease, multiple sclerosis), or a fear of falling.

Although the boundaries of the stability limits will vary according to an individual's inherent biomechanical limitations, the task being performed, or the constraints of the environment, a significant reduction in those limits, particularly in the lateral and backward direction, will place the older adult at a heightened risk for falling. Any small disruption to standing balance in these older adults will quickly move them beyond their limits of stability and require that they reach for something close by or take one or more steps to prevent a fall.

Finally, **mobility** has been defined as the ability to move oneself independently and safely from one place to another (Shumway-Cook & Woollacott, 2001). Adequate levels of mobility are required for many different types of activities we perform in our daily lives. These may include transfers (e.g., rising from a chair, climbing or descending stairs), walking or running, and other types of recreational activities (e.g., gardening, sport, dancing).

reactive postural control—Actions that cannot be planned in advance due to the unexpected nature of an event.

stability limits—The maximum distance an individual is able or willing to lean in any direction without changing the base of support.

sway envelope—The path of the body's movement during a standing balance activity.

mobility—The ability to move independently and safely from one place to another.

Postural Control Strategies Used to Control Balance

ankle strategy—The body moves as a single entity about the ankle joints (i.e., upper and lower body sway in the same direction).

Studies conducted over the years have revealed the existence of at least three distinct postural control strategies that are commonly used to control the amount of body sway. These strategies are referred to as the ankle, hip, and step strategies (see figure 1.2). In the ankle strategy, the body moves as a single entity about the ankle joints as force is exerted against the surface. What you see when you watch a person using an **ankle strategy** is the upper and lower body moving in the same direction, or in phase. Because the amount of force that can be generated by the muscles surrounding the ankle joint is relatively small, this strategy is generally used to control sway when we are standing upright in space or swaying through a very small range of motion. The ankle strategy is also used at a subconscious level to restore balance following a small nudge or push.

hip strategy—The upper and lower body move in opposite directions as a result of the hip muscles being activated to control balance.

In contrast to the ankle strategy, the **hip strategy** involves activation of the larger hip muscles and is used when the COG must be moved more quickly back over the base of support as the speed or distance of the sway increase. When you watch a person using a hip strategy, you will see them move the upper body in a direction that is opposite to the lower body (i.e., out of phase). The hip strategy becomes increasingly important as the speed and distance of sway increase or when we are standing on a surface that is narrower than the length of our feet. In these surface conditions, we can no longer use the ankle strategy because there is not enough surface against which to push in order to generate sufficient force to restore balance using the smaller ankle muscles.

step strategy—Occurs when the COG is displaced beyond the maximal stability limits or sway is too great to use a hip strategy effectively. Requires that a new base of support be established.

The final postural control strategy used to control balance is the **step strategy.** This strategy comes into play when the COG is displaced beyond our maximum limits of stability or the speed of sway is so fast that a hip strategy is insufficient to maintain the COG within the stability limits. In this situation, a new base of support must be

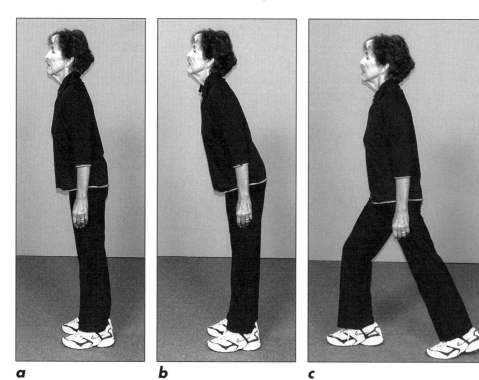

a   **b**   **c**

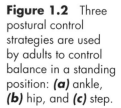

Figure 1.2 Three postural control strategies are used by adults to control balance in a standing position: **(a)** ankle, **(b)** hip, and **(c)** step.

established if we are to prevent a fall. When executing a step strategy, a person takes at least one or more steps in the direction of the loss of balance. Although each of the movement strategies described in this section are represented as distinct movement patterns, it has also been shown that various combinations of these strategies are used to control forward and backward sway in a standing position (Horak & Nashner, 1986).

What factors are likely to limit our ability to use each of these three movement strategies? In the case of the ankle strategy, adequate range of motion and strength within the muscles surrounding the ankle joint are needed. The surface beneath the feet must also be firm and broad, and the individual must have adequate sensation in the feet to be able to feel the surface. Older adults experiencing a significant decline in sensation in the feet or ankles will find it particularly difficult to employ this strategy.

An effective ankle strategy requires

- adequate range of motion and strength in the ankle joints,
- a firm, broad surface below the feet, and
- an adequate level of sensation in the feet and ankles.

Unlike the ankle strategy, our ability to use a hip strategy to control postural sway will be determined more by the amount of muscle strength and range of motion we have in the hip region as opposed to the ankle. Sway in the lateral direction is also controlled by the hip, particularly the adductor and abductor muscle groups. Any weakness in these muscles will adversely affect lateral stability, an important requirement when walking.

An effective hip strategy requires adequate range of motion and strength in the hip region.

As mentioned earlier, the stepping strategy is most likely to be observed when the boundaries of our stability are exceeded. The ability to use this particular movement strategy effectively will be greatly affected by both the amount of lower limb strength available and the speed with which it can be generated (that is, the power) for rapid initiation of the step. Slowed central processing will also adversely affect an older adult's ability to use this strategy effectively. In addition, reduced range of motion at the hip joint will be a factor in determining the length of step we are able to take following a loss of balance.

An effective step strategy requires

- adequate lower body muscle strength, power, and range of motion,
- adequate central processing speed, and
- the ability to move the limb rapidly during step initiation.

The postural strategy training component of the FallProof program (see chapter 6) contains many progressive exercises that are designed to improve the participants' ability to use each of the three movement strategies just described. The primary focus in this component of the program is to help participants learn to select the appropriate movement strategy and scale it in a way that best matches the demands of the task they are being asked to perform and the environment in which it is being performed.

Multiple Systems Contribute to Balance and Mobility

Multiple systems contribute to our ability to maintain balance in standing and moving environments. First, the various sensory systems (i.e., vision, somatosensory, and vestibular) provide us with information arising from the surrounding environment and resulting from our own actions. This information is critical for successful goal-directed action planning as well as the subconscious or automatic adjustments needed to maintain a given position in space or respond rapidly to a change in task or environmental demands. We use our sensory systems to anticipate changes that will affect action, as well as to respond to changes that have already occurred. The many structures within the nervous system that make up the motor system are also critical for action. The motor system acts on the sensory information arising from the external environment as well as other sensory areas within the nervous system. Action is accomplished as a result of the nervous system constraining groups of muscles throughout the body to act together. These are referred to as **muscle response synergies** and are responsible for the many coordinated actions we are able to produce in our daily lives. Finally, the cognitive system plays an important role in helping us appropriately interpret the incoming sensations and plan the ensuing motor response. This system, which encompasses the processes of attention, memory storage, and intelligence, provides us with the collective ability to anticipate or adapt our actions in response to changing task demands and the environment.

muscle response synergies—Groups of muscles constrained to act together.

> Our sensory systems are used to anticipate changes that will affect action as well as respond to changes that have already occurred.
>
> The motor system acts on internally and externally provided sensory information.

As indicated earlier, three sensory systems are particularly important for good postural control and largely determine how well we perceive what needs to be done based on the information presented to us. These are the visual, somatosensory, and vestibular systems. Although no individual system provides us with all the sensory information we need to determine our position in space, each system contributes its own unique and important kind of information about body position and movement to the central nervous system (CNS). Each system also responds to different types of incoming information. Whereas vision responds to light, the somatosensory system is sensitive to touch, vibration, and pain, and the vestibular system responds to movements of the head.

We depend most heavily on the visual system for information about our movements and where we are in space. Not only does this system provide us with a visual layout of the environment around us, but it also provides us with critical information about our spatial location relative to objects within that environment. Once we begin moving through space, vision also helps us to navigate safely, anticipate changes in surfaces we encounter, and avoid obstacles in our path. It is therefore a very important source of mobility information.

In contrast to the visual system, the somatosensory system provides us with information about the spatial location and movement of our body relative to the support surface beneath us. It also informs us about the position and movement of body segments relative to each other. This latter information is provided by important proprioceptors located in the muscles and joints throughout the body (e.g., muscle spindles, joint receptors). In the absence of vision, the somatosensory system becomes our primary source of sensory information for maintaining upright balance and moving about in dark environments.

> The somatosensory system provides us with information about our spatial location and movement of the body relative to the support surface.

The final sensory system that provides us with important balance information is the vestibular system. This delicate balance mechanism is housed in the inner ear and is activated when we move our head. It also works in conjunction with the visual system to help us determine whether the world or we are moving when we turn quickly in space. It becomes particularly important for maintaining upright balance when sensory information usually received by the visual and somatosensory systems is no longer available, distorted, or inaccurate.

> The vestibular system, in conjunction with the visual system, helps us determine whether the world or we are moving.

Once the information derived from each of the three sensory systems has been organized and integrated by the central nervous system, and we have determined where we are in space and what we wish to do, the various structures constituting the motor system, in collaboration with the musculoskeletal system, are responsible for generating the appropriate action plan. As we begin to act, the sensory systems continue to receive additional information from the environment and our own movement response so we can quickly modify our current plan of action, change to an alternative plan, or begin planning the next one. This intricate and continuous interplay between the sensory and motor systems is often referred to as the perception-action cycle. Whereas the sensory systems give rise to a perception that is used to guide our initial action, the results of that initial action generated by the motor system are then used to alter or confirm the accuracy of the original perception. This perception-action cycle is illustrated in figure 1.3.

This dynamic equilibrium model, as it is called, was developed by Nashner (1990) as a means of describing each of the processes occurring in the peripheral and central components of the sensory and motor systems that characterize the perception-action cycle. The visual, somatosensory, and vestibular receptors constitute the peripheral component of the sensory system, and the transmission pathways and specialized areas within the CNS constitute the central components of the sensory system. It is in this central component that the information received from the environment via our visual, somatosensory, and vestibular receptors is compared, selected, and then combined so that we can finally determine the position of our body in space.

Once we have determined where we are in space, we begin the process of determining what we are going to do, if anything, on the basis of the information received. This action-planning process begins within the central component of the motor system with the selection of the various muscle groups we will need to carry out the plan of action, as well as the specific muscle contractile patterns necessary to accomplish the intended movement. That movement may be as simple as standing quietly in space or as complicated as running over uneven terrain. The many different groups of muscles throughout the body that make up the peripheral component of the motor system will ultimately be responsible for generating the desired movement.

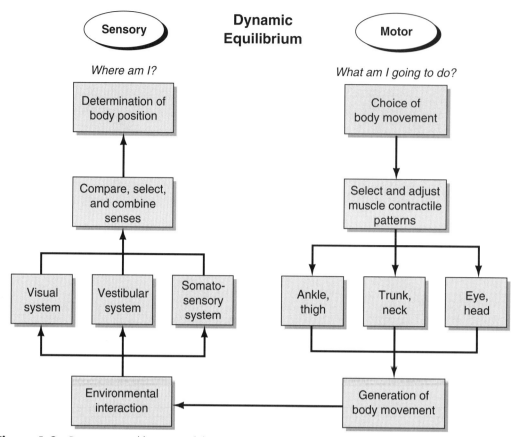

Figure 1.3 Dynamic equilibrium model.
Reprinted from NeuroCom International.

Both the speed and accuracy of the movement generated in response to incoming sensory information will also be influenced by how well we are able to remember what we are supposed to do in a given situation and our ability to allocate our attentional resources, particularly when we are required to perform more than one task at a time. Any impairments in cognition or attention will severely compromise our ability to accurately perceive what type of response is needed and then effectively implement the response, or responses, once selected. Not only has it been well documented that older adults with cognitive impairment experience a more rapid decline in function following an acute illness or hospitalization, but they also experience many more falls than their noncognitively impaired peers (Leape, 2000; van Dijk, Meulenberg, van de Sande & Habbema, 1993).

Several research studies have also demonstrated that older adults must allocate more attention to the task of balancing, particularly when less sensory information is available (Shumway-Cook & Woollacott, 2000). Distributing attention between two cognitive tasks has also been found to be increasingly difficult for older adults, and more so among older adults with identified balance impairments or a history of falls (Shumway-Cook, Baldwin, Polissar & Gruber, 1997; Brauer, Woollacott & Shumway-Cook, 2002).

Older adults must allocate more attention to the task of balancing.

As a balance and mobility instructor, you need to understand not only which body systems contribute to postural stability but also how each system works in collaboration with other systems to solve the many balance problems we are faced with on a daily basis. This knowledge is fundamental to your understanding of the six core components that make up the FallProof™ program. Not only are each of the six program components intended to address the dimensions of balance and mobility just described, but the progression of exercises from an easy to more difficult level of challenge will accommodate the heterogeneous capabilities of participants within each program component.

Age-Associated Changes in the Systems Contributing to Balance and Mobility

Unfortunately, changes in the body systems that contribute to balance and mobility are an inevitable consequence of aging. Although some of the changes occurring in any one of these systems will have no observable effect on how well we perform balance-related tasks across a variety of environments, other changes, particularly those that affect multiple systems, will not only influence the type of strategy we use to perform certain tasks, but even whether we choose to perform those tasks at all. The types of environments in which we are prepared to perform those tasks may also change depending on the severity of the age-associated changes we experience.

> Changes in the body systems that contribute to balance and mobility are an inevitable consequence of aging.

The structural and functional changes that occur within the CNS with advancing age appear to have the most profound and observable effect on motor function as a whole. When older adults are compared to younger adults across a variety of motor tasks, significant differences are evident in the speed with which older adults initiate and execute movements, particularly when the number of response choices available and the complexity of the movement to be performed increase (Spirduso, 1995). Qualitative differences in the strategy used to accomplish the goal of the movement are also evident in some cases.

Despite the many age-associated structural and functional changes occurring within the central and peripheral nervous systems, not all changes occurring within specific regions necessarily result in observable or adverse effects on our behavior. That is because optimal motor function is achieved through the interaction of multiple systems both within and external to the CNS. When multiple systems become impaired, however, the quality of the interaction between the impaired systems declines and results in observable motor dysfunction. For example, although adverse changes occurring in the visual system make it more difficult to use visual information for balance, information from the somatosensory and vestibular systems can be used to compensate for the impaired visual system in most situations. When one or both of the two remaining sensory systems become impaired, however, the ability to organize and integrate sensory information is severely affected. Not only does our perception of the surrounding environment and our position in space become inadequate or inaccurate, but our ability to respond appropriately is also compromised.

> Optimal motor function is achieved through the interaction of multiple systems that are internal and external to the CNS.

At a behavioral level, these cumulative changes in the aging nervous system appear to manifest themselves in a reduced ability to perform a variety of complex movements that require speed and accuracy, balance, strength, or coordination. Let's now describe the age-related changes occurring in the peripheral and central components of the sensory and motor systems illustrated in Nashner's dynamic equilibrium model (see figure 1.3).

Changes in the Peripheral and Central Components of the Sensory System

Age-related changes in the peripheral and central components of the visual, somato-sensory, and vestibular systems can be expected to affect our balance and mobility most adversely because of the interdependency that exists among the processing of incoming sensory information, the selection of an appropriate motor response, and its subsequent control. As illustrated in figure 1.3, the peripheral receptors associated with each sensory system are responsible for the initial reception and transmission of sensory information that arises from our interaction with the environment, whereas the sensory areas constituting the central component of the sensory system are responsible for comparing, selecting, and combining the incoming sensory information from each system so that we can determine where we are in space and what we need to do, if anything, in response to it. This sensory information, once organized and integrated within the central sensory areas of the brain, will then be used to guide the selection of the ensuing motor response.

Age-Related Changes in Vision

Common age-related changes in the peripheral component of the visual system include reduced acuity, depth perception, contrast sensitivity, and narrowing of the visual field, particularly in the peripheral region. These changes will, in turn, alter the quality of the information received within the central component of the system and result in slower processing of the incoming sensory feedback, poor integration of sensory inputs, and an altered perception of the body's position in space.

At a behavioral level, these age-related changes occurring within the visual system can be expected to adversely affect the older adult's ability to accurately perceive or anticipate changes in normal surface conditions and the presence of hazards in the environment. As a result, the ability to avoid obstacles, negotiate curbs and stairs, and efficiently move about in conditions of low or changing light will be adversely affected. Decrements within the visual system, particularly within the peripheral visual field, have also been associated with increased risk for falls among older adults.

> Age-related changes in the visual system will adversely affect an older adult's ability to accurately perceive or anticipate changes in surface conditions or the presence of hazards in the environment.

The increasing prevalence of eye diseases such as cataracts, glaucoma, and macular degeneration among older adults has also been associated with increasing fall rates (Nevitt, Cummings, Kidd & Black, 1989). When combined with normal age-related changes occurring within the visual system, the presence of any of these diseases will further compromise the quality of an older adult's vision. Examples of how these eye diseases affect the quality of what an older adult is able to see are illustrated in figure 1.4.

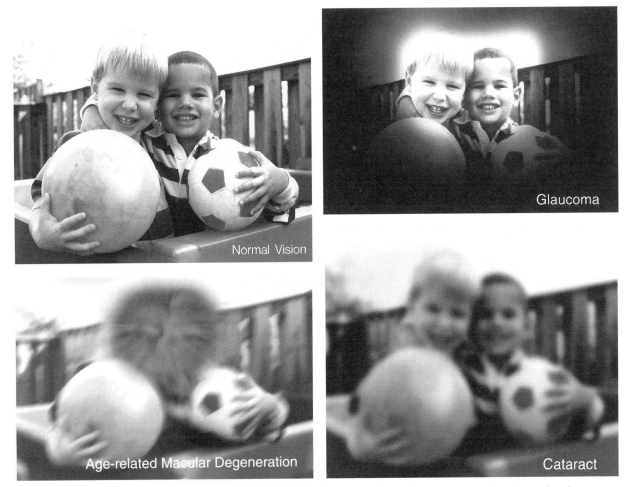

Normal Vision

Glaucoma

Age-related Macular Degeneration

Cataract

Figure 1.4 Normal vision may be adversely affected by diseases such as glaucoma, age-related macular degeneration, or cataracts.
Courtesy of the National Eye Institute, National Institutes of Health.

Age-Related Changes in Somatosensation

Age-related changes within the peripheral component of the somatosensory system have also been shown to directly affect postural stability and the ability to restore upright control following a loss of balance. A two- to tenfold increase in **vibration threshold,** indicating a reduced ability to feel the quality of contact between themselves and the surface beneath them, has been well documented among older adults (Perret & Reglis, 1970). Age-related changes in muscle spindle activity primarily and joint receptor activity to a lesser degree are also believed to influence postural control. As mentioned earlier, proprioceptors found within the muscles and joints provide us with information relative to the static and changing position of our joints in space and are therefore important for optimal balance and mobility.

vibration threshold—The level at which the somatosensory receptor begins to fire in response to the application of a vibratory stimulus.

Age-Related Changes in the Vestibular System

A gradually decreasing density of hair cells within the vestibular system begins as early as age 30 and progresses through older adulthood. These **hair cells** serve as biological sensors of head motion. Therefore, any significant reduction in their number reduces our sensitivity to head movements and will result in increased sway, particularly when vision is no longer available and information from the somatosensory system is distorted. A moderate reduction in the gain of the **vestibulo-ocular reflex**

hair cells—Biologic sensors within the vestibular system that are mechanically deformed (bent) when the head moves, causing neural impulses to be generated.

vestibulo-ocular reflex (VOR)—Reflex responsible for rotating the eyes in a direction that is equal and opposite to the direction of head movement.

(VOR) has also been noted with age. Because this reflex helps us stabilize our vision when we move our heads quickly in space, any impairment in the VOR will affect our ability to accurately determine whether it is the world or we who are moving in certain situations.

In addition to helping us correctly align our head and body with respect to gravity, the vestibular system becomes critical for balance when sensory information from the visual system is absent or when information from the visual and somatosensory systems is distorted or in conflict. For example, we rely heavily on our vestibular system for balance when we are moving around in a very dark environment and on a compliant or unstable surface. The vestibular system also helps resolve the conflict that often arises between the sensory systems when we find ourselves in complex visual environments (e.g., crowded malls, freeway traffic). For example, how often have you found yourself depressing the brake in your stationary car because you have erroneously thought that your car was rolling backward? What has actually happened is that the car next to you has begun to move forward and tricked your visual system into thinking that you are the one moving, even though the somatosensory and vestibular systems are signaling that you are not moving.

> The vestibular system becomes critical for balance when the sensory information from the visual system is absent, or when information from the visual and somatosensory systems is distorted or in conflict.

Older adults who are already experiencing balance problems may often comment on how much they dislike going into crowded malls or grocery stores because they feel increasingly unsteady due to people constantly moving in and out of their visual field. Many older adults compensate for this unsteadiness by pushing a shopping cart through the store to help stabilize them better, whereas others simply avoid these types of sensory environments. They are clearly experiencing difficulty resolving the conflict among the three sensory systems because they are no longer able to identify and then quickly ignore the conflicting input from the visual and somatosensory systems. Older adults with dysfunctional vestibular systems may also frequently report that they are experiencing visual problems, feel dizzy or unsteady, or are experiencing unusual sensory illusions when confronted with a conflicting sensory environment (Wolfson et al., 1997).

> Sensory conflict occurs when information provided by one or more sensory systems is not in agreement with one or both of the other sensory systems.

Changes in the Central and Peripheral Components of the Motor System

Changes in the central component of the motor system as a function of age have been well documented. Chronometric measures (i.e., reaction time, movement time, and response time) used to quantify the time required to plan and execute actions have revealed the most significant age-related declines to be in the action-planning phase (the time when incoming sensory information is processed and an appropriate motor response formulated) (Spirduso, 1995). Many older adults also begin to experience difficulty selecting the appropriate movement strategy to use in a given situation. Inappropriate scaling of the response strategy is also commonly observed in older adults; that is, we see a tendency among older adults to over- or underrespond, particularly when they are perturbed. They might overrespond by immediately taking a step, even though the loss of balance was small, or might underrespond to a larger perturbation by not stepping at all.

Electromyographic (EMG) studies have further revealed significant age-related differences in the temporal sequencing of muscle activation patterns in response to unexpected **perturbations.** Unlike the stereotypical and symmetrical responses of their younger counterparts, healthy older adults apparently exhibit considerably more variable activation patterns and a reduced ability to inhibit inappropriate responses (Stelmach, Phillips, DiFabio & Teasdale, 1989). Inappropriate postural responses are most evident when the functional base of support is reduced, the support surface is compliant or unstable, or visual input is altered (Alexander, 1994).

perturbation—A disturbance to a system. The disturbance may be external or internal in origin.

> The inappropriate scaling of response strategies is commonly observed in older adults.

Finally, older adults appear to lose their ability to anticipate changes in the environment or the demands associated with a task as they age. This loss of anticipatory postural control is no doubt a result of declining processing speeds within both the peripheral and central components of the sensory system and the central component of the motor system. This age-associated change will be most evident when older adults are asked to start or stop quickly, transition between different surfaces (i.e., firm to compliant surface), or negotiate obstacles in their environment. Instead of a smooth and continuous stepping action, you are more likely to see a marked slowing in gait speed as an obstacle is approached and a brief pause before the stepping action is initiated. Be sure to watch for this changing behavior during your initial assessment of the older adult so you can better match the difficulty of the exercise selected to the individual's capabilities.

Age-associated changes in the musculoskeletal component of the motor system also result in longer movement execution times. Decreases in muscular strength, particularly in the lower body, have been well documented. Between the ages of 50 and 70, muscle strength has been shown to decline as much as 30%, with even larger decreases noted after age 80 (Lindle et al., 1997). This decline is thought to be largely due to a decrease in both the size and number of muscle fibers. Physical inactivity also contributes to the loss of muscle strength, particularly in the antigravity or postural muscles required for good upright posture. **Muscle endurance** (i.e., muscle's ability to contract continuously at a submaximal level) also decreases with age. This decrease results in an earlier onset of fatigue during activity that will place an older adult at heightened risk for a loss of balance or a fall. Finally, **muscle power** (i.e., the ability to forcefully contract the muscle in a very short time) also decreases with age. This age-related change in muscle probably has the greatest consequence for the performance of basic activities such as walking, climbing stairs, or rising from a chair because all of these activities require muscle power for their successful completion. Certainly a decline in muscle power is an important contributing factor to an older adult's inability to respond quickly and effectively to an unexpected loss of balance.

muscle endurance—Muscle's ability to contract continuously at a submaximal level.

muscle power—Muscle's ability to forcefully contract in a very short time.

> Between the ages of 50 and 70, muscle strength declines by as much as 30%.

A selective loss of fast-twitch **motor units** has also been observed that will adversely affect the older adult's ability to execute movements quickly. Recent studies have shown that age-related changes in the firing behavior of motor units are also evident (Erim, Beg, Burke & De Luca, 1999). This change in the neuromuscular

motor unit—A motor neuron and all the muscle fibers it innervates.

15

component of the motor system, coupled with the loss of anticipatory postural control abilities due to slower central processing speeds, will place the older adult at greater risk for falling when balance is unexpectedly perturbed.

The loss of muscle strength, combined with structural changes occurring within the joints with age, also leads to a reduction in overall flexibility that can adversely affect postural alignment as well as the quality of an older adult's movement. Specific diseases in the joint such as osteoarthritis and rheumatoid arthritis further influence the joint's integrity and have been strongly associated with impaired balance and mobility. The pain associated with each of these conditions also contributes to a reduction in the functional range of motion. Both of these medical conditions will be discussed in greater depth in chapter 2.

Changes in the Cognitive System

Whereas age-related declines in the sensory and motor systems adversely affect the older adult's balance and mobility, so too do age-associated changes in the cognitive system. In fact, at least 10% of all people over the age of 65 and 50% of those older than 80 have some form of cognitive impairment, ranging from mild deficits to dementia (Yaffe, Barnes, Nevitt, Lui & Covinski, 2001). Adverse changes occurring in the processes of attention, memory, and intelligence are most likely to affect the older adult's ability to anticipate and adapt to changes occurring in the environment.

Older adults find it particularly difficult to store and manipulate information simultaneously in working memory when a second task that also demands cognition is presented. This requirement to divide attention between tasks, particularly when one of the tasks involves balance, is more problematic for healthy older adults than for their younger counterparts (Shumway-Cook, Woollacott, Baldwin & Kerns, 1997; Brown, Shumway-Cook & Woollacott, 1999). Decrements in performance are even more evident when older adults with known balance impairments are compared to healthy younger and older adults (Shumway-Cook et al., 1997; Brauer, Woollacott & Shumway-Cook, 2002).

> At least 10% of all people over 65 years of age and 50% of those over 80 have some form of cognitive impairment.

crystallized intelligence—Refers to verbal, numerical, and spatial abilities.

fluid intelligence—Ability to reason, problem-solve, and form relationships between abstract concepts.

Intelligence comprises two components: **crystallized** and **fluid intelligence.** Crystallized intelligence refers to verbal, numerical, and spatial abilities, whereas fluid intelligence involves the ability to reason, problem-solve, or form relationships between abstract concepts. Although aging does not appear to affect crystallized intelligence, it does have an adverse effect on fluid intelligence. At a practical level, the changes in fluid intelligence are most likely to affect your older adult clients' abilities to quickly find solutions to movement problems that they may not have encountered before or are presented in a different way.

> Changes in fluid intelligence with age are most likely to affect the ability to quickly find solutions to new movement problems.

Can Age-Associated Changes in Balance and Mobility Be Reversed?

Despite the many age-related changes occurring in the multiple systems that contribute to good balance and mobility, there is growing evidence to suggest that we can reverse, or at least slow, the rate of decline occurring in some or all of these systems. Several intervention studies conducted with both healthy older adults and those with existing balance problems have demonstrated moderate to large improvements in balance and mobility and a reduction in fall risk. Interventions that target the source(s) of balance-related problems and repeatedly expose older adults to changing task demands and environmental constraints have been particularly effective (Buchner et al., 1997; Rose & Clark, 2000; Shumway-Cook, Gruber, Baldwin & Liao, 1997; Wolfson et al., 1996). The FallProof program also targets the source(s) of the underlying impairments contributing to postural instability as a result of its comprehensive screening and assessment protocol and multidimensional programming approach. The overall effectiveness of the FallProof program has also been demonstrated and documented across a broad continuum of functional levels (Rose, 2001, 2002; Rose & Clark, 2000; Rose, Jones, Lemon & Bories, 1999; Rose, Jones & Lemon, 2001).

> Interventions that target the source(s) of balance-related problems and repeatedly expose older adults to changing task demands or environmental constraints are particularly effective.

Case Studies

One of the best ways to apply the theoretical information presented in this book is to relate it to an actual person. To help you make the critical connection between theory and practice and also help you develop your problem-solving skills along the way, two case studies are introduced in this section and expanded on in subsequent chapters. Each case study describes an older adult with the types of balance and mobility problems you can expect to encounter in many of the older adults who enroll in a community-based FallProof program. In this chapter, I will provide a general description of their current status and summarize the information each client provided on the health/activity questionnaire completed prior to the start of the program. The completed health/activity questionnaires are presented in figures 1.5 and 1.6 for further review. Both case studies are based on actual people who have participated in the FallProof program at Cal State Fullerton. In addition to the health history provided in this chapter, a complete set of assessment results for Jane Gain and Bill Divine is also provided in chapter 3. It will be important to review these results carefully and use the interpretation tables provided in chapter 3 to identify the possible underlying impairments that are contributing to the changes in balance and mobility indicated by the test results.

Case Study 1: Ms. Jane Gain

Current Status

Ms. Jane Gain is a 73-year-old female who heard about the FallProof program from her primary care physician, who had been treating her for a number of medical conditions over the years. On her first visit to our Center, she described how poor her balance and mobility had become since suffering the latest of several heart attacks in February 2001. Although she had already found it difficult to engage in physical activity because of chronic asthma that she has endured her entire adult life, complications from recent heart surgery (i.e., theophyoline toxicity) had significantly affected her ability to maintain balance and walk confidently.

Figure 1.5

The Health/Activity Questionnaire Used in the *FallProof!* Program

Name __Jane Gain_____ Address _____

_____ City_____ State_____ Zip_____

Home Phone # _____ Gender: Male _____ Female __X__

Age __73_____ Year of birth __1930_____ Height __5' 6"_____ Weight __200 lbs__

1. Have you ever been diagnosed as having any of the following conditions?

	Yes (**X**)	Year of onset (approximate)
Heart attack	X	_____
Transient ischemic attack	☐	_____
Angina (chest pain)	☐	_____
High blood pressure	☐	_____
Stroke	☐	_____
Peripheral vascular disease	☐	_____
Diabetes	☐	_____
Neuropathies (problems with sensations)	X	_____
Respiratory disease	X	_____
Parkinson's disease	☐	_____
Multiple sclerosis	☐	_____
Polio/post polio syndrome	☐	_____
Epilepsy/seizures	☐	_____
Other neurological conditions	☐	_____
Osteoporosis	☐	_____
Rheumatoid arthritis	☐	_____
Other arthritic conditions	X	_____
Visual/depth perception problems	☐	_____
Inner ear problems/recurrent ear infections	X	_____
Cerebellar problems (ataxia)	☐	_____
Other movement disorders	☐	_____
Chemical dependency (alcohol and/or drugs)	☐	_____
Depression	X	_____

3. Do you currently suffer any of the following symptoms in your legs or feet?
   Numbness__X_____ Arthritis __X_____
   Tingling __X_____ Swelling __X_____

4. Do you currently have any medical conditions for which you see a physician regularly? (YES) or NO
   If YES, please describe the condition(s).

Reprinted from the Center for Successful Aging at California State University, Fullerton.
Question 18 reprinted from Rikli & Jones, 1999.

(See Form 3.1 for entire questionnaire.)

From *FallProof!* by Debra J. Rose, 2003, Champaign, IL: Human Kinetics.

Figure 1.5

5. Do you require eyeglasses? YES or NO

6. Do you require hearing aids? (YES) or NO

7. Do you use an assistive device for walking? (circle) (No) Yes Sometimes

   Type? _____

8. List all medications that you currently take (including over-the-counter medications).

Type of medication	For what condition
Albuterol	Gout
Asthma Cort	Hypothyroidism
K-Dur (3x day – 10 meq.)	Bad Knee
Lasix (3x day – 20 mg.)	Asthma
Synthroid (1 day – .175 mg),	CHF
Oyster Shell Calcium (3x day – 500 mg)	
Centrum Silver (1/day)	
Allopurinol (1 day – 300 mg)	
Glucosamine (3x day – 500 mg)	

9. Have you required emergency medical care or hospitalization in the last three years? (YES) or NO

   If YES, please list when this occurred and briefly explain why.

   February 14, 2001—Theophyoline Toxicity - Heart Attacks

10. Have you ever had any condition or suffered any injury that has affected your balance or ability to walk without assistance? (YES) or NO

    If YES, please list when this occurred and briefly explain condition or injury.

    1987 Vertigo

11. How many times have you fallen within the past year? _2_

    Did you require medical treatment? YES or (NO)

    If you answered YES to either question, please list the approximate date of the fall, the medical treatment required, and the reason you fell in each case (e.g., uneven surface, going down stairs).

    Before the heart attacks

12. Are you worried about falling? (circle appropriate number)

1	2	3	4	5	6	(7)
no	a little		moderately	very		extremely

13. How would you describe your health?

    Excellent   Very good   Good   (Fair)   Poor

14. In the past 4 weeks, to what extent did health problems limit your everyday physical activities (such as walking and household chores)?

    Not at all   Slightly   Moderately (Quite a bit) Extremely

15. How much "bodily pain" have you generally had during the past 4 weeks (while doing normal activities of daily living)?

    None   Very little   Moderate (Quite a bit) Severe

16. In general, how much depression have you experienced in the past 4 weeks?

    (None) Very little   Moderate   Quite a bit   Severe

17. In general, how would you rate the quality of your life?

1	2	(3)	4	5	6	7
very low	low	moderate		high		very high

(continued)

Figure 1.5

(continued)

18. Please indicate your ability to do each of the following .

	Can do	Can do with difficulty or with help	Cannot do
a. Take care of own personal needs—such as dressing yourself	(2)	1	0
b. Bathe yourself using tub or shower	2	(1)	0
c. Climb up and down a flight of stairs (e.g., to a second story in a house)	2	(1)	0
d. Walk outside one or two blocks	2	1	(0)
e. Do light household activities—cooking, dusting, washing dishes, sweeping a walkway	2	(1)	0
f. Do own shopping for groceries or clothes	2	(1)	0
g. Walk 1/2 mile (6-7 blocks)	2	1	(0)
h. Walk 1 mile (12-14 blocks)	2	1	(0)
i. Lift and carry 10 pounds (full bag of groceries)	2	(1)	0
j. Lift and carry 25 pounds (medium to large suitcase)	2	1	(0)
k. Do most heavy household chores—scrubbing floors, vacuuming, raking leaves	2	1	(0)
l. Do strenuous activities—hiking, digging in garden, moving heavy objects, bicycling, aerobic dance exercises, strenuous calisthenics, etc.	2	1	(0)

19. In general, do you currently require household or nursing assistance to carry out daily activities?
(YES) or NO

If yes, please check the reasons(s).

Health problems

[X] Chronic pain

[X] Lack of strength or endurance

[X] Lack of flexibility or balance

[ ] Other reasons: _____

20. In a typical week, how often do you leave your house (to run errands, go to work, go to meetings, classes, church, social functions, etc.)?

_____ less than once/week   _____ 3-4 times/week

_____ 1-2 times/week   _X_ almost every day

21. Do you currently participate in regular physical exercise (such as walking, sports, exercise classes, housework or yard work) that is strenuous enough to cause a noticeable increase in breathing, heart rate, or perspiration?   YES or (NO)

If yes, how many days per week? (circle)

One   Two   Three   Four   Five   Six   Seven

22. When you go for walks (if you do), which of the following best describes your walking pace? (check)

_____ Strolling (easy pace, takes 30 minutes or more to walk a mile)

_____ Average or normal (can walk a mile in 20-30 minutes)

_____ Fairly brisk (fast pace, can walk a mile in 15-20 minutes)

_X_ Do not go for walks on a regular basis

23. Did you require assistance in completing this form?

_X_ None (or very little)   _____ Needed quite a bit of help

Reason: _____

Thank You!

Reprinted from the Center for Successful Aging at California State University, Fullerton.
Question 18 reprinted from Rikli & Jones, 1999.

Health/Activity History

In addition to her diagnosis of congestive heart failure and asthma, a review of her completed health/activity questionnaire (see figure 1.5) also revealed that Jane was diagnosed with peripheral neuropathy in both feet in 1996 as well as osteoarthritis in both hips and the right knee that same year. Despite her poor balance and level of conditioning, Jane was highly motivated to improve her balance and mobility. She described her health as good despite her physical limitations and reported no depression in the previous month. She rated her quality of life as moderately low because of her inability to perform a number of basic and intermediate daily activities (e.g., make the bed, vacuum, carry groceries) without requiring some type of assistance and to be as involved socially as she had been in past years. She also indicated that she experiences quite a bit of pain when performing daily activities. Jane is currently taking seven prescription medications for her various medical conditions and five over-the-counter medications. The exact medications are listed in question 8 on Jane's completed health/activity questionnaire in figure 1.5.

Fall History

Jane's fall history indicated that she had fallen twice in the previous year. Both falls occurred outside the home, the first when she was walking across her front lawn at night and the second when she tripped over an obstacle she did not see in her path. She was very fortunate not to break any bones but did sustain some severe bruising in the first fall and lacerations to the arms and legs in the second fall. It is not surprising, then, that she indicated she was extremely worried about falling on her health/activity questionnaire.

Case Study 2: Mr. Bill Divine

Current Status

Mr. Bill Divine is a 69-year-old male who resides in the community with his wife of 34 years. Mr. Divine enrolled in the FallProof program in 2000 because he was experiencing a steady decline in his balance abilities. Although he was a regular participant in an exercise program that operated three days a week at the local senior center, he was looking for a program that specifically focused on improving balance and mobility.

Health/Activity History

Mr. Divine reported five medical diagnoses on his completed health/activity questionnaire (see figure 1.6). He sustained a heart attack in 1993 that resulted in triple bypass surgery, followed by a stroke in 1996 that left him with weakness on the right side. He was also diagnosed with type 2 diabetes in 1996 and osteoarthritis in the back and right knee in 1998. He was first diagnosed with high blood pressure in 1990. The condition is currently being controlled with medication. Although he reports swelling in his legs and feet, he has not been diagnosed with peripheral neuropathy, a common condition secondary to diabetes. Mr. Divine rated his health as good and reported no depression in the previous month. He experiences some difficulty performing daily activities but still rates his quality of life as high.

Mr. Divine currently takes nine prescription medications for his various medical conditions. The exact medications can be reviewed by looking at question 8 on his completed health/activity questionnaire. He wears eyeglasses for reading purposes only, as well as a hearing aid in the right ear. Because of his increasing balance problems, he uses a single-point cane on occasion usually when he is planning to be out in the community for a good portion of the day.

Figure 1.6

The Health/Activity Questionnaire Used in the *FallProof!* Program

Name **Bill Divine**   Address _____

_____ City _____ State _____ Zip _____

Home Phone # _____ Gender: Male **X** Female _____

Age **69** _____ Year of birth **1932** _____ Height **5' 10"** _____ Weight **200 lbs**

1. Have you ever been diagnosed as having any of the following conditions?

	Yes (**X**)	Year of onset (approximate)
Heart attack	X	*1993 (Bypass)*
Transient ischemic attack	☐	
Angina (chest pain)	☐	
High blood pressure	X	*1990*
Stroke	X	*1998*
Peripheral vascular disease	☐	
Diabetes	X	*1996*
Neuropathies (problems with sensations)	☐	
Respiratory disease	☐	
Parkinson's disease	☐	
Multiple sclerosis	☐	
Polio/post polio syndrome	☐	
Epilepsy/seizures	☐	
Other neurological conditions	☐	
Osteoporosis	☐	
Rheumatoid arthritis	☐	
Other arthritic conditions	X	*1998*
Visual/depth perception problems	☐	
Inner ear problems/recurrent ear infections	☐	
Cerebellar problems (ataxia)	☐	
Other movement disorders	☐	
Chemical dependency (alcohol and/or drugs)	☐	
Depression	☐	

3. Do you currently suffer any of the following symptoms in your legs or feet?

   Numbness _____   Arthritis _____

   Tingling _____   Swelling **X** _____

4. Do you currently have any medical conditions for which you see a physician regularly? YES or (NO)

   If YES, please describe the condition(s).

Reprinted from the Center for Successful Aging at California State University, Fullerton.
Question 18 reprinted from Rikli & Jones, 1999.

(See Form 3.1 for entire questionnaire.)

Figure 1.6

5. Do you require eyeglasses? (YES) or NO

6. Do you require hearing aids? (YES) or NO

7. Do you use an assistive device for walking? (circle)   No   Yes   (Sometimes)

   Type? *cane—single point*

8. List all medications that you currently take (including over-the-counter medications).

Type of medication	For what condition
Lanoxin (0.25 mg)	*Heart medication*
Glucophage (500 mg)	*Diabetes*
Lipitor (20 mg)	*Cholesterol*
Furosemide (40 mg)	*Swelling—excess water*
Atenolol (50 mg)	*Blood pressure*
Feldene (20 mg)	*Arthritis*
Plendil (5 mg)	*Blood pressure*
Aspirin (81 mg)	*Blood thinner*
Citracal	*Osteoporosis*

9. Have you required emergency medical care or hospitalization in the last three years? (YES) or NO

   If YES, please list when this occurred and briefly explain why.

   March 1998—Stroke   *Right sided weakness*

10. Have you ever had any condition or suffered any injury that has affected your balance or ability to walk without assistance?   (YES) or NO

   If YES, please list when this occurred and briefly explain condition or injury.

   March 1998—Stroke

11. How many times have you fallen within the past year? *0*

   Did you require medical treatment?   YES or (NO)

   If you answered YES to either question, please list the approximate date of the fall, the medical treatment required, and the reason you fell in each case (e.g., uneven surface, going down stairs).

   Uneven surface

12. Are you worried about falling? (circle appropriate number)

1	2	3	4	(5)	6	7
no	a little	moderately		very		extremely

13. How would you describe your health?

   Excellent   Very good   Good   (Fair)   Poor

14. In the past 4 weeks, to what extent did health problems limit your everyday physical activities (such as walking and household chores)?

   Not at all   (Slightly)   Moderately   Quite a bit   Extremely

15. How much "bodily pain" have you generally had during the past 4 weeks (while doing normal activities of daily living)?

   None   (Very little)   Moderate   Quite a bit   Severe

16. In general, how much depression have you experienced in the past 4 weeks?

   (None)   Very little   Moderate   Quite a bit   Severe

17. In general, how would you rate the quality of your life?

1	2	3	4	(5)	6	7
very low	low		moderate	high		very high

(continued)

Figure 1.6

(continued)

18. Please indicate your ability to do each of the following .

	Can do	Can do with difficulty or with help	Cannot do
a. Take care of own personal needs—such as dressing yourself	(2)	1	0
b. Bathe yourself using tub or shower	(2)	1	0
c. Climb up and down a flight of stairs (e.g., to a second story in a house)	2	(1)	0
d. Walk outside one or two blocks	(2)	1	0
e. Do light household activities—cooking, dusting, washing dishes, sweeping a walkway	(2)	1	0
f. Do own shopping for groceries or clothes	(2)	1	0
g. Walk 1/2 mile (6-7 blocks)	(2)	1	0
h. Walk 1 mile (12-14 blocks)	(2)	1	0
i. Lift and carry 10 pounds (full bag of groceries)	(2)	1	0
j. Lift and carry 25 pounds (medium to large suitcase)	(2)	1	0
k. Do most heavy household chores—scrubbing floors, vacuuming, raking leaves	(2)	1	0
l. Do strenuous activities—hiking, digging in garden, moving heavy objects, bicycling, aerobic dance exercises, strenuous calisthenics, etc.	2	(1)	0

19. In general, do you currently require household or nursing assistance to carry out daily activities? YES or (NO)

If yes, please check the reasons(s).

Health problems

☐ Chronic pain

☐ Lack of strength or endurance

☐ Lack of flexibility or balance

☐ Other reasons: _____

20. In a typical week, how often do you leave your house (to run errands, go to work, go to meetings, classes, church, social functions, etc.)?

_____ less than once/week   _____ 3-4 times/week

_____ 1-2 times/week   _X_ almost every day

21. Do you currently participate in regular physical exercise (such as walking, sports, exercise classes, housework or yard work) that is strenuous enough to cause a noticeable increase in breathing, heart rate, or perspiration? (YES) or NO

If yes, how many days per week? (circle)

One   Two   Three   Four   (Five)   Six   Seven

22. When you go for walks (if you do), which of the following best describes your walking pace? (check)

_____ Strolling (easy pace, takes 30 minutes or more to walk a mile)

_____ Average or normal (can walk a mile in 20-30 minutes)

_____ Fairly brisk (fast pace, can walk a mile in 15-20 minutes)

_X_ Do not go for walks on a regular basis

23. Did you require assistance in completing this form?

_X_ None (or very little)   _____ Needed quite a bit of help

Reason: _____

Thank You!

Reprinted from the Center for Successful Aging at California State University, Fullerton.
Question 18 reprinted from Rikli & Jones, 1999.

Fall History

Mr. Divine reported no falls in the previous year, although he had some near misses, particularly when walking on uneven surfaces. Even though he had not actually fallen in the previous year, he also reported that he was very worried about falling.

Now that you have been introduced to our two case studies and understand a little more about each individual's current status and health history, review each of the completed questionnaires in a little greater detail to learn more about each person. In chapter 2, you will be asked to rate each person's level of physical function and overall risk for falls based on additional information provided on the health/activity questionnaire completed by each client.

Summary

The purpose of this chapter was to introduce you to the important terminology used in the study of balance and mobility as well as provide you with a brief overview of the multiple body systems that contribute to balance and mobility and the types of movement strategies used to control balance. The major age-related changes you are likely to observe in the clients you serve in the FallProof program were also described. As you learned in this chapter, the sensory, motor, and cognitive systems are integral to the development and maintenance of good balance and mobility. Whereas the sensory systems provide us with the information needed to perceive where we are in space, it is the role of the motor system to plan the subsequent action or actions. The cognitive system, which includes the processes of memory, attention, and intelligence, plays a critical role in helping older adults better anticipate changes occurring in the environment as well as adapt their actions in response to changing task or environmental demands.

Although some changes occurring in certain systems may be small (i.e., reduction in visual acuity), others may be so large (i.e., macular degeneration) as to adversely affect an older adult's ability to perform many daily activities that require balance and mobility. The good news is that many of the age-associated changes occurring in the systems that contribute to balance and mobility can be reversed, or at least compensated for, once they are identified. Certainly each of the core exercise components that make up the FallProof program is designed to address each of the dimensions of balance and mobility that, although altered by the aging process, can be positively influenced by a targeted and multidimensional exercise program.

Two case studies were also introduced in this chapter. Each of these case studies is intended to help you better apply the theory presented in this book to actual physical activity settings. They are also intended to sharpen your problem-solving abilities in preparation for leading FallProof classes in the future. Successful instructors of this program must be able to analyze each client's health history thoroughly so they can learn as much about the client as possible even before any baseline tests are administered. Each case study will be further developed during the next two chapters, and practical problems will be presented for you to solve as you begin to acquire the theoretical knowledge needed to design and implement a balance and mobility training program.

TEST YOUR UNDERSTANDING

1. In which of the following situations is anticipatory postural control most likely to be used?

   a. maintaining upright balance
   b. avoiding an obstacle in our path
   c. restoring balance after unexpectedly stepping in a hole
   d. running in the forest at night
   e. sitting on an unstable surface with the eyes closed

2. The boundaries of a person's stability limits are

   a. 12° in the forward, backward, and lateral directions
   b. determined by the task demands
   c. limited by our biomechanical limitations
   d. dependent on the constraints of the environment
   e. b, c, and d

3. Muscle response synergies are

   a. groups of muscles that must be inhibited if movement is to occur
   b. groups of muscles constrained to work together to produce movement
   c. any group of muscles in the body
   d. muscles that are involved in reflexive movements only
   e. a group of muscles that are activated together to produce movement

4. Which sensory system provides us with information about our position in space relative to the surface?

   a. the visual system
   b. the somatosensory system
   c. the vestibular system
   d. the visual *and* somatosensory systems
   e. all three sensory systems

5. The hip strategy is most likely to be used when

   a. the surface beneath the feet is narrow or compliant
   b. the sway distance is small
   c. we exceed our limits of stability
   d. the speed of the sway is slow
   e. the step strategy cannot be used

6. Which of the following is *not* a common age-related change that occurs in the visual system?

   a. reduced visual acuity
   b. reduced contrast sensitivity
   c. narrowing of the visual field
   d. glaucoma
   e. decreased depth perception

7. The primary role of the proprioceptors is to inform us about

   a. the position of the head and body in space
   b. the visual layout of the environment
   c. the changing position of the joints in space

     d. the changing tension of the muscles as they move

     e. the type of surface we are standing on

8. The primary role of the vestibulo-ocular reflex is to

     a. stabilize the head when the eyes are moving

     b. stabilize the body when the head is moving

     c. stabilize the eyes when the head is moving

     d. stabilize the body when the feet are moving

     e. force the head and eyes to move in the same direction

9. A situation of sensory conflict arises when

     a. the visual, somatosensory, and vestibular systems are providing the same information

     b. the information provided by one or more sensory systems is not in agreement with the other sensory systems

     c. information provided to the motor system is not in agreement with the information provided to the sensory systems

     d. the vestibular system is not functioning properly

     e. vision is no longer available

10. The loss of anticipatory postural control that accompanies aging is likely due to

     a. a reduction in muscle strength

     b. cognitive impairment

     c. a decline in central processing speed

     d. impaired memory

     e. improved reactive postural control

PRACTICAL PROBLEMS

This set of age-simulation activities is intended to help you better understand how age-related changes in multiple body systems are likely to affect balance and mobility. You will require the following equipment to complete this set of activities: eyeglasses, petroleum jelly, black tape, athletic tape, gloves, foam-filled shoes, cotton balls or earplugs, and dry macaroni. Although you can perform this activity alone, it is usually best to do it with a partner for safety reasons. After you have made each alteration described below, attempt to navigate an obstacle course and try to follow a set of visual and verbal instructions delivered by your partner as though you were in a physical activity setting.

1. Smear petroleum jelly on a set of clear eyeglasses so that vision is blurred. This simulates age-related changes in visual acuity and also simulates diseases such as macular degeneration or cataracts.

2. Eliminate the peripheral regions of each eyeglass lens with black tape to simulate visual field loss or glaucoma.

3. Insert cotton balls or earplugs in each ear and try to follow a set of softly delivered verbal instructions from your partner.

4. Put dry macaroni in each shoe to simulate the discomfort associated with arthritis.

5. Use the athletic tape to reduce range of motion in key joints (e.g., ankle, knee, and hip). Perform sit-to-stand, walking, and obstacle negotiation activities.

6. Tie a length of resistance band around the ankles to simulate reduced stride length and a narrow base of support.

7. Put on a pair of foam-filled booties to simulate sensation loss in the feet.

Once you have experienced moving about the room with single age-related impairments, combine impairments (e.g., 1 and 3 or 1, 2, and 4) so you can better understand how changes in multiple body systems further influence balance and mobility. Record your thoughts on paper when you have finished each of the activities listed above.

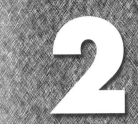

Why Do Many Older Adults Fall?

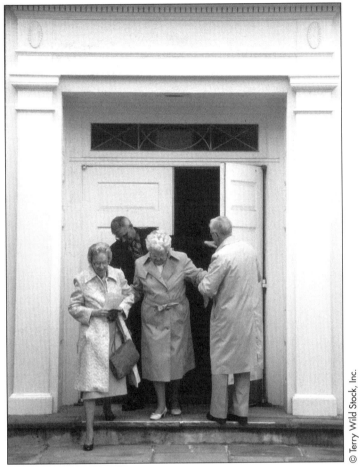

© Terry Wild Stock, Inc.

Objectives

After completing this chapter, you will be able to

- identify the intrinsic and extrinsic risk factors contributing to falls among older adults,
- describe the signs and symptoms associated with common medical conditions evident among older adults,
- understand and be able to modify balance and mobility activities that are contraindicated or likely to exacerbate symptoms associated with a medical condition,
- identify categories of medications that produce side effects likely to adversely affect balance and mobility,
- identify areas in and around the home that are contributing to heightened fall risk, and
- better understand which intrinsic risk factors can be eliminated or reduced through targeted exercise programming.

Falls are common among older adults, often leading to physical injury and psychological trauma. At the national level, falls among the elderly also lead to high rates of morbidity and mortality. In fact, falls are the leading cause of injury death among adults 65 years of age and older (Hoyert, Kochanek & Murphy, 1999). Many possible causes have been attributed to the higher than average fall incidence rates among older adults, and a number of fall-related risk factors have been identified over the past decade. As gloomy as these statistics might appear at first glance, the good news is that many falls are potentially preventable. Educational awareness programs, often combined with home safety inspections and modifications, and exercise-based interventions have all been shown to positively affect fall incidence rates among older adults (Day et al., 2002; Gardner, Robertson & Campbell, 2000; Gillespie et al., 2002).

To better prepare you as a balance and mobility instructor, this chapter is devoted to a discussion of the various risk factors, both intrinsic and extrinsic, that have been shown to be associated with increased fall risk among the elderly. Several strategies will also be presented that you, as an instructor, can employ to help your older adult clients become more aware of the need to make their homes as safe as possible while also improving their own physical capabilities, particularly in the area of balance and mobility. As a result of acquiring more knowledge in this area, you will become better able to identify specific risk factors that are most likely to contribute to each individual client's level of fall risk. This knowledge will also help you develop an individualized exercise plan that targets the specific risk factors identified.

Multiple Factors Cause Falls

intrinsic risk factors—Age- or disease-related changes occurring within the older adult.

First, not all older adults fall for the same reason. In fact, a multitude of reasons and factors contribute to the increased fall rates observed among older adults. These factors may be due to age- or disease-related changes occurring within the older adult **(intrinsic risk factors)** or to factors that are more external in nature, such as the presence of environmental hazards in the home or community that elevate the risk for falls during routine activities associated with daily living **(extrinsic risk factors)**.

extrinsic risk factors—External factors that elevate the risk for falls during the performance of daily activities.

Second, many of the primary causes for falls that occur among community-residing older adults are preventable. Modest safety changes made to the home environment (e.g., installation of grab bars in the bathroom, night-lights in dark corridors, removal of unnecessary clutter) can significantly reduce an older adult's overall risk for falls (see figure 2.1). Impaired balance and gait, identified as another primary cause of increased fall rates, can also be significantly improved with a targeted intervention approach. In fact, many of the exercise progressions you will be introduced to in part II of this instructor guide are intended to target many of the impairments identified as contributors to "accidental" falls among community-residing older adults.

Many of the primary causes for falls among community-residing older adults are preventable.

Extrinsic Risk Factors

Certainly older adults who reside independently within the community are faced with numerous extrinsic risk factors on a daily basis. These may be in the form of environmental hazards in and around the home or in the community itself. Clutter, unsecured floor rugs, poorly designed stairwells, and inadequate lighting in main

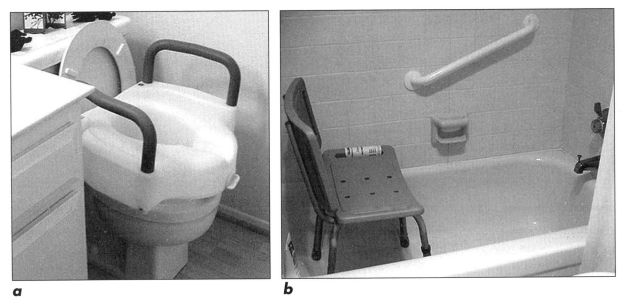

a   *b*

Figure 2.1 Installing devices that raise the height of a toilet *(a)* or provide increased safety during bathing activities *(b)* can reduce the risk of falling during transfer maneuvers.

areas of the home constitute just a few of the many possible external risk factors that have been strongly linked to increased falls. Poorly maintained sidewalks, varying curb heights, or sloping driveways also pose risks for older adults while moving about the community. A list of extrinsic risk factors associated with falls is presented in table 2.1. The list includes environmental, activity-related, and behavioral risk factors.

Table 2.1   Extrinsic Risk Factors Associated With Falls

Home environmental hazards	Outdoor environmental hazards
Ground surfaces	***Ground surfaces***
Throw rugs	Irregular or raised sidewalks
Loose carpets	Wet leaves, ice, or snow on ground
Slippery floors	Uneven, variable surfaces (e.g., holes covered by grass, rocks)
Cords and wires on floor	Oil
Low-lying objects (e.g., toys, pets)	***Home access***
Stairs in poor repair	Entrance stairs in poor repair
Highly polished floors	Raised thresholds
Furniture	Absent or poorly secured handrails
Clutter, especially that obstructs path	***Community***
Unstable furniture	Traffic lights that do not allow sufficient time to cross the street
Low-lying furniture (e.g., coffee table)	
Low chairs without armrests or back support	**Activity related**
Beds that are too high or too low	
Cabinets that are too high or too low	Rising from a chair
Lighting	Walking to the bathroom at night
Glare from uncovered windows or lamps	Navigating unfamiliar environments
Low or dimly lit rooms or corridors	Physical restraint use in long-term care facilities
Absence of night-lights	Hazardous activities (e.g., climbing ladders, hurrying, running)
Bathroom	***Other***
Low toilet seats or absence of secure grab bars	Poorly maintained walking aids and equipment
Absence of nonslip surfaces or secured grab bars in bathtub or shower	Improper shoes (not slip-resistant, high-heeled, too large)

Reprinted from Grisso, Capezuti, and Schwartz, 1996.

Intrinsic Risk Factors

Although many intrinsic risk factors have been identified in the literature as being associated with increased fall incidence rates, the degree of association has been shown to vary across studies (Nevitt, 1997). Those factors shown to be moderately to strongly associated with fall incidence rates are listed in table 2.2. As you can see by reviewing the table, adults over the age of 80 years, females, and older adults with a history of falls, in particular, are likely to fall more often. Difficulty performing a variety of activities of daily living (ADLs) and impaired mobility have also been identified as risk factors for falls (Nevitt, 1997). Poor performance on specific tests of balance and gait are also risk factors known to be strongly associated with increased fall rates.

The presence of certain types of medical conditions such as Parkinson's disease, stroke, arthritis, and dementia have also been shown to be moderately to strongly predictive of increased falls. The increased risk is likely due, at least in part, to the negative effect these diseases have on the various dimensions of balance and mobility, as well as on cognition. The increased joint pain and reduced range of motion that accompany the various arthritic conditions have also been shown to have a strong

Table 2.2 Intrinsic Risk Factors Associated with Falls

Demographic characteristics	Medical conditions
Older age (>80 years) Female White	Postural hypotension Foot problems
Functional level	**Medication and alcohol**
Increased difficulty performing activities of daily living Cane/walker use History of falls	Number of medications used* Hypnotics Sedatives Antipsychotics Antidepressants Antiparkinson drugs Cardiac drugs Diuretics Antihypertensives Alcohol
Gait, balance, strength	**Sensory**
Walking speed Postural sway Lower extremity strength Upper extremity strength Impaired reflexes	Visual acuity Lower extremity sensory perception
Chronic illnesses	**Mental status**
Heart disease Parkinson's disease Other neuromuscular disease Stroke Urinary incontinence Arthritis Acute illness	Cognitive impairment Depression Poor judgment
Low level of physical activity	

Reprinted from Grisso, Capezuti, and Schwartz, 1996.

association with increased falls among the elderly. The common medical conditions observed in the older adult population that are likely to adversely affect balance and mobility are described in more detail in the next section.

Effects of Common Medical Conditions

A large proportion of the older adults enrolled in the FallProof™ program will already have been diagnosed with one or more chronic medical conditions that will influence their ability to perform certain balance and mobility activities. Although the degree to which performance is affected will vary as a function of both the type and severity of the medical condition, become familiar with the signs and symptoms associated with the more common medical conditions so that you can eliminate or adapt any balance and mobility activities that might be contraindicated or harmful to the participants. This section will therefore be devoted to a discussion of selected medical conditions you are likely to observe among your older adult participants. The conditions to be discussed include stroke, cardiovascular disease, arthritis, osteoporosis, Parkinson's disease, diabetes, and vestibular dysfunction. Program considerations related to joint replacement surgery will also be discussed.

Stroke

When an individual experiences a stroke, also known as a cerebrovascular accident (CVA), one of two things has happened; either a blood vessel in the brain has become occluded (blocked) or it has hemorrhaged (a wall has burst). The loss of blood supply that accompanies either of these events causes an **infarction** in the area that was supplied by the blood vessel, causing brain cell death. A less serious medical event, in which the blood supply is reduced (ischemia) but not occluded, is called a **transient ischemic attack (TIA).** A person experiencing a TIA may exhibit symptoms such as weakness, temporary paralysis or loss of speech, or confusion.

Given the prevalence of stroke among the older adult population (approximately 72% of people who suffer a stroke in a given year are 65 or older (American Heart Association, 2002), you are likely to encounter a number of older adults in your community-based class who have experienced a stroke or TIA. Older adults who have experienced a stroke will often demonstrate weakness or even paralysis that affects one or more limbs on one side of the body. Depending on the location of the stroke, speech, cognition, or memory may also be affected. Individuals with impaired cognition are often impulsive or lacking good judgment relative to their abilities. Others experiencing memory loss may find it difficult to complete the health/activity questionnaire without assistance or to follow verbal directions during class. You can expect their progress to be much slower than that of clients without cognitive or memory impairments.

Knowing the exact nature of the deficits each client is experiencing after a stroke will help you decide which exercise progressions are most appropriate and, more important, which exercises should be eliminated. Having this knowledge can provide a safe practice environment for these clients. You will recall that Mr. Divine, the second case study described in chapter 1, experienced a stroke in 1996 that left him with weakness on the right side. His stroke was due to occlusion of a major artery in the left hemisphere of the brain.

Cardiovascular Disease

Because of the high prevalence of cardiovascular disease among older adults (approximately 84% of cardiovascular disease deaths occur in people aged 65 years

infarction—Brain cells die in the area of the brain that is deprived of blood supply following a stroke.

transient ischemic attack (TIA)—Results from temporary interruption of the blood supply to the brain.

hypertension (HTN)—Diagnosed when systolic blood pressure is greater than 140 mmHg and diastolic pressure is greater than 90 mmHg.

and older (American Heart Association, 2002)), many clients in the FallProof program will check one or more of the boxes related to heart disease when they complete their health/activity questionnaires at the outset of the program. Clients who are experiencing heart disease may experience fatigue or shortness of breath when exercising, particularly in the case of congestive heart failure. For individuals with **hypertension (HTN)**, their blood pressure must be medically managed so that they can participate in the program. Check the medications section of the health/activity questionnaire to determine the type of medications prescribed to control their blood pressure. At the same time, look to see if any clients have been prescribed anticoagulant medications designed to prevent blood clots. These clients will be susceptible to excessive bleeding if they sustain a cut, so extra precaution will be needed to ensure their safety during class activities.

Although the program does not involve high-intensity exercise, you will need to monitor clients who have a history of heart disease. Be sure to check with them regularly to find out whether there has been any change in either the type or dose of medication they have been prescribed. Recall that Ms. Gain indicated she suffered from high blood pressure and had a severe heart attack in 2001 that seriously compromised her balance and mobility. She was subsequently diagnosed with **congestive heart failure (CHF)**. Familiarize yourself with this condition so you can better understand how Ms. Gain is likely to respond to the initial assessment and whether you will need to take extra precautions when administering the assessments described in the next chapter.

congestive heart failure (CHF)—Occurs when the heart is unable to adequately deliver oxygen to the metabolizing tissues of the body.

Arthritis

At least 40 million older adults in the United States suffer from one or more types of arthritis, with the two most common forms being osteoarthritis and rheumatoid arthritis (Yelin & Felts, 1990). Osteoarthritis affects approximately 50% of all adults older than 65 years and 80% of those older than 75 (Brandt & Slemenda, 1993). This form of arthritis typically affects the weight-bearing joints, thereby reducing their ability to adequately transmit or absorb the forces associated with impact. Predisposing factors for this form of the disease include obesity, hypermobility, trauma, overuse, infection, inflammation, and genetics. The joint pain that accompanies osteoarthritis invariably leads to higher levels of inactivity and reduced strength, range of motion, and cardiovascular endurance. Although exercise has been shown to be an effective intervention, it will not cure the disease.

Land-based programming consisting of aerobic conditioning, resistance training, and flexibility exercises has resulted in moderate improvements in function, and aquatic-based exercise programs have also produced moderate improvements in strength and flexibility, particularly among older adults with moderate to severe joint damage (Deyle et al., 2000; Ettinger, Burns & Messier, 1999). Improvements ranging from 10% to 18% in strength and range of motion have also been documented following aquatic programs (Danneskiold-Samsoe, Lyngberg, Risum & Telling, 1987; Minor, Hewett, Anderson & Ray, 1989). Both Ms. Gain and Mr. Divine suffer from osteoarthritis in multiple joints. Although Mr. Divine reported that he does not experience much pain on a daily basis, Ms. Gain indicated that she experiences quite a bit of pain that requires her to seek assistance to complete daily chores in the home and community.

In contrast to osteoarthritis, the joint deformities associated with rheumatoid arthritis (RA) are often more severe and affect the entire joint. Because a systemic, inflammatory disease process characterizes RA, it usually affects multiple joints throughout the body. The systemic nature of the disease also produces symptoms that include increased fatigue, sleep disorders, and anemia. As with osteoarthritis, exercise has been demonstrated to be an effective intervention for older adults suffering from rheumatoid arthritis. Moderate gains in aerobic endurance and muscle strength have been reported with no adverse effect on progression of the disease (Van den Ende, Vliet Vieland, Munneke & Hazes, 1998).

The balance and mobility activities presented in the FallProof program have also been shown to be effective for older adults with osteoarthritis or rheumatoid arthritis (Rose, Jones & Lemon, 2001). In addition to significant improvements in their level of strength and flexibility, the older adults with arthritis we have studied also demonstrated improved balance and reduced fall risk after eight weeks of training. The nonrepetitive, low-impact, and multidimensional nature of the FallProof program appears to be an effective method for addressing the special needs of the older adult suffering from arthritis.

The main goal of any exercise program designed for older adults with arthritis is to limit the progression of the existing damage in the affected joint(s). With that in mind, your focus as an instructor should be on selecting activities that promote improved awareness of postural alignment, good body mechanics when performing dynamic activities, and improved strength and flexibility. When conducting any of the strength activities associated with the program, encourage this group of participants to perform a higher number of repetitions (to fatigue) with elastic tubing/bands or hand weights that offer a lower level of resistance. This is particularly important when using elastic tubing because the level of resistance increases as the band is stretched. The greatest resistance is therefore encountered at the end range of the joint's movement when the exercising muscle has exceeded its range of mechanical advantage.

You should also encourage participants with arthritis to stop performing any exercise that causes increased pain. In some cases, you may be able to adapt the exercise, whereas in others, you may have to eliminate it altogether because the plane of motion required is irritating to the joint. Watch these clients carefully during the performance of exercise progressions you suspect might cause pain and ask them regularly during the class whether certain exercises are causing them unnecessary pain. Many older adults may be reluctant to tell you they are experiencing pain during a certain exercise because they want to please you or do not want to be labeled as a complainer. Continually reiterate the mantra "Where there is pain there is *no* gain" to these clients in particular.

> Encourage your participants with arthritis to stop performing any exercise that causes increased pain. Reiterate the mantra "Where there is pain there is *no* gain."

Joint Replacement Surgery

Unfortunately, if more conservative nonoperative approaches fail to improve the function and quality of life for older adults with osteoarthritis and rheumatoid arthritis, it is often necessary to surgically replace a joint with a prosthesis. In fact, more than 120,000 artificial hip joints are being implanted annually in the United States (National Institutes of Health, 1994). Other common conditions that may lead to joint replacement include joint deterioration, the loss of articular cartilage, severe joint pain that compromises functional mobility, significant reduction in joint range of motion, and marked deformity (Kisner & Colby, 1990).

Although participants who have recently undergone successful joint replacement surgery are generally able to perform all of the activities described in this instructor guide, you will need to review the medical release form obtained from the primary care physician to see whether any exercise restrictions have been indicated. An older adult who has delayed the surgery until it was absolutely necessary, resulting in years of living with chronic pain and instability, may exhibit lower levels of self-confidence and a reluctance to "trust" the new hip or knee during some of the more challenging activities. Including balance activities that will foster increased confidence will be particularly important for these clients during the early stages of the program.

Emphasizing good postural alignment and symmetry during standing and walking activities will also be necessary with this group of clients due to their tendency to adopt a misaligned posture (i.e., anterior pelvic tilt, asymmetrical weight bearing) to reduce the amount of pain emanating from the involved joint. Many of the standing balance activities described in the chapter on center-of-gravity control training (chapter 4) that emphasize weight shifting and transfers with the eyes open and closed will be particularly beneficial for participants with joint replacements. Transferring on and off benches of different heights and practicing transfer activities between chairs of different heights will also be beneficial for strengthening the muscle groups surrounding the hip and knee joints. Finally, the activities described in the gait pattern enhancement and variation chapter (chapter 7) should also be practiced regularly.

> Providing balance activities that foster increased confidence will be particularly important for clients who have recently had joint replacement surgery.

Osteoporosis

Osteoporosis is a metabolic bone disease characterized by a progressive loss of bone mass that increases an individual's susceptibility to fractures. In fact, osteoporosis is the major underlying cause of bone fractures in women and older adults. It is estimated that osteoporosis is responsible for more than 1.5 million bone fractures in men and women over the age of 45 (Physicalmind Institute, 2001). Bone mineral density (BMD) levels are measured to determine whether an individual is within a normal range. Individuals with below-normal levels of BMD may be diagnosed with osteopenia (low bone mass) or osteoporosis (see table 2.3; WHO Study Group, 1994).

kyphosis—Increased posterior curvature of the spine.

Individuals with osteoporosis often sustain compression fractures in the thoracic and lumbar regions of the spine. These types of fractures often lead to increased **kyphosis** (rounding of the upper back) and back pain in many older adults. In advanced cases of osteoporosis, fractures can result from the performance of everyday activities such as bending over, lifting objects, and rising from a chair. Although certain compression fractures cause significant pain, many do not and can only be detected following radiographic examination. The lack of any observable symptoms makes it difficult for you as the instructor to select balance and mobility activities that are appropriate for this group of older adults.

Women are at higher risk for osteoporosis than men because of lower bone mass levels in general and an accelerated loss of bone mass following menopause. Underweight women are at greater risk for the disease, as are Caucasian men and women. In addition to medical treatment of the condition, weight-bearing exercise has been strongly recommended as an effective method of preventing further bone loss in individuals diagnosed with osteoporosis. Resistance exercises, both isotonic and iso-

Table 2.3 The World Health Organization Classification of Osteopenia and Osteoporosis

Normal	BMD is within 1 SD of a young normal adult (T-score above −1)
Low bone mass (osteopenia)	BMD is between 1 and 2.5 SD below that of a normal young adult (T-score between −1 and −2.5)
Osteoporosis	BMD is 2.5 SD or more below that of a young normal adult (T-score at or below −2.5)

BMD = bone mineral density; T-scores are derived from measurements provided by dual-energy X-ray absorptiometry (DXA). Values are based on measurements performed on Caucasian women.

Reprinted from the World Health Organization, 1994.

metric, have also been shown to be an effective way of strengthening the muscle and, in turn, strengthening bone.

In considering which activities are most appropriate for the older adult with osteoporosis, you need to review the health/activity questionnaire or interview the participant to ascertain whether a history of compression fractures already exists. Although most of the balance and mobility activities associated with the FallProof program should not place these older adults at undue risk, any exercises that require forward flexion of the spine combined with either stooping or spinal rotation should be avoided (e.g., lifting weighted objects from low levels, toe touching, spine twists). Instead, the emphasis should be on exercises that require spinal extension (e.g., standing backward bends, isometric spinal extension, prone spinal extension exercises for individuals who can tolerate lying on the floor). Upper body resistance exercises are also recommended to induce weight-bearing stress on the spine and wrists. However, begin with a low level of resistance and increase slowly. Standing weight-bearing activities are also desirable for this group. Assigning a set of resistive exercises (isotonic and isometric) as homework will also be particularly beneficial for these participants.

> It is important that older adults with osteoporosis not perform any activities that require forward flexion of the spine combined with either stooping or spinal rotation.

Because of the heightened fear of falling that often accompanies a diagnosis of osteoporosis, you will need to select activities that provide sufficient challenge but also a large dose of success. Being able to perform balance activities that are perceived to be challenging by this group will lead to elevated self-confidence and a reduced fear of falling over the long term. This improved self-confidence should eventually carry over to daily life and lead to increased levels of weight-bearing activity that will delay the progression of the disease.

Parkinson's Disease

Parkinson's disease (PD) is a progressive neurological disease resulting from a reduction in the availability of a vital neurotransmitter called dopamine in the substantia nigra of the basal ganglia. You can expect participants in your program with this disease to exhibit one or more of the following symptoms: resting tremor, **bradykinesia** (slow movements), gait and balance abnormalities, and increasing rigidity. Specific problems you are likely to see include difficulty with the initiation of movements; a slow, shuffling gait pattern with shortened, **festinating** steps (uncontrollable hurrying); reduced arm swing; and a general inability to move the limbs quickly or respond effectively to an unexpected loss of balance.

bradykinesia—Extreme slowness of movement.

festinating gait—An abnormal and involuntary increase in gait speed.

Since balance and mobility are particularly affected by the presence of PD, the risk for falling is extremely high in this group of likely participants and requires that additional safeguards be implemented to ensure a safe practice environment. These participants should use additional support in the form of a chair or wall when performing standing balance exercises, and close supervision should be provided during any of the gait pattern enhancement and variation activities. What makes it even more challenging for the instructor to program effectively for the participant with PD is that the symptoms are likely to fluctuate from class to class and even within a class depending on where in the medication cycle the participant happens to be on a given day. Careful screening of older adults with PD will also be necessary to ensure that they are appropriate candidates for a group exercise class of this type.

Diabetes

The number of older adults diagnosed with diabetes has increased considerably during the past decade, and many clients in your program are likely to be affected by this chronic metabolic disease. Two types of diabetes mellitus have been identified: type 1, or insulin-dependent diabetes, and type 2, or non-insulin-dependent diabetes. Type 1 diabetes is the more serious of the two and requires careful medical management. Exercise, combined with a proper diet designed to control blood glucose levels in the body, has been shown to be particularly beneficial for individuals with diabetes mellitus. The benefits include greater glucose tolerance and a lower insulin response to a glucose challenge. Older adults engaged in vigorous exercise programs are also likely to reduce their overall body fat, which may result in the need for lower doses of insulin or oral medications. In addition to her other medical conditions, Ms. Gain was also diagnosed with type 2 diabetes in 1996. She also has peripheral neuropathy in both feet, which often results from this type of diabetes.

hypoglycemia—Caused by low blood glucose levels. May be caused by too much insulin (or oral medications), insufficient food intake (relative to medication dose), or too much physical activity (relative to medication dose).

As an instructor in the FallProof program, you must understand some of the additional side effects associated with diabetes and the signs and symptoms of **hypoglycemia**. You also will need to know whether any of your program participants with diabetes are experiencing significant vision loss (diabetic retinopathy) or sensation loss, particularly in the feet. Exercises that involve standing or moving on a compliant surface may be problematic for the participant with reduced or absent vision or loss of sensation in the feet as they are no longer able to extract good information from the surface. Participants who have unhealed ulcers on their feet may also need to exercise in a seated position to avoid further complications. Certain head-eye coordination exercises described in chapter 5 may also be ineffective if severe vision loss is evident.

Signs and Symptoms of Hypoglycemia

Anxiety, uneasiness	Sweating, palpitation
Irritability	Headache
Nausea	Loss of motor coordination
Extreme hunger	Strong, rapid pulse
Confusion	Insomnia
Pale, moist skin	Double vision

As a general precaution, always check that participants with diabetes have eaten a light snack before class or have one with them lest any symptoms of hypoglycemia develop during the exercise session. Although the intensity of the balance activities presented in this program often taxes the mind more than the body, you must monitor your diabetic clients carefully and ensure that they remain hydrated at all times while exercising.

Vestibular Disorders

The final set of medical conditions to be discussed in this section are those related to disorders of the vestibular system. Although it is often difficult to identify why an older adult may be experiencing problems in the inner ear system, you must understand how to safeguard a participant who is experiencing dizziness that is not caused by hypertension. In older adults, vestibular dysfunction is caused by specific diseases of the inner ear such as **Ménière's disease** or vascular diseases of the labyrinth, an important area within the vestibular system (Diener & Null, 1997). In some cases, a more temporary disturbance in vestibular function is caused by **benign positional vertigo (BPV)**, a condition that develops as a result of small crystals called **otoconia** falling into the semicircular canals and causing dizziness with certain movements of the head. Although the latter problem can be treated quite easily by a trained physical therapist, it is not uncommon to see older adults who have had the problem for a long time and have not received treatment for it.

Although it is well beyond the scope of your professional boundaries to speculate as to the cause of any dizziness an older adult may be experiencing during class, you must monitor them closely, particularly during activities that require the head to be tilted or turned quickly or activities in which vision is absent and the surface beneath them is compliant or unstable. Older adults with an impaired vestibular system are likely to be at greater risk for a loss of balance during these types of activities. A careful review of the results of selected test items on the Fullerton Advanced Balance (FAB) Scale and the Modified Clinical Test of Sensory Interaction in Balance (M-CTSIB), which will be described in greater detail in the next chapter, will help you identify individuals who may be experiencing difficulties using the information provided by the vestibular system for balance. Although no specific vestibular diagnosis was listed on Ms. Gain's health/activity questionnaire, she did indicate that she experienced a severe bout of vertigo in 1987 that affected her balance and mobility. You will need to monitor her closely when she is performing the M-CTSIB test, particularly condition 4, which requires the person being tested to rely more on the vestibular system to maintain balance.

When working with clients who experience problems with dizziness, encourage them to sit down and rest if a particular activity is making them dizzy to the point that they are at risk of losing balance. In some cases, you can encourage clients to pace themselves during an exercise so that the symptoms do not become too severe. Because some types of dizziness can actually be helped by activities that stimulate the vestibular system, teaching your older adults to move a little more slowly during a particular activity rather than stop altogether can be helpful. It is also a good idea to use a 10-point scale and ask your clients to rate their level of dizziness from 0 (none at all) to 10 (so dizzy they are about to fall down) to get a better sense of how dizzy they are feeling. Generally, if a client reports a dizziness level or 5 or higher, they should sit down and rest. If an activity they are performing results in increased dizziness with each repetition, this is also a sign that the exercise should be discontinued immediately. This might occur during an activity such as "rock hopping," in which the older adult might be bending down to pick up objects as they move down an imaginary creek. If a client is repeatedly experiencing dizziness as a result of activities performed during the class, you should encourage them to talk with their primary care physician about the recurring problem. Some excellent educational

Ménière's disease—A disorder of the inner ear that causes severe disequilibrium that may last anywhere from 30 minutes to 72 hours during an attack.

benign positional vertigo (BPV)—An inner ear condition that produces dizziness or vertigo (illusion of movement) with a rapid change in head position.

otoconia—Calcium carbonate crystals found in the otolithic membranes of the inner ear.

resources are also available that will provide older adults with more information about vestibular disorders. The Vestibular Disorders Association (VEDA) Web site (www.vestibular.org) is just one example.

> If any clients are repeatedly experiencing dizziness during class activities, encourage them to consult with their primary care physician.

Effect of Medication Use on Balance and Mobility

In addition to certain medical conditions being strongly associated with increased fall risk among the elderly, both the type and number of medications prescribed to older adults contribute to heightened fall risk. Specifically, it has been demonstrated that older adults who are taking more than four prescription medications are four times more likely to sustain a fall than their peers who are taking fewer prescription medications (Campbell, Borrie & Spears, 1989). Certain types of medications (i.e., psychotropics, hypnotics/sedatives, and antidepressants) have also been shown to elevate fall risk in older adults (Leipzig, Cumming & Tinetti, 1999a). Side effects such as dizziness, reduced alertness, weakness, fatigue, and postural hypotension that result from taking these types of medications are all likely contributors to heightened fall risk. Finally, other intrinsic risk factors such as impaired visual acuity, foot problems (e.g., loss of sensation, bone deformities), and the presence of depression or anxiety are also known risk factors for falls.

Given that most, if not all, of the clients enrolled in the FallProof program will be taking one or more prescription medications, prospective program participants need to provide you with the names of all their medications and the medical condition for which they were prescribed. Although numerous research studies have identified many individual medications that are known to increase the risk for falling due to their effect on central nervous system function, little is currently known about how the interactive or additive effects of taking multiple medications might further affect balance and mobility. As indicated earlier, certain classes of medications have been positively associated with increased fall risk. These include most classes of psychotropic drugs such as antidepressants, neuroleptics, sedative/hypnotics, and benzodiazepines (both long- and short-acting). A comprehensive listing of these medications and their possible adverse side effects is presented in table 2.4.

Increased risk for falling is particularly associated with the use of antidepressant medications, with new users of these drugs at greater risk for falling than individuals who have been taking them for a while. It has also been demonstrated that older adults taking a higher dosage of an antidepressant drug experience higher fall rates. Little difference in fall rates exists among older adults prescribed different types of antidepressants (Thapa, Gideon, Cost, Milam & Ray, 1998). Older adults at greater risk of falling are those taking more than one psychotropic agent or having other risk factors for falls (Leipzig, Cumming & Tinetti, 1999a). Cardiac and analgesic medications (e.g., Digoxin, type Ia antiarrhythmic, and diuretic drugs) were also studied but were found to be only weakly associated with heightened fall risk (Leipzig, Cumming & Tinetti, 1999b).

> Certain classes of prescription medications are associated with higher fall risk among older adults. These include psychotropics, sedatives/hypnotics, and antidepressant medications.

Table 2.4 Generic and Brand Names of Medications Commonly Prescribed to Older Adults and Their Possible Side Effects

Class of medication	Medical condition	Possible side effects
Benzodiazepines (antianxiety)		
Alprazolam (Xanax) Bromazepam Lectopam Buspirone Clonazepam (Klonopin) Chlorazepate (Tranxene) Chloradiazepoxide (Librium) Diazepam (Valium) Doxepine Estazolam Flurazepam (Dalmane) Halazepam Hydroxyzine Lorazepam (Ativan) Oxazepam Prazepam (Centrax) Quazepam (Doral) Temazepam (Restoril) Triazolam	Nervous tension Panic attacks Moderate anxiety	Instability, light-headedness, dizziness, sedative effect—"hangover effects," decreased central processing/alertness, coordination/impaired balance
Antidepressants		
Amitriptyline (Elavil, Endep) Amoxapine (Asendin) Bupropion (Wellbutrin) Clomapramine (Anafranil) Citalopram Desipramine Doxepine Fluoxetine (Prozac) Mirtazapine Nefazodone Notriptyline Imipramine Paroxetine (Paxil) Phenelzine Sertralin (Zoloft) Venlaxafine	Mild to moderate depression	Headaches, blurred vision, dizziness, memory problems, decreased central processing/alertness, orthostatic hypotension, unsteady gait, weakness
Hypnotics (sedatives)		
Chloral hydrate (Aquachloral, Noctec) Phenobarbital Pentobarnital Temazepam (Restoril) Trazodone Secobarbital Zolpidem	Insomnia, stress	Mild "hangover," drowsiness, lethargy, blurred vision, confusion, depression, dizziness, unsteadiness, altered coordination
Diuretics		
Chlorthalidone (Hygroton) Furosemide (Lasix) HCTZ (Esidrix, Hydrodiuril) Metolazone (Diulo, Zaroxolyn) Triamterene (Dyrenium) Spironolactone (Aldactone)	Hypertension, edema	Drowsiness, temporary nearsightedness, dehydration, light-headedness, orthostatic hypotension, muscle fatigue and cramping, weakness, dizziness, blurred vision

Antidepressant use is higher among older adults living in nursing homes (35.5%) or assisted living facilities (39.8%) when compared to community-dwelling older adults (8%) (Ray & Griffin, 1990). The loss of perceived independence and control over one's life no doubt contributes to the higher use of antidepressants by older adults who are no longer able to live independently within the community. As an individual's level of frailty increases, it is also likely to be accompanied by increased depression. The loss of a spouse or family member is also likely to precipitate the use of these types of drugs.

Are the Risks the Same for All Older Adults?

As mentioned earlier in this chapter, the level of fall risk is not the same for all older adults and has been shown to change over time. With advancing age and declining physical function, not only does the level of risk change, but so too do the types of risk factors contributing to that risk. Older adults who remain physically active as they age and thereby retain a high level of postural competence are at a lower risk for falls than their peers who severely limit or curtail their levels of physical activity as they grow older. These more sedentary older adults are more likely to experience increased difficulty performing activities that require balance and mobility as their level of conditioning declines. Although their risk for falls may decrease in the short term as a function of their reduced exposure, the long-term risk increases significantly as their level of physical function and confidence in their ability to engage in certain activities or venture into more challenging environments declines (Tinetti, Mendes de Leon, Doucette & Baker, 1994).

The level of fall risk is not the same for all older adults and changes over time.

The setting in which an older adult resides has also been shown to influence the type of risk factors associated with increased falls. Frail older adults residing in long-term care settings, for example, rarely fall as a result of environmental factors. Intrinsic risk factors (e.g., general weakness, cognitive impairment, adverse drug events, medical conditions) are much more likely to constitute the primary reasons for increased falls in this group of older adults (Lipsitz, Jonsson, Kelley & Koestner, 1991). In contrast, at least one-third to one-half of all falls sustained by community-residing older adults can be attributed to environmental or extrinsic risk factors (Rubenstein & Josephson, 1992; Tinetti, Speechley & Ginter, 1988).

Researchers who have analyzed fall patterns in the home have identified several known patterns. Collisions with objects in a dark environment, inability to avoid temporary hazards or conditions around the home, experiencing adverse frictional contact with different surface types, careless negotiation or use of the environment are just some of the patterns identified. It has also been demonstrated that older adults who are experiencing a decline in their physical capabilities but continue to be active within their community, take unnecessary personal risks when performing daily activities, or expose themselves to hazardous environments are at especially high risk for falls (Studenski et al., 1994).

Practical Implications for Program Planning

Why is it important that FallProof instructors know about the types of intrinsic and extrinsic risk factors that are most likely to contribute to heightened fall risk? Instructors who know about the risk factors related to increased fall incidence among the elderly will glean vital clues when they review the various sections of a client's completed health and physical activity history that will help them understand the client's initial level of function (e.g., age, gender, number of diagnoses, type and number of medications, self-reported joint pain). This knowledge will also help in designing a more individualized exercise plan that will better address each client's impairments.

Given that falls are often due to many different factors, the exercises you prescribe for your older adult clients must directly address the intrinsic impairments that are most likely contributing to heightened fall risk. For example, an older adult client who demonstrates low levels of muscular strength, particularly at the level of the ankle, knee, and hip, should be provided with balance-related activities, both in the class and at home, that specifically target the strengthening of these muscle groups (see chapter 8 for appropriate exercises). Similarly, an older adult who demonstrates poor mobility skills or impaired gait speed should be prescribed a set of progressive activities that target those impairments. Several activities presented in the gait pattern enhancement and variation section of chapter 7, coupled with activities described in the weight shift and transfer subsections of the center-of-gravity training module, should address these impairments very well.

Although your primary focus as an instructor in the FallProof program is to address the intrinsic risk factors that contribute to increased fall rates among older adults, you may have several opportunities to provide invaluable education about some of the extrinsic risk factors such as environmental hazards and risk-taking behaviors. Additional educational materials can be provided to the client on various topics such as home safety, medication use and abuse, home exercise programs, or community activity resources following a review of the client's health history. It is also a good idea to have each of your clients complete a home safety checklist and return it to you during the first week of class (see the Internet Resources for Medications section at the end of this chapter). Not only will this activity increase the client's awareness of important home safety issues, but it will also let you know if there are hazards in the client's home that are likely to increase the overall fall risk. If the community resources are available, you may even be able to go a step further by contacting a community agency that conducts home safety inspections and repairs. In operating our community outreach programs, we have found that hospitals and home health nursing agencies often provide this type of service.

Have your clients complete a home safety checklist during the first week of class. This activity will raise the client's awareness of important home safety issues and let you know if there are hazards in the home that are likely to increase the client's overall fall risk.

In addition to having clients complete a home safety checklist, consider incorporating role-playing activities into some of your classes as a means of helping your clients make good judgments about how to perform certain daily activities and the types of environments in which they are likely to encounter problems. For example, a client with sensory peripheral neuropathy needs to learn that taking the trash out to the curb at night might not be as prudent as performing the same activity in the morning. The loss of sensation in the feet, coupled with reduced vision at night, places that adult at unnecessary risk for falls when the same activity can be performed much more safely when vision is improved. The Balance Kit Inventory checklist in the appendix lists useful equipment for these activities and for other exercises throughout the book.

Be sure to inquire regularly about any changes in medications or dosage levels so that you can maintain a current list of the various medications being consumed. Because many older adults are using complementary alternative medicines (CAMs), you need to maintain a list of those medications as well (Eisenberg et al., 1993, 1998). Although little is currently known about possible interaction effects between CAMs and more traditional prescription medications, it is a good idea to maintain a record of all prescription medications as well as over-the-counter supplements being taken by your class participants.

> In addition to knowing which prescription medications your clients have been prescribed, maintain a list of any complementary alternative medicines (CAMs) being used by your older adult clients.

Summary

As you have learned from reading this chapter, many factors contribute to an older adult's heightened risk for falls. Although it is not possible for you as an instructor to eliminate certain risk factors known to contribute to increased fall rates, such as advancing age or gender, you can positively affect many intrinsic risk factors through careful program planning. Helping your clients understand which activities and environments they should avoid until their balance improves will also prove invaluable. Having clients complete a home safety checklist as a homework assignment will also make them more aware of potential hazards in and around the home and perhaps lead them to make some changes that are likely to reduce their chances of falling. Of course, your primary goal as an instructor is to improve the balance and mobility of your clients as a means of significantly reducing their overall risk for falls. It is also likely that as their level of postural competence increases, so too will their self-confidence, hopefully to a level that will motivate them to become more physically active on a daily basis.

Internet Resources for Home Safety and Modifications

One of the most comprehensive Web sites addressing home safety and home modification issues is the National Resource Center on Supportive Housing and Home Modification. This nonprofit organization, housed at the University of Southern California, is dedicated to the promotion of aging in place and independent living for people of all ages and disabilities. You will also be able to download a home safety checklist that can be distributed to your class participants when they first join the program. The Web address is www.homemods.org.

Internet Resources for Medications

Information about categories of medications and their known side effects can be obtained by logging onto any of the Web sites listed below:

www.medications-online.com

www.healthsquare.com

www.healthtouch.com

TEST YOUR UNDERSTANDING

1. Which of the following is not an example of an intrinsic risk factor for falls?
   a. medical conditions
   b. level of physical activity
   c. foot problems
   d. unsecured mats/rugs in the home
   e. cognitive impairment

2. Which of the following are symptoms associated with a stroke?
   a. stooped posture
   b. asymmetrical gait pattern
   c. shortness of breath
   d. anemia
   e. shuffling gait

3. A person is diagnosed with hypertension when
   a. systolic blood pressure is greater than 140 mmHg and diastolic blood pressure is less than 90 mmHg
   b. systolic blood pressure is greater than 100 mmHg and diastolic blood pressure is greater than 140 mmHg
   c. systolic blood pressure is greater than 200 mmHg
   d. diastolic blood pressure is greater than 110 mmHg
   e. diastolic blood pressure is greater than 90 mmHg and systolic blood pressure is greater than 140 mmHg

4. A diagnosis of osteoporosis is made once the level of bone mineral density is
   a. between 1 and 2.5 standard deviations (SDs) below normal young adult levels
   b. at least 2.5 SDs above normal young adult levels
   c. within 1 SD of normal young adult levels
   d. a T-score that is at or below −2.5
   e. between 2 and 2.5 SDs below young adult levels

5. Which types of exercises should not be performed by older adults with a diagnosis of osteoporosis?
   a. forward flexion of the spine combined with stooping
   b. lower body strength exercises
   c. spinal extension
   d. weight-bearing activities
   e. a and c

6. Bradykinesia is a symptom associated with Parkinson's disease that is characterized by
   a. an abnormal and involuntary increase in gait speed
   b. extremely slow movements
   c. an unstable movement pattern
   d. increased rigidity
   e. a shuffling gait pattern

7. The following category of medications has been positively associated with increased fall risk:
   a. cardiac drugs
   b. psychotropics
   c. ibuprofen
   d. diuretic drugs
   e. gingko biloba

8. Which of the following is *not* a symptom of hypoglycemia?
   a. strong, rapid pulse
   b. insomnia
   c. pale, moist skin
   d. loss of appetite
   e. nausea

9. An observable characteristic of a condition known as kyphosis is
   a. an increased posterior curvature of the spine
   b. a decreased posterior curvature of the spine
   c. lower than normal levels of BMD
   d. higher than normal levels of BMD
   e. swelling in joint structures

10. At least one-third to one-half of all falls sustained by community-residing adults can be attributed to
    a. intrinsic risk factors
    b. poor judgment
    c. extrinsic risk factors
    d. a low level of physical activity
    e. muscle weakness

PRACTICAL PROBLEMS

Review the completed health/activity questionnaires associated with the two case studies presented in chapter 1. Complete the following tasks:

1. Identify the primary signs and symptoms associated with the medical diagnoses reported by Mr. Divine and Ms. Gain. Indicate whether any special precautions might be necessary when testing either client prior to the program and designing an exercise program for each of them.

2. Research each of the medications listed in the health/activity questionnaires completed by Mr. Divine and Ms. Gain. List the medical condition that each medication is prescribed for and any side effects likely to adversely affect balance and mobility. Also identify any medications on the list that are associated with a heightened risk for falls. Any of the Internet sites listed on page 44 will provide you with additional information about the side effects associated with each medication.

3. Develop a list of the intrinsic risk factors for each individual based on your review of their completed health/activity questionnaires.

PART II

The FallProof Program for Improving Balance and Mobility

3

Screening and Assessment

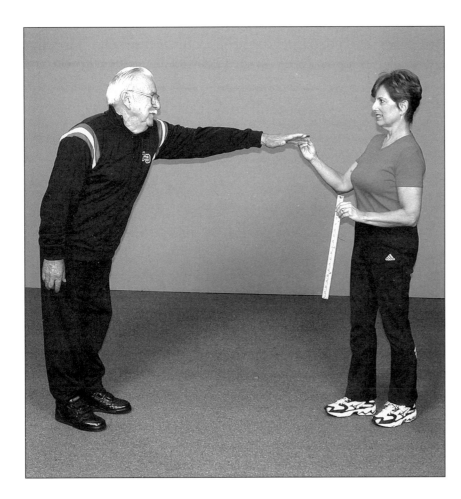

Objectives

After completing this chapter, you will be able to

- identify several tests used to evaluate balance and mobility in older adults,
- screen and evaluate the multiple dimensions of balance and mobility, and
- interpret test results and be able to identify underlying impairments.

Why Screening and Assessment Matter

The assessment of multiple dimensions of physical function (in particular, balance and mobility) assists the instructor in many ways. Not only does assessment facilitate the early identification of older adults who are beginning to experience significant changes in multiple body systems resulting in observable changes in postural stability and mobility, but it also helps you, the instructor, develop an appropriate exercise plan that targets the identified system impairments. When assessments are readministered on a regular basis, the information obtained from these multiple tests can also be used to guide the selection or deletion of certain exercises, help participants set appropriate short- and long-term goals, and motivate them to meet each of those goals. Finally, the overall effectiveness of the program, and your teaching, can be documented.

> A thorough screening and assessment facilitates the early identification of balance problems and helps the instructor develop an exercise plan that targets the identified system impairments.

How to Assess Older Adults With Balance and Mobility Disorders

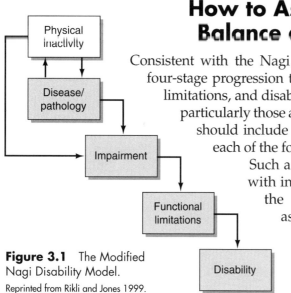

Figure 3.1 The Modified Nagi Disability Model.
Reprinted from Rikli and Jones 1999.

Consistent with the Nagi Disability Model (Nagi, 1991), which describes a four-stage progression to disability (i.e., pathology, impairment, functional limitations, and disability), any screening and assessment of older adults, particularly those already experiencing balance and mobility problems, should include tests designed to assess the level of dysfunction in each of the four stages (shaded boxes) illustrated in figure 3.1.

Such a multistage assessment will provide the instructor with in-depth information that can then be used to select the most appropriate exercise progressions. In the assessment described later in this chapter, information about each of these four stages is obtained as well as important information about lifestyle and physical activity patterns. Recent evidence suggests that lifestyle factors such as physical inactivity and disuse should be considered as important as pathology in contributing to frailty and disability in the later years (Chandler & Hadley, 1996; Di Pietro, 1996; Rikli & Jones, 1997).

Pathology/Disease and Physical Activity Patterns

Information about pathology/disease and physical activity patterns is obtained from the health/activity questionnaire administered prior to the screening (see form 3.1). In addition to providing information about existing medical diagnoses and medications, participants are required to answer three questions related to physical activity and exercise patterns (see questions 20-22 of the health/activity questionnaire). For example, participants are asked how often they leave the house during the week; whether they participate in regular physical exercise that is strenuous enough to cause a noticeable increase in breathing, heart rate, or perspiration; and if so, how many days per week. They are also asked to select, from a list of four options, the pace at which they walk (if they engage in the activity on a regular basis).

The Health/Activity Questionnaire Used in the *FallProof!* Program

Date _____

Name _____ Address _____

_____ City _____ State _____ Zip _____

Home Phone # _____ Gender: Male _____ Female _____

Age _____ Year of birth _____ Height _____ Weight _____

Ethnicity _____ Highest level of education completed _____

Whom to contact in a case of emergency _____ Phone # _____

Name of your physician _____ Phone # _____

1. Have you ever been diagnosed as having any of the following conditions?

	Yes (**X**)	Year of onset (approximate)
Heart attack	☐	_____
Transient ischemic attack	☐	_____
Angina (chest pain)	☐	_____
High blood pressure	☐	_____
Stroke	☐	_____
Peripheral vascular disease	☐	_____
Diabetes	☐	_____
Neuropathies (problems with sensations)	☐	_____
Respiratory disease	☐	_____
Parkinson's disease	☐	_____
Multiple sclerosis	☐	_____
Polio/post polio syndrome	☐	_____
Epilepsy/seizures	☐	_____
Other neurological conditions	☐	_____
Osteoporosis	☐	_____
Rheumatoid arthritis	☐	_____
Other arthritic conditions	☐	_____
Visual/depth perception problems	☐	_____
Inner ear problems/recurrent ear infections	☐	_____
Cerebellar problems (ataxia)	☐	_____
Other movement disorders	☐	_____
Chemical dependency (alcohol and/or drugs)	☐	_____
Depression	☐	_____

(continued)

Reprinted from the Center for Successful Aging at California State University, Fullerton. Question 18 reprinted from Rikli & Jones, 1999.

(continued)

2. Have you ever been diagnosed as having any of the following conditions?

	Yes (**X**)	Year of onset (approximate)
Cancer	☐	_____

    If YES, describe what kind _____

Joint replacement	☐	_____

    If YES, which joint (e.g., knee, hip) and side (left or right)_____

Cognitive disorder	☐	_____

    If YES describe condition _____

Uncorrected visual problems	☐	_____

    If YES, describe type _____

Any other type of health problem?	☐	_____

    If YES, describe condition _____

3. Do you currently suffer any of the following symptoms in your legs or feet?

Numbness _____   Arthritis _____

Tingling _____   Swelling _____

4. Do you currently have any medical conditions for which you see a physician regularly? YES or NO
   If YES, please describe the condition(s).

   _____

5. Do you require eyeglasses? YES or NO

6. Do you require hearing aids? YES or NO

7. Do you use an assistive device for walking? (circle)   No   Yes   Sometimes
   Type? _____

8. List all medications that you currently take (including over-the-counter medications).

Type of medication	For what condition
_____	_____
_____	_____
_____	_____
_____	_____
_____	_____
_____	_____

9. Have you required emergency medical care or hospitalization in the last three years? YES or NO
   If YES, please list when this occurred and briefly explain why.

   _____

10. Have you ever had any condition or suffered any injury that has affected your balance or ability to walk without assistance?   YES or NO
    If YES, please list when this occurred and briefly explain condition or injury.

   _____

11. How many times have you fallen within the past year? _____

       Did you require medical treatment?   YES or NO

   If you answered YES to either question, please list the approximate date of the fall, the medical treatment required, and the reason you fell in each case (e.g., uneven surface, going down stairs).

   _____

   _____

Reprinted from the Center for Successful Aging at California State University, Fullerton. Question 18 reprinted from Rikli & Jones, 1999.

From *FallProof!* by Debra J. Rose, 2003, Champaign, IL: Human Kinetics.

12. Are you worried about falling? (circle appropriate number)

	1	2	3	4	5	6	7
	no		a little	moderately	very	extremely	

13. How would you describe your health?

Excellent   Very good   Good   Fair   Poor

14. In the past 4 weeks, to what extent did health problems limit your everyday physical activities (such as walking and household chores)?

Not at all   Slightly   Moderately   Quite a bit   Extremely

15. How much "bodily pain" have you generally had during the past 4 weeks (while doing normal activities of daily living)?

None   Very little   Moderate   Quite a bit   Severe

16. In general, how much depression have you experienced in the past 4 weeks?

None   Very little   Moderate   Quite a bit   Severe

17. In general, how would you rate the quality of your life? (circle appropriate number)

	1	2	3	4	5	6	7
	very low		low	moderate	high	very high	

18. Please indicate your ability to do each of the following .

	Can do	Can do with difficulty or with help	Cannot do
a. Take care of own personal needs—such as dressing yourself	2	1	0
b. Bathe yourself using tub or shower	2	1	0
c. Climb up and down a flight of stairs (e.g., to a second story in a house)	2	1	0
d. Walk outside one or two blocks	2	1	0
e. Do light household activities—cooking, dusting, washing dishes, sweeping a walkway	2	1	0
f. Do own shopping for groceries or clothes	2	1	0
g. Walk 1/2 mile (6-7 blocks)	2	1	0
h. Walk 1 mile (12-14 blocks)	2	1	0
i. Lift and carry 10 pounds (full bag of groceries)	2	1	0
j. Lift and carry 25 pounds (medium to large suitcase)	2	1	0
k. Do most heavy household chores—scrubbing floors, vacuuming, raking leaves	2	1	0
l. Do strenuous activities—hiking, digging in garden, moving heavy objects, bicycling, aerobic dance exercises, strenuous calisthenics, etc.	2	1	0

19. In general, do you currently require household or nursing assistance to carry out daily activities? YES or NO

If yes, please check the reasons(s).

Health problems

☐ Chronic pain

☐ Lack of strength or endurance

☐ Lack of flexibility or balance

☐ Other reasons: _____

Reprinted from the Center for Successful Aging at California State University, Fullerton. Question 18 reprinted from Rikli & Jones, 1999.   *(continued)*

From *FallProof!* by Debra J. Rose, 2003, Champaign, IL: Human Kinetics.   **53**

20. In a typical week, how often do you leave your house (to run errands, go to work, go to meetings, classes, church, social functions, etc.)?

    ____ less than once/week   ____ 3-4 times/week

    ____ 1-2 times/week   ____ almost every day

21. Do you currently participate in regular physical exercise (such as walking, sports, exercise classes, housework, or yard work) that is strenuous enough to cause a noticeable increase in breathing, heart rate, or perspiration?   YES or NO

If yes, how many days per week? (circle)

                  One   Two   Three   Four   Five   Six   Seven

22. When you go for walks (if you do), which of the following best describes your walking pace? (check)

    ____ Strolling (easy pace, takes 30 minutes or more to walk a mile)

    ____ Average or normal (can walk a mile in 20-30 minutes)

    ____ Fairly brisk (fast pace, can walk a mile in 15-20 minutes)

    ____ Do not go for walks on a regular basis

23. Did you require assistance in completing this form?

          None (or very little)   Needed quite a bit of help

Reason: _____

Thank You!

Reprinted from the Center for Successful Aging at California State University, Fullerton. Question 18 reprinted from Rikli & Jones, 1999.

From *FallProof!* by Debra J. Rose, 2003, Champaign, IL: Human Kinetics.

Let's review the responses that Ms. Gain provided on her health/activity questionnaire so that we can learn more about the nature of her pathology/disease and pattern of physical activity. In answering the question "Have you ever been diagnosed as having any of the following conditions?" Jane indicated that she had been previously diagnosed with a heart attack, respiratory disease (i.e., chronic asthma), peripheral neuropathy, arthritis, inner ear problems, and depression—a total of six medical diagnoses. Her prescription medications include albuterol, Asthmacort, Lasix, Synthroid, Allopurinol, K-Dur, and Beconase—a total of seven prescription medications for her various diagnoses and other conditions (i.e., gout, hypothyroidism).

A review of her responses to questions 20 through 22 indicates that she remains active socially because she reports leaving the house "most every day." She does not, however, engage in any regular physical exercise, nor does she go for walks on a regular basis. Based on her self-report, it is clear that Ms. Gain is a sedentary person who would benefit from being involved in a regular exercise program of low to moderate intensity. Take a moment now to review the same questions on Mr. Divine's completed health/activity questionnaire to learn more about the nature of his pathology/disease and physical activity patterns.

Impairments and Functional Limitations

To assess the level of dysfunction at the impairment and functional limitations stages represented in Nagi's model, several physical performance tests are then administered during the first week of the program. These tests are designed to assess the multiple system impairments (e.g., motor, sensory, cardiovascular, musculoskeletal) that lead to functional limitations in the performance of daily activities requiring balance and mobility. The nature and extent of the functional limitations are also assessed during the same period. Although greater objectivity and sensitivity of measurement is derived by using tests requiring more advanced technology (e.g., computerized dynamic posturography, isokinetic dynamometry, electronystagmography), several clinical and field tests are currently available that provide valid and reliable information, require little or no equipment, and are relatively quick and easy to administer in community-based settings.

Prior to the start of any FallProof™ program, and at regular intervals throughout the program, it is recommended that the following impairment tests be conducted: the Senior Fitness Test (SFT) (Rikli & Jones, 1999a, 1999b), a modified version of the Clinical Test of Sensory Interaction in Balance (M-CTSIB) (Shumway-Cook & Horak, 1986), and the Multidirectional Reach Test (MDRT) (Newton, 1997, 2001). In addition, the Fullerton Advanced Balance (FAB) Scale (Rose & Lucchese, 2003) or Berg Balance Scale (BBS) (Berg, Wood-Dauphinee, Williams & Maki, 1992), the 50-foot walk performed at a preferred and fast speed, and the "walkie-talkie" test (Lundin-Olsson, Nyberg & Gustafson, 1997) should also be administered as the primary tests of functional limitations. Descriptions of how to administer, score, and interpret the results of each of these tests are presented in the next four sections.

> Several clinical and field tests are currently available that provide valid and reliable information, require little or no equipment, and are relatively quick and easy to administer in community-based settings.

Assessment of Physical Impairments Using the Senior Fitness Test

The underlying physical impairments associated with functional mobility in older adults are assessed using the Senior Fitness Test developed by Rikli and Jones (1999a, 1999b). This six-item test battery includes measures of upper and lower body strength and flexibility, aerobic endurance, and dynamic balance and agility. When performed in accordance with the administration guidelines, the results derived from each test item can be compared to norm-referenced standards based on a sample of 7,183 community-dwelling older adults ranging in age from 60 to 94 years. This test has demonstrated reliability and validity and can be performed successfully by older adults ranging from a healthy to physically frail level of function. Although it may be necessary to modify how certain test items are administered in the case of frailer older adults (i.e., allow use of hands during the chair stand or asymmetrical leg lift or use of external support during the 2-minute step test), the results can still be used to identify each participant's immediate program needs and to evaluate progress when administered in the same way at regular intervals throughout the program. A brief description of each of the six test items is provided in table 3.1. The actual test administration procedures and norm-referenced tables are provided in the Senior Fitness Test Manual (Rikli & Jones, 2001).

> A client's performance on the Senior Fitness Test can be compared to norm-referenced standards obtained for community-dwelling older adults ranging in age from 60 to 94 years.

Let's review Jane Gain's test results on the Senior Fitness Test to see how she fared. As her report card indicates (see figure 3.2), Jane was able to complete six arm curls

Table 3.1 Brief Descriptions of the Six Senior Fitness Test Items

Test item	Purpose	Description
30-second chair stand	To assess lower body strength needed for numerous tasks such as climbing stairs, walking, and getting out of a chair, tub, or car. Also reduces the chance of falling.	Number of full stands that can be completed in 30 seconds with arms folded across chest.
Arm curl	To assess upper body strength needed for performing household and other activities involving lifting and carrying things such as groceries, suitcases, and grandchildren.	Number of biceps curls that can be completed in 30 seconds holding a hand weight of 5 lb (2.27 kg) for women; 8 lb (3.63 kg) for men.
6-minute walk or 2-minute step test	To assess aerobic endurance—important for distance walking, stair climbing, shopping, sightseeing while on vacation, etc. Alternate aerobic endurance test for use when space limitations or weather prohibit giving the 6-minute walk test.	Number of yards/meters that can be walked in 6 minutes around a 50-yd (45.7-m) course (5 yd = 4.57 m). Number of full steps completed in 2 minutes, raising each knee to a point midway between the patella (kneecap) and iliac crest (top hip bone). Score is number of times right knee reaches the required height.
Chair sit-and-reach test	To assess lower body flexibility, which is important for good posture, for normal gait patterns, and for various mobility tasks such as getting into and out of a bathtub or car.	From a sitting position at the front of the chair with one leg extended and hands reaching toward toes, the number of inches (cm) (+ or –) between the extended fingers and the tip of toe.
Back scratch	To assess upper body (shoulder) flexibility, which is important in tasks such as combing one's hair, putting on overhead garments, and reaching for a seat belt.	With one hand reaching over the shoulder and one up the middle of the back, the number of inches (cm) between the extended middle fingers (+ or –).
8-foot up-and-go	To assess agility/dynamic balance, important in tasks that require quick maneuvering such as getting off a bus in time or getting up to attend to something in the kitchen, go to the bathroom, or answer the phone.	Number of seconds required to get up from a seated position, walk 8 ft (2.44 m), turn, and return to a seated position.

Adapted, by permission, from Rikli and Jones 2001.

using the right arm within the 30-second test period. A quick review of the national norms for women between 70 and 74 years of age indicates that Jane is below the 5th percentile for her age group on this measure of upper body strength. Her score of 4 on the 30-second chair stand test item also places her in the lowest 5th percentile for her age group. This score indicates that she has very poor lower body strength. On the two test items that measure flexibility, Jane was placed in the lowest 10th percentile based on her performance on the scratch test (–7 inches), a measure of upper body flexibility, and below the 5th percentile on the chair sit-and-reach (–6.5 inches), a measure of lower body flexibility. As was the case for strength, Jane also demonstrates a very low level of flexibility in the upper and lower body.

Jane's performance on the 8-foot up-and-go test, a measure of functional mobility, also placed her below the 5th percentile for her age and gender. Her best score of 11 seconds on the two recorded test trials also indicates that she is at high risk for falls (Rose, Jones & Lucchese, 2002). Any individual who requires more than 8.5 seconds to complete this test item is considered at high risk for falls. Finally, Jane was able to complete 53 unassisted steps in place on the 2-minute step test. Once

Figure 3.2

FallProof Program Report Card for Jane Gain

Name: *Jane Gain*   **Center:** *Dingley Senior Center*

Balance test	Baseline score	Rating	Additional comments
Fullerton Advanced Balance (FAB) Scale	16/40	Very low	Scored poorly on all items requiring vestibular inputs, strength and flexibility, and dynamic COG control.
M-CTSIB	110/120 sec	Good	Lost balance on trial 1 only—condition 4. Poor initial use of vestibular inputs. Provide close supervision when working on foam with eyes closed. Review MST component for appropriate exercises.
8-foot up-and-go	Trial 1 11.9 sec Trial 2 11.0 sec	<5th percentile, high fall risk	Mobility is poor. Need to focus on GPEV, dynamic COG exercises, and strength components.
"Walkie-talkie" test* *(circle one)*	Positive (Negative)	Good	Jane is able to divide attention between walking and talking.
50-foot walk (preferred speed) (fast speed)	2.4 ft/sec 3.6 ft/sec	Below average Below average	Gait speed needs to be improved. Review GPEV component for appropriate exercises. Also strength and flexibility.
Multidirectional Reach Test (measured in inches reached)	FWD: 8.0 in., BWD: 1.0 in. RLAT: 4.0 in., LLAT: 6.0 in.	Below average in backward direction	Review standing COG section: dynamic weight shifts for appropriate exercises. Need to increase LOS in backward direction.
Arm curl (left) right) *(circle one)*	6	<5th percentile	Score indicates very poor upper body strength. Review strength component for appropriate exercises.
30-second chair stand	4	<5th percentile	Score indicates very poor lower body strength. Possible dynamic COG problems also. Review strength and COG components for appropriate exercises.
Sit-and-reach test	−6.5 in.	<5th percentile	Very poor lower body flexibility. See flexibility section for appropriate exercises.
Scratch test	−7.0 in.	<10th percentile	Poor upper body flexibility. See flexibility component for appropriate exercises.
2-minute step	53 steps	<5th percentile	Score indicates very low aerobic endurance. Will need to rest during class sessions to maximize safety. Encourage short walks with partner between classes.
Balance Efficacy Scale	40/100	Below average	Score indicates Jane has low self-confidence in balance-related abilities. Requires high dose of success in exercises presented early in program.

*"Walkie-talkie": Positive = participant had to stop in order to respond to question; Negative = participant was able to continue walking while talking.

Note: COG = center of gravity; GPEV = gait pattern enhancement and variation; LOS = limits of stability; MST=multisensory training

again, her performance placed her below the 5th percentile for her age and gender. This indicates that her aerobic endurance is very poor.

Bill scored higher on most of the SFT test items than Jane. He completed 14 arm curls and 10 chair stands in separate 30-second test intervals. On the two trials of the sit-and-reach, he reached a distance of –8 inches and –7.5 inches. On the back scratch test he scored –6.5 inches on both test trials. All tests were performed using the right arm or leg. Bill's fastest time on the 8-foot up-and-go test was 9 seconds (trial 1 = 10 seconds), just a little slower than the 8.5-second cut-off score for high risk. Finally, during the 2-minute step test he completed 57 steps at the required height. Several steps were not counted because of his inability to repeatedly raise the right leg to the required step height.

To determine how Bill compared to the national norms on each of the test items consult the *Senior Fitness Test Manual* (Rikli & Jones, 2001). Once you have compared his scores to those of similarly-aged men, you will have a better idea of which components of his physical fitness are in need of improvement during the program.

Jane's test results clearly show that she has several physical impairments that will need to be addressed immediately if she is to make any significant gains in balance and mobility. She will clearly benefit from activities designed to improve her strength and flexibility, as well as activities designed to improve her level of aerobic endurance and functional mobility. The fact that she scored low on all items of the SFT also suggests that she will need to start with activities that are not too challenging for her and that specifically target each of the physical impairments identified by the SFT. Now review Bill Divine's performance on the SFT and identify the areas he needs to improve, considering his physical abilities.

Assessment of Sensory System Impairments Using the M-CTSIB

A modified version of the Clinical Test of Sensory Interaction in Balance (Shumway-Cook & Horak, 1986) is used to evaluate the older adult's ability to use different sensory strategies. Although unable to distinguish between different sensory system impairments, this test can be used to identify whether the use of sensory information in different sensory environments is normal or abnormal. In the modified version of the test used in the FallProof program, participants are required to stand quietly for 30 seconds with feet shoulder-width apart and arms folded across the chest in each of four different sensory conditions: (a) eyes open, stable surface (EOSS), (b) eyes closed, stable surface (ECSS), (c) eyes open, foam surface (EOFS), and (d) eyes closed, foam surface (ECFS). Each of the four test conditions is pictured in figure 3.3.

As a time-saving measure, if the person is able to maintain balance for the duration of the first trial, the tester can proceed to the next sensory condition. If the person lifts the arms from the chest or loses balance during the first trial, however, you should repeat the trial as a way of determining whether the person can "learn" to maintain balance if exposed to the particular sensory environment a little longer. To maintain a total test score of 120 seconds, repeated trial scores are averaged. Increased sway or loss of balance observed in the eyes closed, stable surface condition indicates poor use of somatosensory inputs for balance, whereas increased sway or loss of balance in the two foam surface conditions may indicate poor use of visual-vestibular (i.e., eyes open, foam surface) inputs or vestibular inputs alone (i.e., eyes closed, foam surface). Test administration instructions and a scoring form are provided in the box on the following page and form 3.2, respectively.

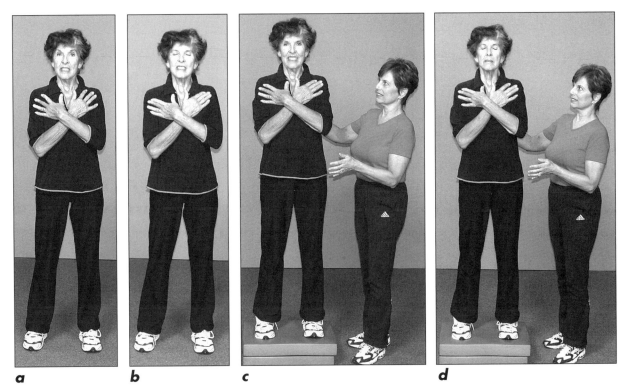

a   b   c   d

Figure 3.3 The four sensory conditions associated with the modified version of the Clinical Test of Sensory Interaction in Balance: **(a)** condition 1 (EOSS); **(b)** condition 2 (ECSS); **(c)** condition 3 (EOFS); **(d)** condition 4 (ECFS).

Test Administration Instructions for the Modified Clinical Test of Sensory Interaction in Balance (M-CTSIB)

Purpose: Evaluate how well an individual is able to use the three primary sensory inputs contributing to postural control (i.e., visual, somatosensory, vestibular)

Equipment: Two foam balance pads, two 12-inch lengths of nonslip material, stopwatch

Testing procedures: The individual is required to stand quietly for 30 seconds in each of four different sensory conditions: (a) eyes open, stable surface (EOSS); (b) eyes closed, stable surface (ECSS); (c) eyes open, foam surface (EOFS); (d) eyes closed, foam surface (ECFS). The person being tested should adopt a consistent standing position when performing this test. When testing older adults, ask them to stand with their feet shoulder-width apart and their arms folded across the chest. Stop the trial immediately if the person (a) lifts the arms from the chest, (b) requires manual assistance due to loss of balance, (c) prematurely opens the eyes prior to completion of the trial, or (d) moves the feet from the original starting position. Record the time in seconds. If the person is able to maintain balance for the duration of the first 30-second trial in a particular sensory condition, proceed to the next sensory condition. Allow the participant to perform up to two additional trials if unsuccessful on the first trial. The total score possible on this test is 120 seconds. If multiple trials are performed in certain conditions, the mean of those trials should be averaged to calculate the total score.

Although no cutoff scores have been developed for this test relative to fall risk, an instructor can use the information derived from each test condition to determine

Form 3.2

Scoring Form for the Modified Version of the Clinical Test of Sensory Interaction in Balance (M-CTSIB)

Condition 1: Eyes open, stable surface

    Trial 1   Total Time: _____ /30 sec

Condition 2:   **Eyes closed, stable surface**

    Trial 1   Total time: _____ /30 sec

    Trial 2   Total time: _____/30 sec

    Trial 3   Total time: _____/30 sec

                                     Mean: _____

Condition 3: Eyes open, foam surface

    Trial 1   Total time: _____ /30 sec

    Trial 2   Total time: _____/30 sec

    Trial 3   Total time: _____/30 sec

                                     Mean: _____

Condition 4: Eyes closed, foam surface

    Trial 1   Total time: _____ /30 sec

    Trial 2   Total time: _____ /30 sec

    Trial 3   Total time: _____/30 sec

                                     Mean: _____

*Complete additional trials in conditions 2, 3, and 4 if unable to complete previous trial. Average scores in case of additional trials.

From *FallProof!* by Debra J. Rose, 2003, Champaign, IL: Human Kinetics. Adapted from Shumway-Cook and Horak 1986.

whether the individual's ability to use sensory inputs for maintaining upright balance is normal or abnormal. For example, abnormal use of sensory inputs would be indicated if an individual required two or more trials to successfully maintain balance for the allotted time of 30 seconds on any of the four test conditions or was unable to complete any of the trials in any or all of the test conditions. From a program-planning perspective, knowing which sensory conditions pose the greatest difficulty for the participant can also help the instructor select the most appropriate multisensory activities (described in chapter 5) for each individual as well as the initial level of difficulty. An instructor guide to interpreting the results of this test is provided in table 3.2.

> The information obtained from each test condition on the M-CTSIB can be used to determine whether the use of sensory inputs for maintaining upright balance in different sensory conditions is normal or abnormal.

Jane's performance on the M-CTSIB was actually very good. She scored a total of 110 seconds out of a possible 120 seconds. Despite having been diagnosed with peripheral neuropathy, she performed very well in the eyes closed, stable surface condition (a test of somatosensory system impairment). She was able to complete the

Table 3.2 Interpreting the M-CTSIB Test Results

Test condition	Possible impairments	Recommended exercises
1. Eyes open, stable surface (3/3 systems available)	1. Poor gaze stabilization	Teach visual "spotting."
	2. Poor use of surface cues	Balance activities with reduced/ engaged/absent vision.
	3. Lower body weakness	Lower body exercises against resistance (i.e., gravity/ resistance band/weights).
2. Eyes closed, stable surface (2/3 systems available) No vision available	1. Poor use of surface cues*	Increase awareness of surface information through verbal cueing during standing exercises. Balance activities with reduced/engaged/absent vision.
	2. Lower body weakness	Lower body exercises against resistance (i.e., gravity/ resistance band/weights).
	3. Fear of falling	Confidence-building activities.
3. Eyes open, foam surface (2/3 systems available) Somatosensory information reduced	1. Poor use of vision	Gaze stabilization techniques. Balance activities performed on compliant or moving surfaces seated, standing, moving (do not add visual task).
	2. Lower body weakness	Lower body exercises against resistance (i.e., gravity/ resistance band/weights).
	3. Poor COG control	Standing COG activities on compliant surfaces of different thicknesses.
4. Eyes closed, foam surface (1/3 systems available) Somatosensory reduced and vision unavailable	1. Poor use of vestibular inputs**	Balance activities performed on compliant/moving surfaces. Vision reduced/engaged/absent.
	2. Fear of falling in high-sway conditions	Voluntary sway activities to build confidence.
	3. Lower body weakness	Lower body exercises against resistance (i.e., gravity/ resistance band/weights).

*Review medical history to determine if any medical condition exists indicating progressive or permanent loss of sensation in foot or ankle region.

**Review medical history to determine if any chronic or progressive medical condition affecting vestibular system (i.e., Ménière's disease) exists before performing first set of exercises.

first 30-second trial successfully, indicating that she was able to use somatosensory inputs to maintain balance in the absence of vision. The only difficulty she experienced was on the first trial of condition 4. She was only able to maintain balance with her eyes closed while standing on the foam surface for 10 seconds. On the second trial, however, she was able to maintain her balance for the full 30-second test period. Although she initially experienced difficulty maintaining balance when vision was removed and the somatosensory system was distorted as a result of having to stand on a foam surface, she was able to "learn" how to maintain balance on the second trial. As you will recall, this test condition is designed to force greater use of the vestibular system for maintaining balance. Bill Divine also performed very well on the M-CTSIB. He successfully maintained balance in all test conditions, yielding the best possible score of 120 seconds.

Although her performance was good on this test, Jane will benefit from multisensory training activities that are designed to improve her use of the vestibular system and also the visual system, given that her peripheral neuropathy is likely to progress as she ages. Despite his perfect score, Bill should also continue to fine tune each of the sensory systems for balance; the level of balance challenge can be increased based on his test scores. You will learn how to improve the use of each of these sensory systems in chapter 5 of this instructor guide.

Assessment of Motor Impairments Using the Multidirectional Reach Test (MDRT)

Possible motor impairments related to the voluntary planning and execution of movements are identified using the Multidirectional Reach Test (Newton, 1997, 2001). This test is an expanded version of the functional reach test (Duncan, Weiner, Chandler & Studenski, 1990) used to measure the distance an individual is able or willing to lean in a forward direction only. The MDRT measures how far individuals are able to lean through their region of stability in the forward, backward, and lateral directions without altering the base of support (figure 3.4). The participant extends the preferred arm and fingers and attempts to lean as far as possible in each of the four directions without moving the feet or rising up onto the toes. The distance leaned in each direction is recorded in inches. The procedures for administering this test are presented in the box on the following page; use form 3.3 to score the test.

This test provides the instructor with information about the size of each individual's region of stability and the type of postural strategy (i.e., ankle or hip) used to achieve maximal lean. Although the distance leaned will be affected by the age and height of the participant, Newton (2001) suggests that the mean values obtained from her evaluation of 254 older adults can be used to determine above- and below-average performance on this test. The mean values recorded were 8.9 inches in a forward direction, 4.6 inches in a backward direction, and 6.2 and 6.6 inches in the right and left lateral directions, respectively. Above and below average scores for each direction are provided in table 3.3.

Jane also completed this test of motor impairment and recorded the following scores: 8 inches on the forward lean, 1 inch on the backward lean, 4 inches on the right lateral lean, and 6 inches on the left lateral lean. A comparison of her scores to the mean values presented in table 3.3 indicates that her ability to lean in the forward and left lateral directions was within the average range but her ability to lean in the backward and right lateral directions was below average. These results indicate that she has reduced limits of stability in the backward and right lateral directions. These areas of stability limits will need to be improved to reduce her risk for falling. It is perhaps not surprising that her ability to lean in a right lateral direction is compromised, given that she has severe arthritis in the right knee. This orthopedic condition makes it more difficult for her to shift her weight onto the right side due to the increased pain and lack of confidence she feels in the capabilities of this joint. Her extreme fear of falling may also account for her reluctance to lean in a backward direction.

Bill's scores on the MDRT yielded lean scores of 9.6 inches in the forward direction, 2 inches in the backward direction, 7 inches in the left lateral direction, and 4 inches in the right lateral direction. Compare his scores to the mean values in table 3.3 to see if his scores fall within the acceptable mean range in all directions.

The Multidirectional Reach Test can be used to identify possible motor impairments related to the voluntary planning and execution of movements.

Test Administration Instructions for Multidirectional Reach Test (MDRT)

Purpose: To measure the distance a person is able or willing to lean in a forward, backward, and lateral direction.

Equipment: Yardstick; wall

Forward reach

- Position yardstick on wall at height of acromion.
- Instruct the individual to stand in a comfortable position with feet shoulder-width apart.
- Instruct the individual to raise one arm in front to shoulder height (hand extended, palm turned to face medially) and not to touch the yardstick.
- Instruct the individual to reach forward as far as possible without raising the heels from the floor. Record the location of the middle fingertip.
- Now instruct the individual to stop reaching and return to the starting position.
- Subtract the end number from the starting position number to obtain the length reached.
- Pause before the next trial.
- Provide one practice trial before the start of the three test trials.

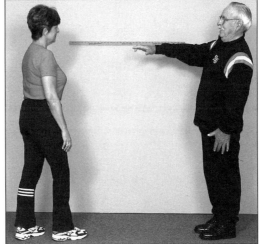

Figure 3.4 Older adult performing Multidirectional Reach Test.

Backward reach

Repeat all instructions, but this time ask the individual to lean backward as far as possible without raising the toes from the floor. Record the location of the middle fingertip.

Lateral reach to the right

- Position yardstick on wall at height of acromion.
- Instruct the individual to stand in a comfortable position with feet shoulder-width apart.
- Instruct the individual to raise one arm horizontally to shoulder height (hand extended, palm turned to face medially) and not to touch the yardstick.
- Instruct the individual to reach sideways to the right as far as possible. Record the location of the middle fingertip.
- Now instruct the individual to stop reaching and return to the starting position.
- Subtract the end number from the starting position number to obtain the number of inches reached.
- Pause before the next trial.
- Provide one practice trial before the start of the three test trials.

Lateral reach to the left

Repeat all previous instructions, but this time ask the individual to reach sideways to the left as far as possible. Record the location of the middle fingertip.

(Newton 1997)

Scoring Form for Multidirectional Reach Test (MDRT)

FORWARD REACH

Distance reached	Movement strategy

Trial 1 _____

hip ____ ankle ____ trunk rotation _____

scapular protraction _____ other _____

Trial 2 _____

hip ____ ankle ____ trunk rotation _____

scapular protraction _____ other _____

Trial 3 _____

hip ____ ankle ____ trunk rotation _____

scapular protraction _____ other _____

Mean: _____

BACKWARD REACH

Distance reached	Movement strategy

Trial 1 _____

hip ____ ankle ____ trunk rotation _____

scapular protraction _____ other _____

Trial 2 _____

hip ____ ankle ____ trunk rotation _____

scapular protraction _____ other _____

Trial 3 _____

hip ____ ankle ____ trunk rotation _____

scapular protraction _____ other _____

Mean: _____

LATERAL REACH TO THE RIGHT

Distance reached	Movement strategy

Trial 1 _____

hip ____ ankle ____ trunk rotation _____

scapular protraction _____ other _____

Trial 2 _____

hip ____ ankle ____ trunk rotation _____

scapular protraction _____ other _____

Trial 3 _____

hip ____ ankle ____ trunk rotation _____

scapular protraction _____ other _____

Mean: _____

LATERAL REACH TO THE LEFT

Distance reached	Movement strategy

Trial 1 _____

hip ____ ankle ____ trunk rotation _____

scapular protraction _____ other _____

Trial 2 _____

hip ____ ankle ____ trunk rotation _____

scapular protraction _____ other _____

Trial 3 _____

hip ____ ankle ____ trunk rotation _____

scapular protraction _____ other _____

Mean: _____

From *FallProof!* by Debra J. Rose, 2003, Champaign, IL: Human Kinetics.

Table 3.3   Multidirectional Reach Test (MDRT) Reference Values

On the basis of recommendations forwarded by Newton (2001), the following values for each direction can be used as the basis for evaluating an individual's performance:

Forward direction	Above average	>12.2 in.
Mean: 8.9 in.) (SD: ±3.4 in.)	Below average	<5.6 in.
Backward direction	Above average	>7.6 in.
(Mean: 4.6 in.) (SD: ±3.1 in.)	Below average	<1.6 in.
Right lateral direction	Above average	>9.4 in.
(Mean: 6.2 in.) (SD: ±3.0 in.)	Below average	<3.8 in.
Left lateral direction	Above average	>9.4 in.
(Mean: 6.6 in.) (SD: ±2.9 in.)	Below average	<3.8 in.

Assessment of Functional Limitations

The tests used to measure functional limitations associated with the performance of daily activities requiring balance include the Fullerton Advanced Balance Scale (Rose & Lucchese, 2003) or Berg Balance Scale (Berg et al., 1992), whereas limitations in functional mobility are measured using a 50-foot walk test performed at a preferred and fast speed. Finally, limitations in the allocation of attention are evaluated using the "walkie-talkie" test (Lundin-Olsson, Nyberg & Gustafson, 1997).

The FAB Scale is a new test designed to measure changes in balance occurring in higher-functioning older adults. It is therefore considered appropriate for use with the community-residing older adults who are most likely to enroll in your community-based programs. The FAB Scale is composed of 10 items that are scored using a 0- to 4-point **ordinal scale**. The scale includes a combination of static and dynamic balance activities performed in different sensory environments. Items include standing on foam with eyes closed, walking with head turns, stepping over an obstacle, and jumping for distance. Detailed test administration procedures and a scoring form are provided in the box on the following page and in form 3.4, respectively.

The test has demonstrated high test-retest reliability and inter- and intra-rater reliability when conducted by experienced clinicians. Scores on the FAB Scale also correlate well with scores obtained using the Berg Balance Scale (r = .75), another measure of balance-related abilities. The FAB Scale was developed as an alternative measure of functional limitations because of the tendency of the BBS to produce ceiling effects (i.e., very high scores on repeated tests) when administered to higher-functioning older adults with impaired balance. The FAB Scale also includes items intended to better identify older adults who may be experiencing increased fall risk as a result of sensory system impairments. The BBS has been criticized for its lack of sensitivity in identifying sensory system impairments (Allison & Rose, 1998). An individual's performance on each of the FAB Scale test items can also be evaluated and the possible underlying impairments identified so that exercise progressions that specifically target those impairments can be selected. Table 3.4 provides a list of the possible underlying impairments associated with poor performance on each of the 10 test items and a set of recommended exercises to address the identified impairments.

ordinal scale—A numerical ranking of performance from best (e.g., 4 points) to worst (e.g., 0 points). The difference between two adjacent scores is not the same throughout the scale.

The Fullerton Advanced Balance Scale is designed to measure changes in multiple dimensions of balance in higher functioning community-dwelling older adults.

Test Administration Instructions for the Fullerton Advanced Balance (FAB) Scale

1. Stand with feet together and eyes closed

Purpose: Assess ability to use ground cues to maintain upright balance while standing with a reduced base of support

Equipment: Stopwatch

Testing procedures: Demonstrate the correct test position and then instruct the participants to move the feet independently until they are together. If some participants are unable to achieve the correct position due to lower extremity joint problems, encourage them to bring their heels together even though the front of the feet are not touching. Have participants adopt a position that will ensure their safety as the arms are folded across the chest and they prepare to close the eyes. Begin timing as soon as the participant closes the eyes. (Instruct participants to open the eyes if they feel so unsteady that a loss of balance is imminent.)

Verbal instructions: "Bring your feet together, fold your arms across your chest, close your eyes when you are ready, and remain as steady as possible until I instruct you to open your eyes."

2. Reach forward to retrieve an object (pencil) held at shoulder height with outstretched arm

Purpose: Assess ability to lean forward to retrieve an object without altering the base of support; measure of stability limits in a forward direction

Equipment: Pencil and 12-inch ruler

Testing procedures: Instruct the participant to raise the preferred arm to 90° and extend it with fingers outstretched. (Follow with a demonstration of the correct action.) Use the ruler to measure a distance of 10 inches from the end of the fingers of the outstretched arm. Hold the object (pencil) horizontally and level with the height of the participant's shoulder. Instruct the participant to reach forward, grasp the pencil, and return to the initial starting position without moving the feet, if possible. (It is acceptable to raise the heels as long as the feet do not move while reaching for the pencil.) If the participant is unable to reach the pencil within 2-3 seconds of initiating the forward lean, indicate to the participant that it is okay to move the feet in order to reach the pencil. Record the number of steps taken by the participant in order to retrieve the pencil.

Verbal instructions: "Try to lean forward to take the pencil from my hand and return to your starting position without moving your feet from their present position." After allowing 2-3 seconds of lean time: "You can move your feet in order to reach the pencil."

3. Turn 360° in right and left directions

Purpose: Assess ability to turn in a full circle in both directions in the fewest number of steps without loss of balance

Equipment: None

Testing procedures: Verbally explain and then demonstrate the task to be performed, making sure to complete each circle in four steps or less and pause briefly between turns. Instruct the participant to turn in a complete circle in one direction, pause, and then turn in a complete circle in the opposite direction. Count the number of steps taken to complete each circle. Allow for a small correction in foot position before a turn in the opposite direction is initiated.

Verbal instructions: "Turn around in a full circle, pause, and then turn in a second full circle in the opposite direction."

4. Step up onto and over a 6-inch bench

Purpose: Assess ability to control center of gravity in dynamic task situations; also a measure of lower body strength and control

Equipment: 6-inch-high bench (18- by 18-inch stepping surface)

Testing procedures: Verbally explain and demonstrate the step up onto and over the bench in both directions before the participant performs the test item. Instruct the participant to step onto the bench with the right foot, swing the left leg directly up and over the bench, and step off the other side, then repeat the movement in the opposite direction with the left leg leading the action. During performance of the test item, watch to see that the participant's trailing leg (a) does not make contact with the bench or (b) swing around, as opposed to directly over, the bench.

Verbal instructions: "Step up onto the bench with your right leg, swing your left leg directly up and over the bench, and step off the other side. Repeat the movement in the opposite direction with your left leg as the leading leg."

5. Tandem walk

Purpose: Assess ability to dynamically control center of mass with an altered base of support

Equipment: Masking tape

Testing procedures: Verbally explain and demonstrate how to perform the test item correctly before the participant attempts to perform it. Instruct the participant to walk on the line in a tandem position (heel-to-toe) until you tell them to stop. Allow the participant to repeat the test item *one time* if unable to achieve a tandem stance position within the first two steps. The participant may elect to step forward with the opposite foot on the second trial. Score as interruptions any instances where the participant (a) takes a lateral step away from the line when performing the tandem walk or (b) is unable to achieve correct heel-to-toe position during any step taken along the course. Do not ask the participant to stop until 10 steps have been completed.

Verbal instructions: "Walk forward along the line, placing one foot directly in front of the other such that the heel and toe are in contact on each step forward. I will tell you when to stop."

6. Stand on one leg

Purpose: Assess ability to maintain upright balance with a reduced base of support

Equipment: Stopwatch

Testing procedures: Instruct the participant to fold the arms across the chest, lift the preferred leg off the floor, and maintain balance until instructed to return the foot to the floor. Begin timing as soon as the participant lifts the foot from the floor. Stop timing if the legs touch, the preferred leg contacts the floor, or the participant removes the arms from the chest before the 20 seconds has elapsed. Allow the participant to perform the test a second time with the other leg if they are unsure as to which is the preferred limb.

Verbal instructions: "Fold your arms across your chest, lift your preferred leg off the floor (without touching your other leg), and stand with your eyes open as long as you can."

7. Stand on foam with eyes closed

Purpose: Assess ability to maintain upright balance while standing on a compliant surface with eyes closed

Equipment: Stopwatch; two Airex pads, with a length of nonslip material placed between the two pads and an additional length of nonslip material between the floor and first pad if the test is being performed on an uncarpeted surface

Testing procedures: Instruct the participant to step onto the foam pads without assistance, fold the arms across the chest, and close the eyes when ready. (Demonstrate the correct standing position on foam.) Make sure the position adopted ensures the safety of the participant. Position the foam pads close to a wall in all cases and in a corner of the room if the participant appears unsteady. Begin timing as soon as the eyes close. Stop the trial if the participant (a) opens the eyes before the timing period has elapsed, (b) lifts the arms off the chest, or (c) loses balance and requires manual assistance to prevent falling. (Instruct participants to open their eyes if they feel so unsteady that a loss of balance is imminent.)

Verbal instructions: "Step up onto the foam and stand with your feet shoulder-width apart. Fold your arms over your chest, and close your eyes when you are ready. I will tell you when to open your eyes."

8. Two-footed jump for distance

Purpose: Assess upper and lower body coordination and lower body power

Equipment: 36-inch ruler

Testing procedures: Instruct the participant to jump as far but as safely as possible while maintaining a two-footed stance. Demonstrate the correct movement prior to the participant performing the jump. (Do not jump much more than twice the length of your own feet when demonstrating.) Observe whether the participant leaves the floor with both feet and lands with both feet. Use the ruler to measure the length of the foot and then multiply by two to determine the ideal distance to be jumped.

Verbal instructions: "Try to jump as far but as safely as you can with both feet."

9. Walk with head turns

Purpose: Assess ability to maintain dynamic balance while walking and turning the head

Equipment: Metronome set at 100 beats per minute

Testing procedures: After first demonstrating the test item, allow the participant to practice turning the head in time with the metronome while standing in place. Encourage the participant to turn the head at least 30° in each direction (i.e., "Turn your head to look into each corner of the room."). Observe how far the participant is able to turn the head during the standing head turns. A 30° head turn is required during the walking trial. Instruct the participant to walk forward while turning the head from side to side and in time with the auditory tone. Begin counting steps as soon as the participant attempts to turn the head to the beat of the metronome. Observe whether the participant deviates from a straight path while walking or is unable to turn the head the required distance to the timing of the metronome

Verbal instructions: "Walk forward while turning your head from left to right with each beat of the metronome. I will tell you when to stop."

10. Reactive postural control

Purpose: Assess ability to efficiently restore balance following an unexpected perturbation

Equipment: None

Testing procedures: Instruct the participant to stand with his or her back to you. Extend your arm with the elbow locked and place the palm of your hand against the participant's back between the scapula. Instruct the participant to lean back slowly against your hand until you tell him or her to stop. Quickly flex your elbow until your hand is no longer in contact with the participant's back at the moment you estimate that a sufficient amount of force has been applied to require a movement of the feet to restore balance. You may actually begin releasing your hand while you are still giving the instructions. This release should be unexpected, so do not prepare the participant for the moment of release.

Verbal instructions: "Slowly lean back into my hand until I ask you to stop."

Score Sheet for
Fullerton Advanced Balance (FAB) Scale

Name: _____ Date of Test: _____

1. Stand with feet together and eyes closed

( ) 0 Unable to obtain the correct standing position independently

( ) 1 Able to obtain the correct standing position independently but unable to maintain the position or keep the eyes closed for more than 10 seconds

( ) 2 Able to maintain the correct standing position with eyes closed for more than 10 seconds but less than 30 seconds

( ) 3 Able to maintain the correct standing position with eyes closed for 30 seconds but requires close supervision

( ) 4 Able to maintain the correct standing position safely with eyes closed for 30 seconds

2. Reach forward to retrieve an object (pencil) held at shoulder height with outstretched arm

( ) 0 Unable to reach the pencil without taking more than two steps

( ) 1 Able to reach the pencil but needs to take two steps

( ) 2 Able to reach the pencil but needs to take one step

( ) 3 Can reach the pencil without moving the feet but requires supervision

( ) 4 Can reach the pencil safely and independently without moving the feet

3. Turn 360° in right and left directions

( ) 0 Needs manual assistance while turning

( ) 1 Needs close supervision or verbal cueing while turning

( ) 2 Able to turn 360° but takes more than four steps in both directions

( ) 3 Able to turn 360° but unable to complete in four steps or fewer in one direction

( ) 4 Able to turn 360° safely taking four steps or fewer in both directions

4. Step up onto and over a 6-inch bench

( ) 0 Unable to step up onto the bench without loss of balance or manual assistance

( ) 1 Able to step up onto the bench with leading leg, but trailing leg contacts the bench or leg swings around the bench during the swing-through phase in both directions

( ) 2 Able to step up onto the bench with leading leg, but trailing leg contacts the bench or swings around the bench during the swing-through phase in one direction

( ) 3 Able to correctly complete the step up and over in both directions but requires close supervision in one or both directions

( ) 4 Able to correctly complete the step up and over in both directions safely and independently

5. Tandem walk

( ) 0 Unable to complete 10 steps independently

( ) 1 Able to complete the 10 steps with more than five interruptions

( ) 2 Able to complete the 10 steps with five or fewer interruptions

( ) 3 Able to complete the 10 steps with two or fewer interruptions

( ) 4 Able to complete the 10 steps independently and with no interruptions

(continued)

Form 3.4

6. **Stand on one leg**

( ) 0 Unable to try or needs assistance to prevent falling

( ) 1 Able to lift leg independently but unable to maintain position for more than 5 seconds

( ) 2 Able to lift leg independently and maintain position for more than 5 but less than 12 seconds

( ) 3 Able to lift leg independently and maintain position for 12 or more seconds but less than 20 seconds

( ) 4 Able to lift leg independently and maintain position for the full 20 seconds

7. **Stand on foam with eyes closed**

( ) 0 Unable to step onto foam or maintain standing position independently with eyes open

( ) 1 Able to step onto foam independently and maintain standing position but unable or unwilling to close eyes

( ) 2 Able to step onto foam independently and maintain standing position with eyes closed for 10 seconds or less

( ) 3 Able to step onto foam independently and maintain standing position with eyes closed for more than 10 seconds but less than 20 seconds

( ) 4 Able to step onto foam independently and maintain standing position with eyes closed for 20 seconds

8. **Two-footed jump for distance**

( ) 0 Unable to attempt or attempts to initiate two-footed jump, but one or both feet do not leave the floor

( ) 1 Able to initiate two-footed jump, but one foot either leaves the floor or lands before the other

( ) 2 Able to perform two-footed jump, but unable to jump farther than the length of their own feet

( ) 3 Able to perform two-footed jump and achieve a distance greater than the length of their own feet

( ) 4 Able to perform two-footed jump and achieve a distance greater than twice the length of their own feet

9. **Walk with head turns**

( ) 0 Unable to walk 10 steps independently while maintaining 30° head turns at an established pace

( ) 1 Able to walk 10 steps independently but unable to complete required number of 30° head turns at an established pace

( ) 2 Able to walk 10 steps but veers from a straight line while performing 30° head turns at an established pace

( ) 3 Able to walk 10 steps in a straight line while performing 30° head turns at an established pace but head turns less than 30° in one or both directions

( ) 4 Able to walk 10 steps in a straight line while performing required number of 30° head turns at established pace

10. **Reactive postural control**

( ) 0 Unable to maintain upright balance; no observable attempt to step; requires manual assistance to restore balance

( ) 1 Unable to maintain upright balance; takes two or more steps and requires manual assistance to restore balance

( ) 2 Unable to maintain upright balance; takes two or more steps but is able to restore balance independently

( ) 3 Unable to maintain upright balance; takes one to two steps but is able to restore balance independently

( ) 4 Unable to maintain upright balance but able to restore balance independently with only one step

Table 3.4 Interpretation of the Individual Test Items on the Fullerton Advanced Balance (FAB) Scale for Possible Underlying Impairments

Item	Possible impairments	Recommended exercises
1. Stand with feet together and eyes closed	1. Weak hip abductors/adductors	Lateral weight shifts against resistance; side leg raises against gravity/resistance
	2. Poor COG control	Seated/standing balance activities emphasizing weight shifts in multiple directions
	3. Poor use of somatosensory cues	Standing balance activities with eyes closed (controlled sway in A-P and lateral directions)
2. Reach forward to object	1. Reduced limits of stability	Seated/standing COG control activities
	2. Reduced ankle ROM	Ankle circles, heel lifts, and drops from height
	3. Fear of falling	Confidence-building activities—high success
	4. Lower body muscle weakness	Wall sits; LB exercises with resistance
3. Turn in a full circle	1. Poor dynamic COG control	Standing weight transfer activities; gait pattern enhancement (turns, directional changes)
	2. Possible vestibular impairment (e.g., dizziness)	Head and eye movement coordination exercises
	3. Lower body weakness	LB exercises with resistance; emphasize hip and knee flexion; hip abduction/adduction
4. Step up and over	1. Poor dynamic COG control	Seated/standing balance activities emphasizing backward weight shifts
	2. Lower body weakness	LB exercises with resistance (own body/resistance band; emphasize sustained unilateral stance positions)
	3. Reduced ROM at ankle, knee, hip	Flexibility exercises emphasizing hip/knee/ankle flexion; seated and standing
5. Tandem walk	1. Poor dynamic COG control	Standing/moving COG control activities; emphasize A-P control during weight shifts
	2. Poor use of vision	Activities emphasizing gaze-stabilization techniques
	3. Weak hip abductors/adductors	Side leg raise against gravity/resistance; lateral weight shift and lunge activities
6. Stand on one leg	1. Poor COG control	Standing A-P weight shifts and transfers; reduced BOS activities
	2. Lower body muscle weakness	LB exercises with resistance (body/resistance band); emphasize hip abductors/adductors
	3. Poor use of vision	Activities emphasizing gaze stabilization
7. Stand on foam with eyes closed	1. Poor use of vestibular inputs for balance	Seated/standing activities performed with reduced/absent vision on altered surfaces
	2. Lower body muscle weakness	LB exercises with resistance (body/resistance band); emphasize quadriceps, gastrocnemius/soleus muscles
	3. Heightened fear of falling when vision absent	Confidence-building activities with progressive reduction in availability of vision
8. Two-footed jump	1. Poor dynamic COG control	Standing/moving COG activities emphasizing leaning away from and back to midline
	2. Poor upper and lower body coordination	Selected exercises to improve UB and LB coordination; multiple task activities
	3. Lower body muscle weakness	LB exercises with resistance (body/resistance band) performed at progressively faster speeds
9. Walk with head turns	1. Possible vestibular impairment	Head and eye movement coordination exercises; gait pattern enhancement (turns, directional changes)
	2. Poor use of vision	Activities emphasizing gaze stabilization
	3. Poor dynamic COG control	Standing/moving activities with head turns; progressively increase speed and frequency of head turns
10. Reactive postural test	1. Absent postural strategy (i.e., step)	Activities emphasizing step strategy (i.e., resistance band release activity)
	2. Poor COG control	Standing COG control activities; volitional stepping activities in multiple directions
	3. Lower body muscle weakness	LB exercises with resistance; emphasize hip and knee flexion; hip abduction/adduction

Note: A-P=anterior-posterior direction; BOS=base of support; COG=center of gravity; LB=lower body; UB=upper body.

An alternative measure for assessing functional limitations is the BBS, a test that has also been shown to be highly reliable and valid when used across a broad continuum of functional levels. This test represents an effective means of assessing each participant's ability to perform a series of functional tasks that require balance. Many of the tasks presented in this test simulate activities likely to be encountered by older adults in their daily lives (e.g., transfers, object retrieval, turning). The procedures for administering and scoring this test are presented in the box below.

Test Administration for the Berg Balance Scale (BBS)

Purpose: Evaluate functional limitations associated with the performance of daily activities requiring balance

Equipment: Stopwatch; two straight-backed chairs, one with armrests and one without; 12-inch ruler; slipper; 6-inch bench

Test procedures: Conduct each test item in the order described on the test form. Demonstrate each test item or read instructions aloud (as written) to each participant. Record the score on the test form after completion of each test item, recording any additional form-related comments next to each test item (e.g., "Tended to look down as she attempted to rise from chair"; "Very unstable immediately after rising from chair"). This is not intended to be a test of endurance, so allow participants to rest as needed.

Interpreting test results: The total score possible on the full version of the test is 56. A score of 45 or below is associated with a high risk for falls (Thorbahn & Newton, 1997). A more recent study, however, suggests that a cut-off score of 50/56 improves the test's ability to predict which older adults are more likely to fall (Riddle & Stratford, 1999). In the modified version, a total score of 36 is possible. Remember, however, that you will learn more about each participant and be able to identify more specific limitations in function if you review each of the individual test item scores in addition to the total score.

In addition to providing valuable information about the types of balance activities that are most difficult to perform, this test can be used to identify older adults who are appropriate for intervention (Harada, Chiu, Fowler, Lee & Reuben, 1995); however, many practitioners argue that it is less useful as a tool for identifying who will actually fall (Thorbahn & Newton, 1996; Chandler, 1996). It is recommended that older adults who score less than 46 out of a possible 56 points on the BBS would benefit from immediate intervention. This test measure, as opposed to the FAB Scale, is recommended when assessing lower-functioning older adults (i.e., those who score lower than 14/24 on the composite physical function scale question on the health/activity questionnaire).

The Berg Balance Scale is recommended when assessing low-functioning older adults.

To save time, a modified version of the test can also be used with higher-functioning community-dwelling older adults. The first five items are eliminated on the modified version, reducing the test to nine items in total. The new score for the modified test is 36. This version of the test has been demonstrated as reliable and valid as the longer version (Daschle et al., 1999). The items that are retained on the modified version are identified with an asterisk (*) on the original BBS test form (form 3.5). Although no cutoff score for fall risk has been established for the shortened version

Berg Balance Scale

Name: _____ Date of Test: _____

1. Sit to stand

Instructions: "Please stand up. Try not to use your hands for support."

Grading: Please mark the lowest category that applies.

(   ) 0   Needs moderate or maximal assistance to stand

(   ) 1   Needs minimal assistance to stand or to stabilize

(   ) 2   Able to stand using hands after several tries

(   ) 3   Able to stand independently using hands

(   ) 4   Able to stand with no hands and stabilize independently

2. Standing unsupported

Instructions: "Please stand for 2 minutes without holding onto anything."

Grading: Please mark the lowest category that applies.

(   ) 0   Unable to stand 30 seconds unassisted

(   ) 1   Needs several tries to stand 30 seconds unsupported

(   ) 2   Able to stand 30 seconds unsupported

(   ) 3   Able to stand 2 minutes with supervision

(   ) 4   Able to stand safely for 2 minutes

If person is able to stand 2 minutes safely, score full points for sitting unsupported (item 3). Proceed to item 4.

3. Sitting with back unsupported with feet on floor or on a stool

Instructions: "Sit with arms folded for 2 minutes."

Grading: Please mark the lowest category that applies.

(   ) 0   Unable to sit without support for 10 seconds

(   ) 1   Able to sit for 10 seconds

(   ) 2   Able to sit for 30 seconds

(   ) 3   Able to sit for 2 minutes under supervision

(   ) 4   Able to sit safely and securely for 2 minutes

4. Stand to sit

Instructions: "Please sit down."

Grading: Please mark the lowest category that applies.

(   ) 0   Needs assistance to sit

(   ) 1   Sits independently but has uncontrolled descent

(   ) 2   Uses back of legs against chair to control descent

(   ) 3   Controls descent by using hands

(   ) 4   Sits safely with minimal use of hands

Reprinted from Berg, 1992.

(continued)

5. **Transfers**

   Instructions: "Please move from chair to chair and back again." (Person moves one way toward a seat with armrests and one way toward a seat without armrests.) Arrange chairs for pivot transfer.

   Grading: Please mark the lowest category that applies.

   (   ) 0   Needs two people to assist or supervise to be safe

   (   ) 1   Needs one person to assist

   (   ) 2   Able to transfer with verbal cueing and/or supervision

   (   ) 3   Able to transfer safely with definite use of hands

   (   ) 4   Able to transfer safely with minor use of hands

6. ***Standing unsupported with eyes closed**

   Instructions: "Close your eyes and stand still for 10 seconds."

   Grading: Please mark the lowest category that applies.

   (   ) 0   Needs help to keep from falling

   (   ) 1   Unable to keep eyes closed for 3 seconds but remains steady

   (   ) 2   Able to stand for 3 seconds

   (   ) 3   Able to stand for 10 seconds with supervision

   (   ) 4   Able to stand for 10 seconds safely

7. ***Stand unsupported with feet together**

   Instructions: "Place your feet together and stand without holding on to anything."

   Grading: Please mark the lowest category that applies.

   (   ) 0   Needs help to attain position and unable to hold for 15 seconds

   (   ) 1   Needs help to attain position but able to stand for 15 seconds with feet together

   (   ) 2   Able to place feet together independently but unable to hold for 30 seconds

   (   ) 3   Able to place feet together independently and stand for 1 minute with supervision

   (   ) 4   Able to place feet together independently and stand for 1 minute safely

The following items are to be performed while standing unsupported.

8. ***Reaching forward with outstretched arm**

   Instructions: "Lift your arm to 90°. Stretch out your fingers and reach forward as far as you can." (Examiner places a ruler at end of fingertips when arm is at 90°. Fingers should not touch the ruler while reaching forward. The recorded measure is the distance forward that the fingers reach while the person is in the most forward lean position.)

   Grading: Please mark the lowest category that applies.

   (   ) 0   Needs help to keep from falling

   (   ) 1   Reaches forward but needs supervision

   (   ) 2   Can reach forward more than 2 inches safely

   (   ) 3   Can reach forward more than 5 inches safely

   (   ) 4   Can reach forward confidently more than 10 inches

9. ***Pick up object from the floor from a standing position**

   Instructions: "Please pick up the shoe/slipper that is placed in front of your feet."

   Grading: Please mark the lowest category that applies.

   (   ) 0   Unable to try/needs assistance to keep from losing balance or falling

( ) 1 Unable to pick up shoe and needs supervision while trying

( ) 2 Unable to pick up shoe but comes within 1-2 inches and maintains balance independently

( ) 3 Able to pick up shoe but needs supervision

( ) 4 Able to pick up shoe safely and easily

10. ***Turn to look behind over left and right shoulders while standing**

Instructions: "Turn your upper body to look directly over your left shoulder. Now try turning to look over your right shoulder."

Grading: Please mark the lowest category that applies.

( ) 0 Needs assistance to keep from falling

( ) 1 Needs supervision when turning

( ) 2 Turns sideways only but maintains balance

( ) 3 Looks behind one side only; other side shows less weight shift

( ) 4 Looks behind from both sides and weight shifts well

11. ***Turn 360°**

Instructions: "Turn completely in a full circle. Pause, then turn in a full circle in the other direction."

Grading: Please mark the lowest category that applies.

( ) 0 Needs assistance while turning

( ) 1 Needs close supervision or verbal cueing

( ) 2 Able to turn 360° safely but slowly

( ) 3 Able to turn 360° safely to one side only in less than 4 seconds

( ) 4 Able to turn 360° safely in less than 4 seconds to each side

12. ***Place alternate foot on bench or stool while standing unsupported.**

Instructions: "Place each foot alternately on the bench (or stool). Continue until each foot has touched the bench (or stool) four times". (Recommend use of 6-inch-high bench.)

Grading: Please mark the lowest category that applies.

( ) 0 Needs assistance to keep from falling/unable to try

( ) 1 Able to complete fewer than two steps; needs minimal assistance

( ) 2 Able to complete four steps without assistance but with supervision

( ) 3 Able to stand independently and complete eight steps in more than 20 seconds

( ) 4 Able to stand independently and safely and complete eight steps in less than 20 seconds

13. ***Stand unsupported with one foot in front**

Instructions: "Place one foot directly in front of the other. If you feel that you can't place your foot directly in front, try to step far enough ahead that the heel of your forward foot is ahead of the toes of the other foot." (Demonstrate this test item.)

Grading: Please mark the lowest category that applies.

( ) 0 Loses balance while stepping or standing

( ) 1 Needs help to step but can hold for 15 seconds

( ) 2 Able to take small step independently and hold for 30 seconds

( ) 3 Able to place one foot ahead of the other independently and hold for 30 seconds

( ) 4 Able to place feet in tandem position independently and hold for 30 seconds

Reprinted from Berg, 1992.

(continued)

From *FallProof!* by Debra J. Rose, 2003, Champaign, IL: Human Kinetics.

14. *Standing on one leg

Instructions: "Please stand on one leg as long as you can without holding onto anything."

Grading: Please mark the lowest category that applies.

(   ) 0   Unable to try or needs assistance to prevent fall

(   ) 1   Tries to lift leg, unable to hold 3 seconds, but remains standing independently

(   ) 2   Able to lift leg independently and hold up to 3 seconds

(   ) 3   Able to lift leg independently and hold for 5 to 10 seconds

(   ) 4   Able to lift leg independently and hold more than 10 seconds

Total score   /56

Note: Perform only items 6 through 14 (*) in the modified version of the scale. Maximum score for modified version is 36 points.

From *FallProof!* by Debra J. Rose, 2003, Champaign, IL: Human Kinetics. Reprinted from Berg, 1992.

of the test, the total score can still be valuable in identifying a baseline performance level against which later test performance can be compared. As with the FAB Scale, a review of the individual test item scores on either version of this test will help you identify possible underlying impairments that can be addressed using exercise progressions described in one or more of the FallProof program components. An appropriate set of exercises can then be selected to address the identified impairments (see table 3.5).

Table 3.5   Interpretation of Individual Test Item Results on the Berg Balance Scale (BBS)

Item	Possible impairments	Recommended exercises
1. Sit to stand	1. Lower and/or upper body weakness	Wall sits; UB and LB exercises with resistance (quadriceps, biceps/triceps, hip abductors/adductors)
	2. Poor dynamic COG control	Seated/standing balance activities emphasizing forward weight shifts
	3. Abnormal weight distribution	Standing balance activities with eyes closed (controlled sway in A-P and lateral directions)
2. Stand for 2 minutes	1. Poor gaze stabilization	Teach gaze fixation and stabilization techniques
	2. Lower body weakness	Wall sits; LB exercises with resistance
	3. Abnormal weight distribution in standing	COG standing balance activities
3. Sit for 2 minutes	1. Poor trunk stabilization and/or UB weakness	UB exercises with resistance (own body); seated balance activities on compliant surfaces
	2. Abnormal perception of true vertical	Standing against wall with eyes closed; somatosensory cues
4. Stand to sit	1. Poor dynamic COG control	Seated/standing balance activities emphasizing backward weight shifts
	2. Lower and/or upper body weakness	UB and LB exercises with resistance (own body/resistance band; emphasize eccentric component)
	3. Poor trunk flexibility	Flexibility exercises emphasizing trunk rotation/flexion; seated and standing
5. Transfer (chair to chair)	1. Poor dynamic control of COG	Seated/standing balance activities emphasizing multidirectional weight shifts
	2. Lower and/or upper body weakness	UB and LB exercises with resistance

Table 3.5

6. Stand with eyes closed (10 sec)	1. Poor use of somatosensory inputs; visual dependency and/or fear of falling	Seated/standing balance activities with eyes closed. Verbally emphasize use of surface cues
	2. Lower body weakness	Wall sits; LB exercises with resistance
7. Stand with feet together (1 min)	1. Poor COG control	Standing balance activities with reduced BOS
	2. Weak hip abductors/adductors	Lateral leg raises/weight shifts against resistance
8. Standing forward reach	1. Poor dynamic COG control (reduced limits of stability)	Seated/standing COG activities emphasizing leaning away from and back to midline
	2. Lower body weakness	LB exercises with resistance (body/resistance band); emphasize dorsiflexors; gastrocnemius/soleus muscles
	3. Reduced ankle ROM	Flexibility exercises (emphasize dorsiflexion)
9. Pick up object	1. Poor dynamic COG control	Seated/standing COG activities emphasizing leaning away from and back to midline
	2. Poor upper and lower body flexibility	Selected exercises to improve UB and LB flexion
	3. Lower body weakness	LB exercises with resistance (body/resistance band)
	4. Vestibular impairment (dizziness)	Head and eye movements: habituation exercises
10. Turn to look behind	1. Poor dynamic COG control	Standing weight shifts in lateral direction
	2. Poor neck and/or trunk flexibility	Selected exercises emphasizing rotation of neck, shoulders, and hips
	3. Lower body weakness	LB exercises with resistance; ball movement exercises in standing position
11. Turn in a circle	1. Poor dynamic COG control	Standing weight transfer activities; gait pattern enhancement (turns, directional changes)
	2. Possible vestibular impairment (e.g., dizziness)	Head and eye movement coordination exercises
	3. Lower body weakness	LB exercises with resistance; emphasize hip and knee flexion; hip abduction/adduction
12. Dynamic toe touch	1. Poor dynamic COG control	Standing weight shifts in lateral/A-P directions
	2. Lower body weakness	LB exercises with resistance; emphasize hip and knee flexion; hip abduction/adduction
13. Tandem stance	1. Poor static and dynamic COG control	Standing A-P weight shifts and transfers; reduced BOS activities
	2. Lower body weakness	LB exercises with resistance (body/resistance band); emphasize hip abkuctors/adductors
	3. Poor gaze stabilization	Practice focusing on visual targets in front of and at head height during standing and moving activities
14. Stand on one leg	1. Poor static and dynamic COG control	Standing A-P weight shifts and transfers; reduced BOS activities
	2. Lower body weakness	LB exercises with resistance (body/resistance band); emphasize hip abductors/adductors
	3. Poor gaze stabilization	Practice focusing on visual targets during standing and moving activities

Key: A-P = anterior-posterior direction; BOS = base of support; COG = center of gravity; LB = lower body; UB = upper body.

Despite Jane's medical history and poor performance on the two tests of sensory and motor impairment, the FAB Scale was the functional limitations test administered to her prior to the start of the FallProof program. The decision to administer the FAB Scale was based on the fact that Jane was still residing in the community and maintained an active social life. Jane's total score on the FAB Scale was 16 out of a possible 40 points. Although there currently are no established cutoff scores, Jane's performance was clearly well below average. She experienced the greatest difficulties on the following items: turning 360° in a right and left direction (2/4); stepping up onto and over a 6-inch bench (0/4); tandem walking (1/4); standing on one leg (1/4); standing on foam with eyes closed (0/4); jumping with two feet for distance (1/4); walking with head turns (1/4); and reactive postural control (1/4). As you review the types of activities performed in each test item and what types of physical abilities they require, a clear pattern of impairment begins to emerge for Jane. She scored poorly on all items that require (a) good vestibular function, (b) strength and flexibility, (c) the ability to manipulate the center of gravity in static and dynamic situations, and (d) the ability to use the compensatory step strategy effectively following an unexpected loss of balance. Take a moment now to review Bill Divine's scores on the FAB Scale in table 3.6 to identify any underlying impairments that can account for the functional limitations observed on his completed test.

Table 3.6 Fullerton Advanced Balance (FAB) Scores for Bill Divine

Item Number	Description	Score
1.	Stand with feet together (eyes closed)	4
2.	Reach forward to retrieve an object	4
3.	Turn 360 degrees to right and left	2
4.	Step up and over 6-in bench	4
5.	Tandem Walk	1
6.	Stand on One Leg	1
7.	Stand on Foam with Eyes Closed	4
8.	Two-Footed Jump for Distance	2
9.	Walk With Head Turns	1
10.	Reactive Postural Control	3
	TOTAL SCORE:	26/40

Although you would administer only one of the two functional limitations tests to clients prior to the start of the FallProof program, we also administered the BBS to Jane and Bill so you could compare the final scores achieved on each test. In contrast to the FAB Scale, Jane scored 48 out of a possible total score of 56 on the BBS. What is surprising about this score is that Jane would not be categorized at high risk for falls because she scored above the cutoff value of 46 points. In terms of possible improvement, she can only improve by 8 points on the BBS, whereas her score of only 16/40 on the FAB Scale leaves her with considerable room for improvement prior to the next administration of the test. The same was true for Bill, who scored only 26/40 on the FAB scale but as high as 51/56 on the BBS. He has even less room for improvement on the BBS scale, but considerably more on the FAB scale.

In addition to the up-and-go test (Senior Fitness Test item), a second test used to identify functional limitations in mobility is the 50-foot (approximately 15 meters) walk test performed at both a preferred and fast speed. Participants are required to walk a total distance of 70 feet (first at preferred speed and then at maximal speed) with the distance between 10 and 60 feet being timed for the purpose of calculating gait velocity. Counting the number of steps recorded by each participant over the same 50-foot distance can also be used to calculate the additional measure of stride length. Test administration and scoring procedures are described below and on the next page respectively. This test serves as both a useful measure of overall gait speed and an indication of whether older adults are able to adapt their walking speed to accommodate a change in task demands (i.e., walk at maximal speed). Gait speed values can also be compared to a limited set of reference values presented in table 3.7. The reference values for preferred and maximal speeds were based on data collected on 78 healthy older adults ranging in age from 60 to 79 years. The results of the 50-foot walk test provide the instructor with additional information needed to select the most appropriate gait pattern enhancement and variation activities for each participant.

> The 50-foot walk test is a useful measure of gait speed and an indication of whether an older adult is able to adapt their gait speed to accommodate a change in task demands.

Test Administration Instructions for 50-Foot Walk at Preferred and Maximum Speed

Purpose: Measure gait speed at preferred and fast speeds; stride length can also be calculated by counting the number of steps taken over the test distance. Slow gait speeds have been associated with increased risk for falls.

Equipment: Stopwatch; measuring tape (at least 100 feet); masking tape or chalk to mark starting, 10-, 60-, and 70-foot marks

Test Procedures: Measure a 70-foot distance and place small markers at the start and at 10, 60, and 70 feet along the course. Instruct the participant to begin walking at a comfortable speed until you ask them to stop. Begin recording the time as soon as the person's foot crosses the 10-foot line. Stop recording the elapsed time once either foot crosses the 60-foot marker. An additional 10 feet are included at the start and end of the walkway to ensure that the person has reached a relatively consistent walking velocity after accelerating from a standing position. The additional 10 feet at the end of the 50-foot walkway are included to ensure that participants do not begin to slow down as they reach the 50-foot marker.

Stride length can also be calculated by counting the number of steps the participant takes while between the 10- and 60-foot markers. Begin counting as soon as the first foot crosses the 10-foot marker and stop counting as soon as either foot crosses the 60-foot marker. Stride length is calculated by dividing the number of steps recorded over the 50-foot test distance (i.e., number of steps/50). Make sure that you walk slightly behind the person performing the test so as not to influence their walking speed.

Perform the 50-foot walk at preferred speed and then at maximum speed to see whether the person is able to change gait speed noticeably on command. Instruct the person to "walk as quickly but as safely as possible." Assistive devices may be used to perform this test. Be sure to indicate what type of device was used so that the same device is used on subsequent tests.

Reprinted from the Center for Successful Aging at California State University, Fullerton.

Form 3.6

Scoring Form for 50-Foot Walk

Test scores

Walk at preferred speed   Time: _____ (in seconds)   Gait velocity: _____ (in feet/second)

                        (Formula: 50/time in seconds)

                        Stride length: _____(in feet)

                        (Formula: number of steps/2)

Walk at maximum speed   Time: _____ (in seconds)   Gait velocity: _____ (in feet/second)

                        (Formula: 50/time in seconds)

                        Stride length: _____(in feet)

                        (Formula: number of steps/2)

From *FallProof!* by Debra J. Rose, 2003, Champaign, IL: Human Kinetics.

Table 3.7   **Reference Values for the 50-Foot Walk Performed at Preferred and Maximum Speeds**

Age	Preferred (ft/sec)		Maximum (ft/sec)	
	Men	**Women**	**Men**	**Women**
60s	4.46 (.074)	4.25 (.063)	6.34 (.106)	5.82 (.10)
70s	4.36 (.073)	4.17 (.069)	6.82 (.114)	5.74 (.10)
Age	**Preferred (m/sec)**		**Maximum (m/sec)**	
	Men	**Women**	**Men**	**Women**
60s	1.36 (.023)	1.30 (.019)	1.93 (.032)	1.77 (.029)
70s	1.33 (.022)	1.27 (.021)	2.08 (.035)	1.75 (.029)

Note: Reference values for gait speed based on small sample sizes (60s: 18 men and 18 women; 70s: 20 men and 22 women).

Reprinted from Bohannon, 1997.

Jane was able to complete the 50-foot walk test at preferred speed in a time of 21 seconds (50/21 = 2.4 feet/second), whereas the time required for her to complete the maximal speed condition of the test was 14 seconds (50/14 = 3.6 feet/second). Based on the reference values presented in table 3.7, Jane is well below average in terms of gait speed for both test conditions. The average preferred speed for females in their 70s is 4.17 feet/second and the maximum speed for the same age group is 5.74 feet/second. Including a number of activities described in the gait pattern enhancement and variation training component of the program will be important if Jane is to improve both the speed and flexibility of her gait pattern (see chapter 7). Improving her level of strength and flexibility will also be important.

Bill completed the 50-foot walk test at both the preferred and maximum speed considerably faster than Jane. His preferred speed time was 12 seconds (50/12 = 4.17 feet/second) and his time for the maximum speed condition was 10 seconds (50/10

= 5.00 feet/second). Comparing Bill's scores to the reference values provided in table 3.7, we find that Bill is just below the mean of 4.36 feet/second for men aged between 70 and 79 years in the preferred speed condition but further below in the maximum speed condition, where the mean equals 6.82 feet/second.

Finally, the "walkie-talkie" test is used to measure an older adult's ability to divide attention between tasks (see box below). This quick test can be administered as the instructor or assistant walks with the participant to the location where the 50-foot walk begins. A conversation is initiated by the instructor in the form of an open-ended question that requires more than a yes or no response from the participant. A positive score is recorded if the participant stops walking in order to respond to the question posed. Alternatively, if a person is able to continue walking while respond-ing to the question, a negative score is recorded. A positive score on this test suggests that the person is unable to divide attention their between the tasks of walking and talking (see form 3.7). The results of this test can be used to determine the nature of the task demands introduced during the early stages of the program. For example, an individual who records a positive score on this test would be best suited to perform activities with a single goal (i.e., standing quietly on a foam surface while fixating on a point in space), whereas a person recording a negative score would be able to engage in tasks with multiple task demands (i.e., reaching for or catching objects while standing on a foam surface) much earlier in the program.

> The "walkie-talkie" test is used to measure an older adult's ability to divide attention between two tasks.

In contrast to all previous tests performed by Jane, she actually recorded a nega-tive score on the "walkie-talkie" test, indicating that she is able to divide her atten-tion between two tasks. On the basis of this test, it would appear that Jane is more limited physically than cognitively. Although it will still be important to have her perform the lower-level exercise progressions in each component of the program, her ability to divide attention between a task that requires balance and a second cogni-tive task means that you will be able to introduce additional tasks once she is able to perform the various balance and gait activities correctly. Bill Divine also recorded a negative score on this test.

Test Instructions for Administering the "Walkie-Talkie" Test

Purpose: Evaluate ability to divide attention between multiple tasks, in this case, the task of talking while walking

Testing procedures: As you walk to the location where you plan to start the 50-foot walk, begin a conversation with the individual you are testing. If the person stops walk-ing in order to respond to you, it is a sign that they are unable to divide their attention adequately between the tasks of walking and talking. It is important to ask open-ended questions that require more than a yes or no response.

Interpreting test results: A "positive" score is recorded if the person stops walking in order to respond to your question. Alternatively, if the person is able to continue walking while conversing with you, a "negative" score is recorded. A "positive" score on this test suggests that the person needs to direct their attention to the task of balancing while walk-ing and will therefore not be ready to perform multiple tasks in the class until they have developed better overall balance abilities.

Form 3.7

Scoring Form for "Walkie-Talkie" Test

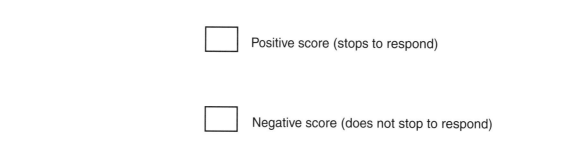

Positive score (stops to respond)

Negative score (does not stop to respond)

Assessment of Balance-Related Self-Confidence

The Balance Efficacy Scale (BES) is designed to evaluate how confident the older adult feels when performing various activities of daily living that require balance. Participants are asked to rate, on a scale from 0 to 100, how confident they are that they could successfully perform a given task (i.e., rise from a chair) without losing their balance. The scale consists of 18 questions that assess an individual's perceived confidence when performing a variety of daily activities with or without assistance. The total score obtained on the test is then divided by 18 to yield a mean BES score. This scale should be completed by program participants *before* they perform any of the physical performance tests so that the evaluation of their abilities is not influenced by their performance on a physical test that might have been administered before they completed the BES. This form is generally included with other program materials that participants bring to the first class session. Alternatively, participants could be asked to complete the form (preferably away from the testing area and with an assistant present to answer questions) while they are waiting to perform the other physical tests associated with the program. Participants who score below 50 on the scale should be considered to have low self-confidence, and every effort should be made to present activities early in the program that foster confidence through success. Decisions on how much to challenge participants should be guided by how confident they feel in their balance abilities. A copy of the BES is presented in form 3.8.

The Balance Efficacy Scale (BES) should be completed by program participants before they perform any of the physical tests associated with the FallProof program.

Consistent with Jane's response to question 11 of the health/activity questionnaire, which asks how worried a person is about falling, she also scored very low on the Balance Efficacy Scale, a self-report measure of balance-related self-confidence. Not only is she extremely worried about falling in general, but she demonstrates very low self-confidence on the BES as indicated by her score of 40/100. She exhibits the highest lack of self-confidence when she is asked how confident she would feel if she had to perform activities of daily living requiring balance *without* assistance.

The Balance Efficacy Scale

Listed below are a series of tasks that you may encounter in daily life. Please indicate how confident you are, *today,* that you can complete each of these tasks without losing your balance. Your answers are confidential. *Please answer as you feel, not how you think you should feel.*

(Circle one number from 0 to 100%)

1. **How confident are you that you can get up out of a chair (using your hands) without losing your balance?**

    0%   10%   20%   30%   40%   50%   60%   70%   80%   90%   100%

    not at all   somewhat   absolutely
    confident   confident   confident

2. **How confident are you that you can get up out of a chair (*not* using your hands) without losing your balance?**

    0%   10%   20%   30%   40%   50%   60%   70%   80%   90%   100%

    not at all   somewhat   absolutely
    confident   confident   confident

3. **How confident are you that you can walk up a flight of 10 stairs (using the handrail) without losing your balance?**

    0%   10%   20%   30%   40%   50%   60%   70%   80%   90%   100%

    not at all   somewhat   absolutely
    confident   confident   confident

4. **How confident are you that you can walk up a flight of 10 stairs (*not* using the handrail) without losing your balance?**

    0%   10%   20%   30%   40%   50%   60%   70%   80%   90%   100%

    not at all   somewhat   absolutely
    confident   confident   confident

5. **How confident are you that you can get out of bed without losing your balance?**

    0%   10%   20%   30%   40%   50%   60%   70%   80%   90%   100%

    not at all   somewhat   absolutely
    confident   confident   confident

6. **How confident are you that you can get into or out of a shower or bathtub (*with* the assistance of a handrail or support wall) without losing your balance?**

    0%   10%   20%   30%   40%   50%   60%   70%   80%   90%   100%

    not at all   somewhat   absolutely
    confident   confident   confident

7. **How confident are you that you can get into or out of a shower or bathtub (with *no assistance* from a handrail or support wall) without losing your balance?**

    0%   10%   20%   30%   40%   50%   60%   70%   80%   90%   100%

    not at all   somewhat   absolutely
    confident   confident   confident

8. **How confident are you that you can walk down a flight of 10 stairs (using the handrail) without losing your balance?**

    0%   10%   20%   30%   40%   50%   60%   70%   80%   90%   100%

    not at all   somewhat   absolutely
    confident   confident   confident

(continued)

9. **How confident are you that you can walk down a flight of 10 stairs (*not* using the handrail) without losing your balance?**

0%	10%	20%	30%	40%	50%	60%	70%	80%	90%	100%

not at all   somewhat   absolutely
confident   confident   confident

10. **How confident are you that you can remove an object from a cupboard *located at a height that is level with your shoulder* without losing your balance?**

0%	10%	20%	30%	40%	50%	60%	70%	80%	90%	100%

not at all   somewhat   absolutely
confident   confident   confident

11. **How confident are you that you can remove an object from a cupboard *located above your head* without losing your balance?**

0%	10%	20%	30%	40%	50%	60%	70%	80%	90%	100%

not at all   somewhat   absolutely
confident   confident   confident

12. **How confident are you that you can walk across uneven ground (with assistance) when good lighting is available without losing your balance?**

0%	10%	20%	30%	40%	50%	60%	70%	80%	90%	100%

not at all   somewhat   absolutely
confident   confident   confident

13. **How confident are you that you can walk across uneven ground (with *no* assistance) when good lighting is available without losing your balance?**

0%	10%	20%	30%	40%	50%	60%	70%	80%	90%	100%

not at all   somewhat   absolutely
confident   confident   confident

14. **How confident are you that you can walk across uneven ground (with assistance) at night without losing your balance?**

0%	10%	20%	30%	40%	50%	60%	70%	80%	90%	100%

not at all   somewhat   absolutely
confident   confident   confident

15. **How confident are you that you can walk across uneven ground (with *no* assistance) at night without losing your balance?**

0%	10%	20%	30%	40%	50%	60%	70%	80%	90%	100%

not at all   somewhat   absolutely
confident   confident   confident

16. **How confident are you that you could stand on one leg (with support) while putting on a pair of trousers without losing your balance?**

0%	10%	20%	30%	40%	50%	60%	70%	80%	90%	100%

not at all   somewhat   absolutely
confident   confident   confident

17. **How confident are you that you could stand on one leg (with *no* support) while putting on a pair of trousers without losing your balance?**

0%	10%	20%	30%	40%	50%	60%	70%	80%	90%	100%

not at all   somewhat   absolutely
confident   confident   confident

Reprinted from the Center for Successful Aging at California State University, Fullerton.

Form 3.8

18. How confident are you that you could complete a daily task *quickly* without losing your balance?

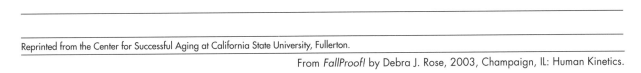

| 0% | 10% | 20% | 30% | 40% | 50% | 60% | 70% | 80% | 90% | 100% |

not at all
confident

somewhat
confident

absolutely
confident

Last, we are interested in understanding what factors affect your confidence levels. On the lines below, please provide reasons for answering the way you did on questions 1 through 18. For example, if you answered that you were "not very" confident, why do you feel that way? If you were "not very" confident about an activity because you no longer do it very often (e.g., climb stairs, walk on uneven ground), we would like to know that also.

_____

_____

_____

On each item of the scale that asked Jane to rate how confident she would feel performing a certain activity (e.g., climbing or descending stairs, getting into and out of a shower or bathtub, putting on a pair of trousers) without assistance, she indicated that she was "not at all confident," a response that equates to a score of 0 on a 0 to 100 response scale.

Bill Divine stated he was very worried about falling (that is, 5/7) on question 12 of the health/activity questionnaire, and scored a 53 on the BES. Although not as low a score as Jane's, Bill also demonstrated low levels of self-confidence (0 to 20%) when asked to rate how confident he would feel performing any of the daily activities *without* assistance. On the items of the scale that described activities in which assistance was available, however, he generally indicated that he was "absolutely confident." This response equated to scores ranging between 90 to 100% on the BES scale.

Assessing the Level of Disability

The health/activity questionnaire in form 3.1 also includes a self-report composite physical function (CPF) scale (question 18) that assesses a wide range of functional abilities ranging from those associated with basic activities of daily living (e.g., bathing, dressing oneself) to instrumental or intermediate-level ADLs, or IADLs (e.g., housework, shopping). This scale is an expanded version of three previously published scales and was developed by Rikli and Jones (1998). Participants are placed in an advanced (>22/24), moderate (16-22/24), or low functioning (<16/24) category based on their responses. This score is used to assess the participant's level of disability, not only at the time of entering the program, but also at regular intervals during the program (refer to question 18 on the health/activity questionnaire in form 3.1). It is a good idea to ask program participants to complete the CPF scale periodically (every 3 to 6 months) to see whether any improvements you have documented on the physical tests of balance and mobility are positively influencing their perceived ability to perform basic, intermediate, and advanced activities associated with daily living.

The composite physical function (CPF) scale should be used to assess a participant's level of disability at the time of entering the program but also at regular intervals (i.e., every three to six months) during the program.

As you can see by reviewing the results of question 18 on Jane's health/activity questionnaire, she scored 14 out of a total of 24 points on the CPF scale. This score places her just above the low functioning category. A closer look at her individual responses reveals that, with the exception of dressing, Jane requires assistance to complete all other basic and intermediate activities of daily living and is unable to do any of the advanced activities described (e.g., strenuous activities, most heavy household chores, lift and carry 25 pounds). Now look at the same question on Bill Divine's completed questionnaire and calculate his CPF score.

Why Should Testing Be Conducted on a Regular Basis?

Before the start of the program

- To help participants better understand the specific nature of their balance and mobility problems
- To help establish a starting point for all participants in each program component
- To individualize program content based on the identified impairments and functional limitations

During the program

- To determine whether each participant's balance and mobility problems are being adequately addressed
- To determine the program's effectiveness
- To provide valuable feedback to participants about their progress
- To motivate participants to continue in the program

Summary

The goal of this chapter was to introduce you to each of the screening and assessment tools administered as part of the FallProof program. By using the modified Nagi model as the theoretical framework for test selection, the instructor will obtain a better understanding of each client's level of disability, as well as the nature of the pathology and physical activity patterns, impairments, and functional limitations that contribute to the disability observed. Collectively, the test results then serve as the basis for developing a balance and mobility program that addresses the individual needs of each participant.

Retesting participants at regular intervals (i.e., every two to three months) is also a means of determining both the overall effectiveness of the program and whether each participant's balance and mobility problems are being adequately addressed. Regular testing also provides valuable feedback to participants as to their progress and may serve as a motivating tool as well. Each of the tests described in this chapter is intended to help you, the instructor, learn more about the various dimensions of the balance system and provide more targeted instruction as a result.

A review of the health/activity questionnaire and various test results of our first case study, Jane Gain, provided you with a wealth of information that you can now use to design a program that will meet her specific needs. As the health/activity questionnaire revealed, Jane has several medical conditions that adversely affect her balance and mobility. The physical impairments associated with the various medical conditions reported (e.g., heart attack, diabetes, chronic asthma, arthritis) have resulted in a number of functional limitations that necessitate the need for assistance to accomplish many of the activities associated with daily living. These functional limitations, in turn, have so limited her participation in regular exercise and other social and recreational activities as to move her into the final stage of disability described in the Nagi model. As a result of her declining abilities and fall history, Jane also has a very high fear of falling and very low level of balance-related self-confidence that will need to be addressed immediately if any significant improvement is to occur with respect to her physical impairments.

Bill will also benefit from participation in the program. Although his functional abilities are higher than Jane's, he could improve in several areas and thereby lower his overall fall risk. You will be able to select higher-level exercises for Bill earlier in the program, so that the level of balance challenge is better matched to his capabilities.

Can Jane benefit from participation in the FallProof balance and mobility program? Absolutely! Although she must contend with a number of permanent impairments that cannot be ameliorated (e.g., peripheral neuropathy, asthma, arthritic joints), the more temporary impairments she is experiencing can be significantly improved (e.g., strength, flexibility, dynamic balance). A targeted program of exercises that specifically address each of the temporary impairments and compensate for the permanent impairments will lead to significant improvements in her ability to engage in daily activities that require balance and mobility and a better overall quality of life as a result.

TEST YOUR UNDERSTANDING

1. The Nagi model describes a multistage progression to disability. The stages identified include
   a. pathology/disease, functional limitations, disability
   b. disease/pathology, impairments, functional limitations, disuse
   c. physical inactivity, disease/pathology, impairments, functional limitations, disability
   d. disease/pathology, impairment, functional limitations, disability
   e. disease/pathology, physical inactivity, functional limitations, disability

2. Your client has difficulty performing the sit-to-stand item on the Berg Balance Scale. All of the following could be potential impairments *except*
   a. lower body muscle weakness
   b. poor sensory integration
   c. poor dynamic center-of-gravity control
   d. abnormal weight distribution during transfer to standing
   e. upper body muscle weakness

3. The primary purpose of the Berg Balance Scale is to determine if your client
   a. has a gait problem
   b. has lower body muscle weakness

c. needs further medical testing

d. has the ability to perform functional tasks associated with daily living that require balance

e. is appropriate for your community balance program

4. Which of the following is *not* true regarding the Fullerton Advanced Balance Scale?

a. It is composed of 10 items that measure multiple dimensions of balance.

b. It is a standardized test with good reliability and validity.

c. It is designed to measure impairments in balance and gait.

d. It addresses functional limitations contributing to balance problems.

e. It does not require specialized equipment.

5. If a client performs poorly on item 10 of the FAB Scale, an appropriate interpretation would be that the client

a. has reduced limits of stability

b. has poor anticipatory postural control

c. has poor reactive postural control

d. does not use surface information adequately to maintain balance

e. has poor lower body flexibility

6. The Senior Fitness Test is used to measure the following physical impairments associated with functional mobility:

a. lower and upper body strength and flexibility, aerobic endurance, dynamic balance and agility

b. lower body strength and flexibility, upper body strength and flexibility, aerobic endurance

c. aerobic endurance, dynamic balance and agility, lower body strength, and upper body flexibility

d. lower and upper body strength, dynamic balance and agility, and lower and upper body flexibility

e. lower and upper body strength, lower and upper body flexibility, gait speed, and aerobic endurance

7. Your client is unable to successfully complete three consecutive trials on condition 2 of the M-CTSIB. The correct interpretation is that the client may be

a. visually dependent

b. unable to use vestibular inputs for balance

c. weak in the lower body musculature

d. unable to use visual inputs for balance

e. an inappropriate candidate for the FallProof program

8. The Multidirectional Reach Test is used to measure a client's ability to

a. automatically respond to a perturbation

b. anticipate a postural disturbance

c. voluntarily plan and execute movements

d. reach for an object in space

e. coordinate the upper and lower body when reaching

9. The "walkie-talkie" test measures a client's ability to
   a. divide attention between two tasks
   b. ask and answer a question while walking
   c. walk while carrying on a conversation
   d. hear another person ask a question while walking
   e. respond quickly to a question that is asked of them while walking

10. Which of the following is *not* true of the Senior Fitness Test?
   a. It is quick and easy to administer.
   b. It requires very little equipment to administer.
   c. It has norm-referenced standards that can be used for comparison.
   d. It is a highly valid and reliable test.
   e. It can only be used to measure older adults who are relatively healthy.

PRACTICAL PROBLEMS

1. Familiarize yourself with the instructions associated with each of the physical performance tests described in this chapter and administer at least three of the tests to an older adult so you can practice administering them.

2. Complete a report card for Case Study 2: Bill Divine. Use the completed report card for Case Study 1: Jane Gain as a guide. Develop a prioritized list of problems for both Jane and Bill that you plan to address first during the program. Be sure to indicate which impairments you think are changeable or temporary (e.g., strength) and those you think are more permanent or less amenable to change (e.g., peripheral neuropathy). This may help you better prioritize your efforts during the early stages of the FallProof program.

Center-of-Gravity (COG) Control Training

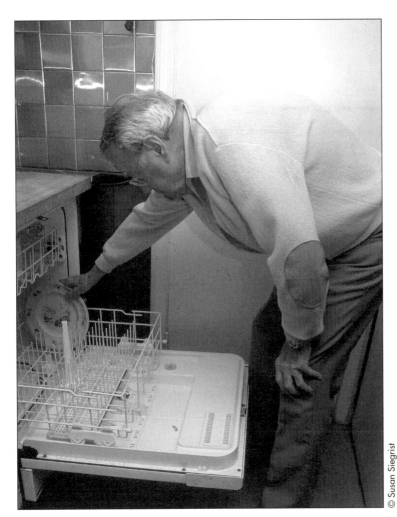

© Susan Siegrist

Objectives

After completing this chapter, you will be able to

- understand how center-of-gravity control influences balance,
- develop a set of exercise progressions designed to improve center-of-gravity control in seated, standing, and moving task situations,
- manipulate the difficulty of a balance activity by altering the task demands or environmental constraints, or both, and
- manipulate the task demands or the environment, or both, to ensure safety.

4

The balance and mobility activities presented in this chapter are designed to improve your participant's ability to (a) maintain a better upright position in space, whether seated or standing; (b) lean away from and return to the midline with improved postural control; and (c) move the body through space more quickly and confidently. In addition, the exercises are intended to improve selected physical and motor-skill-related fitness parameters (e.g., aerobic endurance, strength, power, coordination, flexibility) that are essential to good balance and mobility. To accomplish each of these movement goals, participants must first understand where the COG is relative to their base of support (i.e., feet and buttocks when sitting or feet when standing) and how to move it relative to that base (e.g., rising from a chair, walking up a flight of stairs). These exercises are often labeled the "belly button" control exercises because they readily conjure up an image in the participant's mind of the approximate location of the COG when standing and what part of the body must be manipulated to maintain postural control while performing a variety of daily tasks in various environmental contexts.

Older adults who are experiencing a decline in postural stability often develop inaccurate perceptions of true vertical and begin to adopt abnormal standing postures as a result (see figure 4.1). A commonly observed maladaptive standing posture is one with a forward head position, rounded upper back, and backward tilt of the pelvis. Asymmetrical standing postures are also observed wherein the older adult tends to place more weight on one side of the body. This posture is common among older adults who have experienced a stroke, suffer from arthritis-related pain in certain joints, or have an uncorrected leg-length discrepancy.

> Older adults who are experiencing a decline in postural stability often develop inaccurate perceptions of true vertical and begin to adopt abnormal standing postures as a result.

The exercises described in this chapter progress from seated to standing to moving task situations. In a seated position, for example, participants learn to sit in an upright position, shift their weight to various positions in space, or restore an upright seated position following small perturbations (e.g., pushing or pulling of the body) that are either expected or unexpected. After the core exercise progressions are described for each level of balance challenge, you will learn how to further manipulate the level of balance challenge associated with a set of exercise progressions by varying either the demands of the task being performed or the environment in which it is performed.

Ideas for increasing the overall challenge of each set of exercise progressions are described in two summary tables, one at the end of the seated balance section and one at the end of the standing balance section. For example, a simple way to increase the balance challenge associated with a set of seated or standing exercise progressions would be to instruct participants to repeat each exercise they were able to perform successfully with their eyes open, but this time wearing dark glasses so that vision is reduced or with their eyes closed. This simple environmental manipulation will encourage participants to rely more on actually feeling where the various body parts are in space and thereby develop a more correct internal representation of true vertical that is not reliant on vision for maintenance or correction.

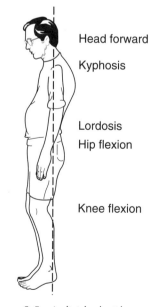

Head forward

Kyphosis

Lordosis
Hip flexion

Knee flexion

Figure 4.1 Individual with maladaptive posture.

Finally, a set of culminating activities is presented following the seated, standing, and moving balance exercise sections that combines several different core exercises previously practiced in isolation. For example, a culminating activity such as "shift around the clock" combines seated dynamic weight shifts in multiple directions as individuals shift weight to different numbers on an imaginary clock face on verbal command.

Seated Balance Activities

The type of support surface initially selected for the seated center-of-gravity control exercises will depend on the *individual capabilities* of the participant. Although more frail participants may need to begin the exercise progressions while seated on a chair with a firm support surface and back support, most participants in a community-based program will be ready to begin exercising while seated on a chair with no back support and a compliant surface added (i.e., easiest level of difficulty). The next levels of difficulty would involve the client being seated on a balance ball with a ball holder beneath it (more difficult) and then, finally, without a ball holder supporting the ball (most difficult). Where the hands are placed during each exercise will also help establish the level of challenge. The easiest position involves the hands being placed on the chair or ball surface. Resting the hands on the thighs results in a more difficult hand position, and asking participants to fold their arms across their chest results in the most difficult hand position. Figure 4.2, a through c, shows three examples of seated support surfaces and hand positions illustrating the three levels of relative difficulty: easiest, more difficult, and most difficult.

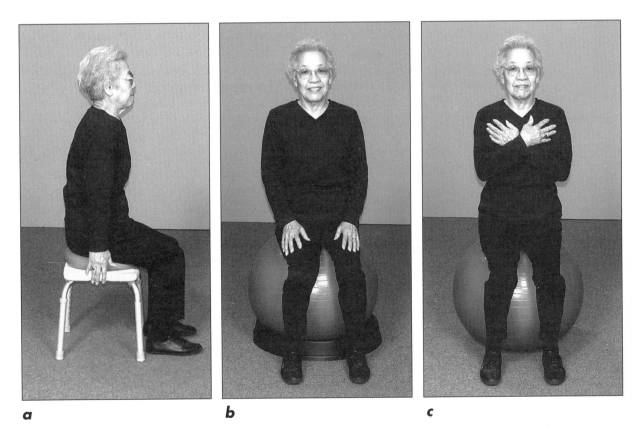

a   b   c

Figure 4.2 Different levels of balance challenge can be introduced by manipulating the type of seated support surface and position of the hands during an exercise: *(a)* easiest, *(b)* more difficult, *(c)* most difficult.

General Safety Tips

- Following a review of your initial test results, identify participants who are likely to experience difficulty with certain exercises, recommending modifications where appropriate. If you have assistants, tell them as well.

- Instruct assistants to closely supervise participants who are likely to encounter difficulties with an exercise, particularly when sitting on the balance ball without a ball holder. Two methods of supervising participants are illustrated in figure 4.3.

- When too few assistants are available to guard less stable participants, use chairs or the wall to help stabilize them. If you are working with a large group, you might consider moving participants to less difficult seated support surfaces.

- When a participant is using a balance ball, select a size that allows the person to sit in the middle of the ball and still have the feet flat on the floor. Ideally, the knees should be flexed at a 90° angle to the floor. Unless otherwise instructed, the feet should also be hip-width apart.

- Increase the angle of knee flexion for participants who have artificial joints, severe lower body weakness, or medical conditions that cause pain in the hip or knee joints by having them sit on a slightly larger ball or higher chair with a Dyna-Disc™ beneath their buttocks.

- Do not ask participants to perform the next level of a task until they can *safely* perform the previous exercise progression.

- Do not ask participants to perform an exercise with their eyes closed if they are not able to perform the task safely with their eyes open. Increasing a participant's postural stability by altering the hand position (i.e., hands on support surface versus thighs) or moving them to an easier seated support surface may be sufficient to facilitate better performance.

- Instruct participants to open their eyes immediately if they feel they are about to lose balance.

- When introducing arm, trunk, or leg movements, select a seated support surface that is challenging but safe so participants can still perform the exercises successfully.

- Instruct participants to avoid grabbing other participants if they feel unstable.

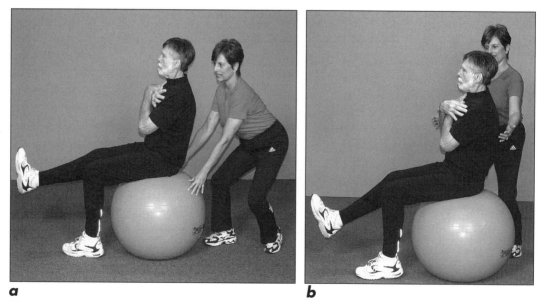

a *b*

Figure 4.3 Two methods of supervising participants: **(a)** assistant stabilizing ball while participant performs exercise; **(b)** assistant spotting participant seated on balance ball.

Level 1: Maintaining Seated Balance

The activities described in level 1 are designed to teach participants how to (a) develop a more upright seated posture, (b) use vision to improve seated balance, (c) develop a better sensory awareness of the body's position in space, and (d) strengthen the muscles of the trunk. Select the support surface and hand position that is best suited to each individual's capabilities before beginning any of the seated exercises described in this section. The support surface and hand position should require active stabilization of the trunk muscles but should not be so difficult that the participant is unable to maintain balance during the eyes-closed sensory awareness activity in level 1. This introductory activity will also help you plan for subsequent activities after observing how well participants perform the sequence of exercises while seated on the different support surfaces and with the hands in different starting positions.

Before beginning any of the seated COG balance activities, demonstrate the correct sitting posture for your class participants and then have them practice while they are seated in a straight-back chair. The following verbal cues should be provided to your participants as they practice:

- "Sit tall with your back resting against the chair and your feet flat on the floor."
- "Relax your arms and place your hands on your thighs or lap."
- "Hold your head erect with your eyes focused on a forward target, and tuck in your chin by gently pulling it straight back (as though it is sliding on a tray held directly beneath it) until your ears are directly above your shoulders."
- "Pull your abdominal muscles up and in—try to flatten your stomach."
- "Straighten your upper back and raise your chest while moving your shoulders back and down against the chair back."
- "Maintain this position for 15 seconds, breathing normally and relaxing the rest of your body at the same time. Relax (but not too much), and repeat the exercise again."

This is an excellent exercise that you can also assign as homework during the early stages of the program. Introducing this exercise before starting any of the seated balance activities will also help you establish the initial level of balance challenge for each individual client. Participants who are unable to achieve a correct sitting posture while seated on a stable surface will not be ready to sit on the more challenging balance ball surface without further compromising their posture.

Matching the Size of the Balance Ball to the Height of the Client

Carefully match the size of the balance ball to the height of your clients (see figure 4.4). As a general rule of thumb, the following ball sizes are recommended:

Height	Size of balance ball
Below 5' 5"	45-cm ball
5' 5" to 5' 8"	55-cm ball
5' 9" to 6' 3"	65-cm ball
6' 4" to 6' 9"	75-cm ball
6' 10" and taller	85-cm ball

Additional Reminders

- Always check that the ball is fully inflated to the specified dimension (check with measuring tape after inflation, or use a ball-measuring device).
- Check for any scratches or deep cuts on the balance ball that might render it unsafe. (Deflate damaged balls, render them unusable, and then discard them appropriately.)
- Check to see whether you need to alter the size of the balance ball when using a ball holder or when using an Airex™ pad as a support surface (elevates feet by 2 inches). Using an Airex pad in this way changes the relative angles of the knee and hip joints.
- Consider having clients with total hip replacements use a balance ball that is one size larger than recommended for their height (particularly if they are at the high end of the height range) to increase the angle at the hip joint. This will increase their level of comfort during certain activities.

Exercise Progressions

■ SEATED BALANCE

Hands in one of three starting positions.

a. With feet hip-width apart and flat on the floor, the participant should maintain an upright, seated position for 30 seconds with the eyes open (figure 4.4).

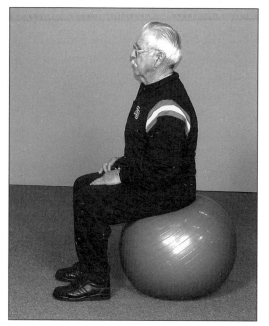

b. The eyes should be directed forward and fixed on a visual target immediately in front of the participant and at eye level. Vertical targets (e.g., door or window jambs, vertical lines on a wall) are particularly helpful for reinforcing an upright postural alignment.

c. Repeat the exercise with the eyes closed. Instruct participants to move the hands to an easier position during the first repetition.

d. Repeat the exercise with the hands in a more difficult position if the participant was stable on the previous repetition.

Figure 4.4 Older adult seated on correct-height balance ball.

Important Sensory Awareness Cues

The following sensory awareness cues should be presented to participants during level 1 seated balance activities, particularly during eyes-closed repetitions:

- "Imagine there is a string connected to the top of your head that is being pulled toward the ceiling."
- "Can you sense that your ears are directly above your shoulders?"
- "Can you sense that your shoulders are directly above your hips?"
- "Can you feel that you have equal weight on both sides of your buttocks?"

- "Can you sense the angle of your knees?"
- "Can you feel your feet in contact with the floor?"
- "Can you feel that the pressure is evenly distributed under both feet?"

Level 2: Seated Balance With Voluntary Arm Movements

Different arm movements are introduced in level 2 seated balance activities to further challenge each participant's seated balance abilities. Subtle movements of the COG are now required as the arms are moved in different directions. At the same time, trunk and lower body muscles are being used more actively for stabilization, thereby improving strength. The movements in this section also help improve flexibility, particularly at the shoulder joints, as participants are encouraged to move their arms through as complete a range of motion as possible. The development of a good breathing pattern is also emphasized during this set of exercise progressions.

Important Reminders

- Sit tall on the chair or ball.
- Inhale as the arms move away from the body and exhale as the arms return to the starting position.
- Keep the eyes directed forward and focused on a visual target at eye level unless otherwise instructed.
- Move the arms through as complete a range of motion as possible while maintaining upright balance.
- Perform each exercise slowly.

Exercise Progressions

■ **1. SINGLE ARM RAISES**

a   Raise one arm to as close to a vertical position as possible (figure 4.5).

b. Hold for three slow counts, then lower the arm back to the starting position.

c. Repeat with the opposite arm.

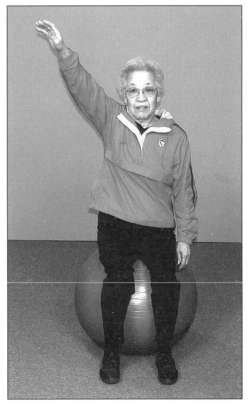

Figure 4.5 Single arm raises.

■ 2. DOUBLE-ARM RAISES

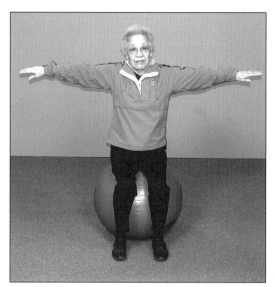

a. With palms facing down, raise both arms to a lateral and horizontal position and hold for three counts (inhale)(figure 4.6).

b. Turn the palms up and continue raising the arms until they reach a vertical position with palms touching (exhale).

c. Hold for three counts (inhale), then lower the arms to the starting position, pausing briefly at the intermediate position to turn the palms down again (exhale).

Figure 4.6 Double-arm raises.

■ 3. DIAGONAL ARM RAISES

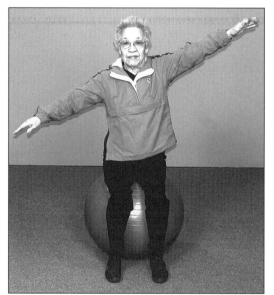

a. Raise one arm diagonally out to the side of the body and toward the ceiling (figure 4.7).

b. Hold for three counts, then lower the arm to the starting position.

c. Repeat with the opposite arm.

d. Repeat the exercise with both arms moving simultaneously, one arm moving diagonally upward and the other arm moving diagonally downward.

Figure 4.7 Diagonal arm raises.

Once participants become familiar with the movements associated with each of the core exercise progressions in level 2, you can begin to manipulate either the demands associated with the task or the environment in which the task is performed to further increase the level of balance challenge. Several ideas are presented on page 110 of this chapter.

Level 3: Seated Balance With Voluntary Trunk Movements

Balance is further challenged in these level 3 exercises by asking participants to move the trunk in different directions. The movements of the COG will increase as a result of moving a larger segment of the body, requiring more effort on the part of the participant to maintain balance during each movement. These exercises are also designed to improve the strength of the trunk, hip, and lower body muscles by requiring larger and controlled movements away from the midline and against gravity. Flexibility, particularly in the hip and trunk regions, will also be improved during each of these exercise progressions, as participants are encouraged to move through as complete a range of motion as possible. Do not hesitate to reduce the level of difficulty associated with the starting hand position or move participants to less challenging seated support surfaces if you feel they are not ready to perform these exercises on a more difficult surface.

Important Reminders

- Sit tall with the feet flat on the floor before beginning each trunk movement.
- Inhale as the trunk moves away from a midline position and exhale as the trunk returns to midline.
- Keep the eyes directed forward and focused on a visual target at eye level unless otherwise instructed.
- Perform each trunk movement through as complete a range of motion as possible while maintaining balance.
- Perform each exercise slowly.

Exercise Progressions

■ 1. LATERAL TRUNK ROTATIONS

a. Rotate the trunk *slowly* to one side, keeping the hips directed forward (figure 4.8). (The goal should be to look over the turning shoulder at the wall behind.)

b. Hold the position for three counts, then return to the starting position at the midline.

c. Repeat in the opposite lateral direction.

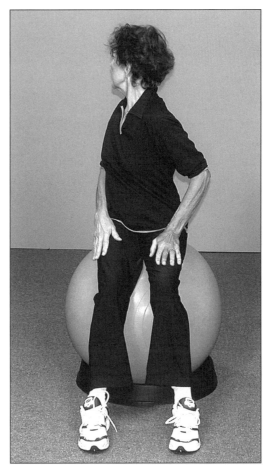

Figure 4.8 Lateral trunk rotations.

■ 2. TRUNK LEAN IN FORWARD AND BACKWARD DIRECTIONS

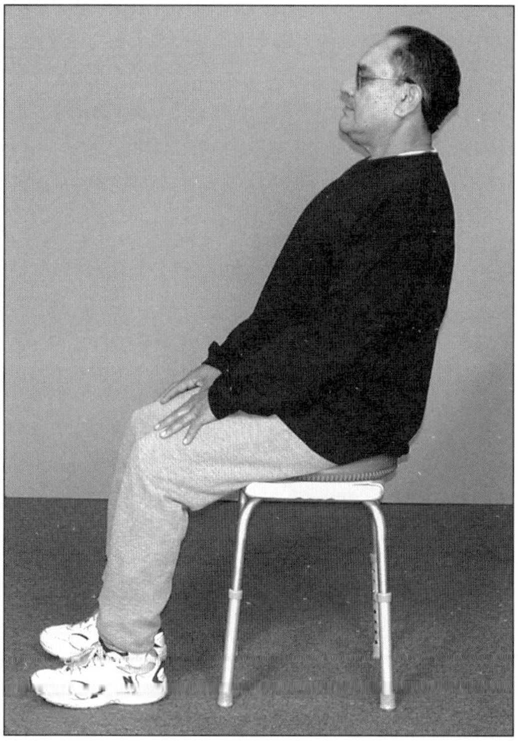

a. Lean the trunk forward, beginning at the hips, until the nose is above the knees. The eyes should be directed forward and focused on a target at eye level throughout the lean.

b. Maintain an extended upper body position throughout the lean.

c. Hold for three counts, then return to an upright starting position.

d. Lean the trunk backward while keeping the upper body extended (figure 4.9).

e. Hold for three counts, then return to an upright starting position.

Figure 4.9 Trunk lean in backward direction.

■ 3. TRUNK LEAN IN DIAGONAL FORWARD AND BACKWARD DIRECTIONS

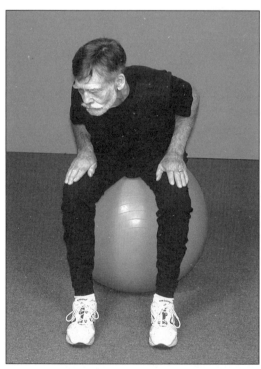

a. Lean the trunk diagonally forward until the nose is above one knee. The eyes should be directed forward and focused on a target at eye level throughout the lean (figure 4.10).

b. Maintain the upper body in an extended position throughout the lean.

c. Hold for three counts, then return to an upright starting position.

d. Repeat the movement in the opposite forward diagonal direction.

e. Repeat the diagonal trunk movements to both sides of the body, but this time lean the trunk in a backward direction. Keep the eyes directed forward and focused on a target.

Figure 4.10 Diagonal forward lean on balance ball.

Once again, refer to page 110 of this chapter for additional ideas on how to manipulate the level of balance challenge associated with each set of exercise progressions presented in level 3. Following completion of these core exercises, you might also consider incorporating one of the culminating activities that are described on pages 112 through 114 at the end of the seated balance section. Each culminating activity is designed to reinforce the many skills that have been acquired at each skill level. These activities can be performed in small groups and provide a fun way to practice a combination of skills in a gamelike setting. The most appropriate culminating activities to introduce after your class participants have practiced the first four levels would be one of the following: (a) seated bunny hop, (b) "Pass the potato, please," (c) "Hot potato!" or (d) balloon volleyball. Each culminating activity is presented in order of balance challenge, from the lowest to the highest.

Level 4: Seated Balance With Voluntary Leg Movements

Level 4 activities increase the challenge to maintain seated balance by having participants perform various movements with the legs as opposed to the arms and trunk. These lower body movements are also excellent activities for strengthening the muscles of the trunk, legs, and feet. Requiring movements to be performed through as complete a range of motion as possible also improves hip, knee, and ankle joint flexibility.

Important Reminders

- Sit tall on the chair or ball.
- Return the foot to the floor immediately if you start to lose balance.
- Keep the eyes directed forward and focused on a visual target at eye level unless otherwise instructed.
- Perform each exercise through as complete a range of motion as possible while maintaining seated balance and an upright trunk.
- Perform each exercise slowly.

Exercise Progressions

■ 1. HEEL LIFTS

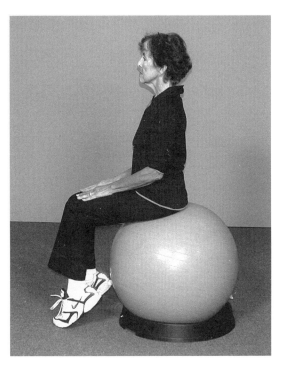

a. Perform continuous heel lifts with both feet simultaneously (weight should shift to the ball of the feet as the heels leave the floor). Perform 10 repetitions (figure 4.11).

b. Perform alternating heel lifts with each foot 10 times.

c. Perform double and single heel lifts on verbal commands ("Double," "Single").

Figure 4.11 Double heel lifts.

■ 2. TOE LIFTS

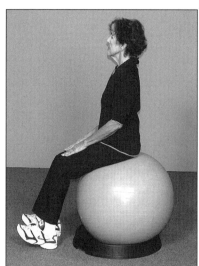

a. Perform continuous toe lifts with both feet (weight should shift to the heels of the feet as the toes lift up from the floor). Perform 10 repetitions (figure 4.12).

b. Perform alternating toe lifts with each foot 10 times.

c. Perform double and single toe lifts on verbal command.

Figure 4.12 Toe lifts.

■ 3. COMBINATION HEEL AND TOE LIFTS

a. Combine continuous heel and toe lifts with both feet (weight should first shift to the ball of the feet as the heels leave the floor, then back to the heels as the toes are lifted off the floor).

b. Perform 10 repetitions.

c. Perform alternating heel and toe lifts with each foot 10 times.

d. Perform double and alternating heel and toe lift combinations on verbal command.

■ 4. ANKLE CIRCLES

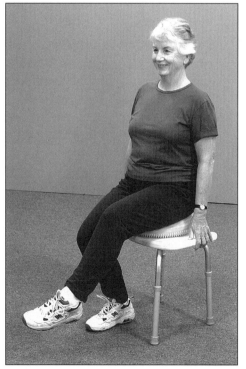

a. Lift one foot slightly off the floor (figure 4.13). (*Note:* Less stable participants may need to circle the ankle with the heel in contact with the floor during early repetitions or hold on to the chair or ball).

b. Circle the ankle in a clockwise direction. Perform the exercise five times, then reverse the direction for the same number of repetitions.

c. Repeat the exercise with the other foot.

Figure 4.13 Ankle circles.

■ 5. SEATED MARCHES

a. March in place by alternating knee lifts (height of knee lift depends on individual capabilities).

b. Perform 10 repetitions while maintaining an upright seated position.

c. Repeat the exercise but vary the height of the knee lifts (e.g., low, medium, high).

■ 6. SINGLE LEG RAISES

a. Extend one leg out until it is as close to horizontal to the floor as possible (figure 4.14). (Height will be determined by participant's ability to maintain an erect trunk position.)

b. Hold for three counts, then lower the leg to the starting position.

c. Repeat with the other leg until the exercise has been performed 10 times with each leg.

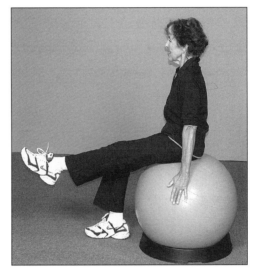

Figure 4.14 Single leg raises.

Refer again to page 110 of this chapter for ideas on how to increase the balance challenge by manipulating the task and environmental demands associated with the exercise. A fun culminating activity that can be introduced after sufficient practice of the core exercise progressions in this level is seated soccer (see page 114 for a description).

Level 5: Seated Balance While Resisting Perturbations

Level 5 activities further increase the challenge to maintain seated balance through the application of small and quick perturbations (pushes/pulls) to the hips or shoulders of the participant in various directions (i.e., forward, backward, lateral, diagonal). At this level, you are now working on the participants' anticipatory *and* reactive postural control abilities. Participants are seated on a support surface (e.g., chair with no back, Dyna-Disc, balance ball with holder) that matches their individual capabilities while adopting one of the three starting arm positions (i.e., hands resting on the chair or ball, hands resting on the thighs, or arms folded across the chest) described at the beginning of this section.

When the participant is perturbed, muscles of the trunk and lower body are also being strengthened as the participant tries to maintain a seated balance position. These activities challenge each participant to react quickly and efficiently to the perturbation. Look for the participant to respond with the appropriate countermovement (i.e., body movement in a direction that is opposite to the perturbation). Note how quickly each participant begins moving in the opposite direction after the perturbation and the amount of countermovement used. Ideally, the amount of countermovement should be proportional to the size of the perturbation.

Important Safety Guidelines to Follow When Performing Seated Perturbation Activities

- Inform assistants of any participant who should not be perturbed due to an existing medical condition.
- Begin with small perturbations (pushes or pulls) applied to the hip region. The push or pull movement should be administered quickly and the force gradually increased on each subsequent repetition. You also need to consider the type of surface on which the participant is seated when deciding how much force to apply. For example, an older adult who is seated on a chair with no backrest and a Dyna-Disc below the buttocks will be able to tolerate more force being applied than an individual who is seated on a balance ball with no ball holder beneath it.
- Do not increase the size of the perturbation if the participant is slow to initiate the countermovement or responds with too small or too large a countermovement for the size of perturbation applied.
- Wait until the participant recovers appropriately from the pushing or pulling action before initiating the next perturbation.
- Be prepared to provide manual support at this advanced stage of the exercise progression.

Exercise Progressions

■ 1. PREDICTABLE PERTURBATIONS

a. Inform participants in advance that you (or your assistants) are going to try to disrupt their seated balance by saying "Don't let me pull/push you off balance." By verbally warning participants in advance of applying the perturbation, you are testing how well they are able to stabilize the body in anticipation of being pushed or pulled off balance. Predictable perturbations are designed to test a participant's level of *anticipatory postural control.*

b. Begin by quickly pushing or pulling each participant's hips in a forward or backward direction. Progress to lateral and diagonal pushes and pulls once the participant is able to respond appropriately to the forward and backward perturbations.

■ 2. UNPREDICTABLE PERTURBATIONS

a. With no advance warning, provide unexpected perturbations of different sizes. In this situation, you are observing how well the participant is able to respond automatically to the disruption of balance. Unpredictable perturbations are designed to test a participant's level of *reactive postural control.*

b. Stand behind the participant so it is more difficult for them to predict the direction of the perturbation. Note the ability of participants to scale the response appropriately for the size of the perturbation (e.g., small push, small response in the opposite direction). Also check whether the participant is adapting to repeated perturbations of similar force by applying more muscular force in advance of the perturbation. If this is the case, they will not move as far from the midline following the perturbation. This reduced movement indicates that they are able to establish a good "postural set" for this activity.

c. Repeat the perturbations, but this time simultaneously push/pull one hip and shoulder in different directions using different levels of intensity (small and medium pushes or pulls). Do not provide advance warning of the perturbations. Vary the interval between perturbations in an effort to increase the level of unpredictability.

Level 6: Seated Balance With Dynamic Weight Shifts Through Space

Seated balance activities requiring self-initiated weight shifts improve dynamic center-of-gravity control because participants must now shift their weight away from the midline by moving the hips in various directions while maintaining balance. At the same time, the trunk, hip, and lower body muscles are being strengthened during these isotonic exercises. In addition, these exercises help increase flexibility, particularly at the hip joint. As with the exercises described previously, the type of seated support surface (e.g., chair with backrest, chair with no backrest, chair with Dyna-Disc, balance ball with or without holder) and arm position (e.g., holding seated surface, hands resting on thighs, arms folded across chest) should match each participant's individual capabilities.

Important Reminders

- Sit tall on the chair or ball.
- Position the feet hip-width apart and flat on the floor.
- Keep the shoulders relaxed and level throughout the exercises.
- Keep the eyes directed forward and focused on a visual target at eye level unless otherwise instructed.
- Inhale as the weight shifts away from the midline and exhale as the weight shifts back to the midline.
- Perform all exercises slowly and through as complete a range of motion as possible.

Exercise Progressions

■ **1. LATERAL WEIGHT SHIFTS**

a. Shift weight in a lateral direction through the hip and away from the midline (figure 4.15).

b. Return to a midline position, then shift weight laterally in the other direction.

c. Repeat the exercise with the eyes closed.

d. Repeat the lateral weight shift, but this time move from right to left without stopping at the midline position.

e. Repeat the previous lateral weight shift exercise with the eyes closed.

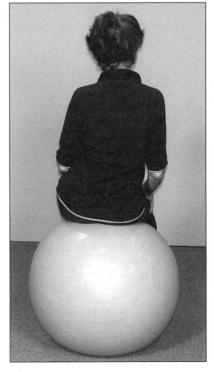

Figure 4.15 Lateral weight shifts on balance ball.

105

Important Tactile Cues

- "Can you feel yourself shifting the weight from one hip to the other as you move? Imagine you are sliding your hips on a tray beneath you."
- "Can you feel that your shoulders are relaxed and level as you move?"
- "Can you feel the pressure increase under the foot of the hip that is leading the action?"
- On diagonal weight shifts: "Can you feel the pressure increase under the foot of the hip that is leading the action?"

■ 2. FORWARD AND BACKWARD WEIGHT SHIFTS

a. Shift weight by moving the hips in a forward direction, hold for three counts, and return to the midline (figure 4.16a).

b. Shift weight by moving the hips backward, hold for three counts, and return to the midline (figure 4.16b).

c. Repeat the exercise with the eyes closed.

d. Repeat the forward and backward weight shifts, but move through the midline without stopping.

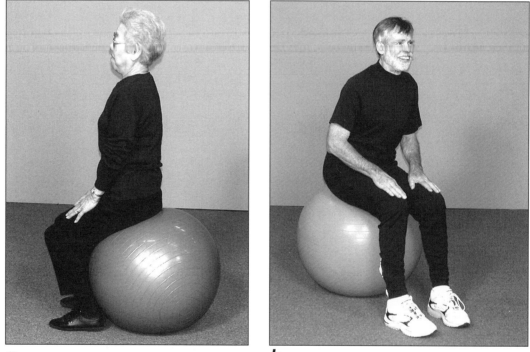

a   *b*

Figure 4.16 Forward *(a)* and backward *(b)* weight shifts on balance ball.

■ 3. DIAGONAL WEIGHT SHIFTS

a. Shift weight in a diagonal and forward direction (figure 4.17a).

b. Return to a midline position, then shift weight diagonally and backward (figure 4.17b).

c. Repeat the exercise with the eyes closed.

d. Repeat the diagonal weight shifts, but this time move diagonally forward and back without stopping at the midline.

e. Repeat the previous diagonal weight shifts with the eyes closed.

f. Repeat diagonal weight shifts in each of the four directions without stopping at the midline between movements.

g. Repeat the diagonal weight shifts in all four directions with the eyes closed.

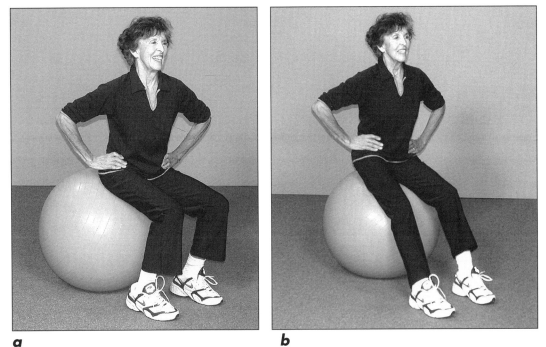

a   **b**

Figure 4.17 Diagonal forward **(a)** and backward **(b)** weight shifts on balance ball.

One task demand that is appropriate to introduce following adequate practice of each of the core progressions in level 6 is the addition of resistance (figure 4.18). This can be accomplished by wrapping a length of resistance band of a given tension low around each participant's hips that you then gently pull in a direction opposite to the intended weight shift. In addition to adding more challenge to the activity, the resistance band also serves as an excellent tactile feedback device. Participants will be able to feel the band's resistance increase against their hips as they shift weight in each direction. If they do not feel the increased tension, they will know they are not initiating the weight shift through the hips. Some general guidelines for using resistance bands are presented in the box below.

Use of Resistance Bands for Exercise

- Use a resistance band that is at least 6 feet in length.
- Determine the resistance most appropriate for the participant (the color of the band and the amount of pull in the opposite direction are associated with a given tension).
- For all dynamic weight shift exercises, place the resistance band low around the hips of the participant.
- Apply resistance by gently pulling the band in a direction exactly opposite to the direction in which the participant is shifting weight. Be sure to distribute the tension evenly across the band by keeping it flat against the hips.
- Instruct participants to position the hands on the thighs or fold them across the chest.
- Be sure to select a seated support surface (e.g., chair with no backrest, chair with Dyna-Disc, balance ball with or without holder) that allows participants to perform the exercises safely.

- Resistance bands also serve as excellent tactile cueing devices, reinforcing the importance of initiating the weight shift through the hips.

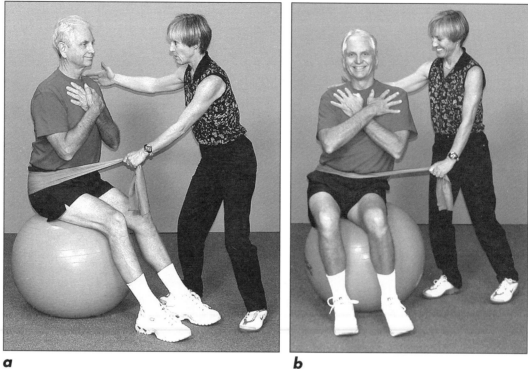

a   ***b***

Figure 4.18 Moving against a resistance band in backward **(a)** and lateral **(b)** directions.

Refer to page 110 for other ideas on how to increase the balance challenge related to this set of exercise progressions. An excellent culminating activity to introduce after each of the core progressions are practiced is "shift around the clock." This activity is described in further detail in the Culminating Activities section on page 114.

Level 7: Seated Balance With Dynamic Weight Shifts Against Gravity

The exercise progressions described in level 7 shift from practicing weight shifts through space to introducing weight shifts that are performed against gravity. These exercise progressions are intended to further challenge the balance system and teach class participants how to dynamically control the center of gravity when they are required to bounce in a vertical, horizontal, or diagonal direction. The exercises also work to strengthen and increase the power of the lower body muscles, especially the hip flexors and extensors, quadriceps, and plantar and dorsiflexor muscle groups.

General Instructions and Safety Guidelines for Performing Dynamic Weight Shifts Against Gravity

- Instruct participants to position the hands on the thighs or fold them across the chest.
- Provide less stable participants with a support holder for the balance ball and position them close to a wall or place a chair in proximity to the ball. (Dyna-Disc support surfaces are not appropriate for these activities.)

- Have participants position their feet hip-width apart and flat on the floor.
- Instruct participants to sit tall and focus their eyes on a visual target in front of them and at eye level while bouncing.
- The goal is to gradually increase the size of the vertical bounce until the buttocks leave the ball on each bounce.
- Instruct participants to stop bouncing if any discomfort is experienced in the hip or knee joints or they begin to experience any dizziness.
- Check the level of dizziness in all participants following each exercise progression using the 0 to 10 scale described on page 39 in chapter 2. Remember that the level of dizziness reported should not exceed a rating of 4 to 5.
- Encourage participants to reduce the height of the bounce or stop bouncing if they begin to feel unstable on the ball.
- This is an advanced activity and requires good dynamic postural control to perform.
- Gradually increase the number of repetitions you ask your participants to perform over several classes. This is a more demanding balance activity, and your more deconditioned class participants will fatigue quickly. Participants with arthritis or total joint replacements should be instructed to bounce at lower heights during all exercise progressions.

Exercise Progressions

■ 1. VERTICAL BALL BOUNCES

a. Push against the floor with the feet to initiate the vertical bounce. The top of the head moves upward toward the ceiling. Repeat the bounce 10 times.

b. Increase the size of the vertical bounce by gradually increasing the speed and force applied against the floor with the feet. The buttocks will begin to lose contact with the ball on the upward bounce. Complete 10 repetitions, increasing the height of the bounce on each repetition.

c. Repeat low bounces with the eyes closed.

■ 2. BOUNCES IN FORWARD AND BACKWARD DIRECTIONS

a. Push against the floor with the feet to initiate the bounce while shifting the weight (through the hips) forward and backward during the bounce. Repeat the exercise 10 times.

b. Increase the size of the forward and backward movement by increasing the force applied against the surface with the feet and the range of motion at the hips. Complete 10 repetitions.

c. Repeat the forward and backward bounces at a low level with the eyes closed.

■ 3. BOUNCES IN LATERAL DIRECTIONS

a. Push against the floor with the feet to initiate the bounce while shifting the weight through the hips in the right and left lateral directions during the bounce. Repeat the exercise 10 times at a low bounce height.

b. Repeat the exercise, but gradually increase the size of each lateral movement by increasing the force applied against the surface with the feet and increasing the range of motion at the hips on each repetition. Complete 10 repetitions.

■ 4. BOUNCES IN FORWARD AND BACKWARD DIAGONAL DIRECTIONS

a. Push against the floor with the feet to initiate the bounce while shifting the weight through the hips in the forward and backward diagonal directions during the bounce. Repeat the exercise 10 times.

b. Increase the size of the forward and backward diagonal movement on each subsequent repetition by using more force against the surface with the leading foot and increasing the range of motion at the hip. Complete 10 repetitions.

Once participants have mastered each of the exercise progressions in level 7, you can again begin to manipulate the task and environmental demands as described in the box below. Because these exercise progressions are relatively difficult in and of

Increasing the Seated Balance Challenge by Manipulating the Task and Environmental Demands

Task demands

- Change the difficulty level of the seated support surface (e.g., Dyna-Disc to ball with ball holder to ball with no ball holder).
- Require a more difficult starting arm position (e.g., hands on chair or ball to hands on thighs to arms folded across chest).
- Reduce or alter the base of support (e.g., feet together, semi- or full tandem, one-legged stance).
- Increase the number of repetitions of each exercise.
- Increase or decrease the speed at which the exercise must be performed.
- Follow arm movement with eyes and head (level 2).
- Combine arm and leg movements on certain activities.
- Coordinate arm, trunk, or leg movements to music of various tempos.
- Perform trunk movements (level 3) while holding a weighted object.
- Introduce resistance to selected activities in the form of hand or ankle weights or resistance band of different tensions (levels 2 and 4).
- Alter the shape and weight of objects being manipulated during an exercise.
- Develop a sequence of movements that must be performed in the correct order (also improves memory skill).
- Perturb participants (level 4) simultaneously at hips and shoulders and in opposite directions (e.g., pull left or right hip as left or right shoulder is pushed).
- Increase the size of the perturbation (level 4).
- Introduce a second task to be performed simultaneously with a balance activity (e.g., in order of difficulty, counting backward, reading aloud, reaching for objects, catching objects).

Environmental constraints

- Perform selected exercises with vision reduced (lower room lighting or have participants wear dark glasses) or absent (have participants close eyes).
- Alter the type of support surface beneath the feet (e.g., foam squares, rocker board, Dyna-Disc).
- Reduce or remove vision *and* alter the support surface beneath the feet.
- Perform certain exercises in a busy visual environment (e.g., in front of a striped curtain or while following a checkerboard being moved in front of the face).

themselves, use caution when selecting a particular task or environmental demand to manipulate when presenting them in class.

Now that you have been introduced to each level associated with the seated component of COG training, let's consider which exercise progressions would be most appropriate to present to our first case study subject, Jane Gain, during the initial week of classes. Reviewing her initial test results once again will help you make an informed guess as to the appropriate starting level for her and the types of balance challenges that can be added to the basic exercise progressions. Table 4.1 lists the exercise progressions I would recommend for Jane, as well as important verbal cues and reminders that would be helpful to share with her as she practices each exercise progression. Once you have reviewed the list of recommended exercises, try to develop a similar set of recommendations for Bill Divine.

Table 4.1 Sample Set of Seated Center-of-Gravity Control Exercises for Case Study 1: Jane Gain

Balance activity	Level of challenge	Comments
Level 1: Seated balance	Sitting on Dyna-Disc with feet hip-width apart. Arms on thighs with eyes open; arms on chair with eyes closed.	Emphasize somatosensory cues—pressure under buttocks and feet, good alignment of body. Close supervision when eyes are closed.
Level 2: Voluntary arm movements	Sitting on Dyna-Disc with feet hip-width apart. Perform all movements with eyes open only. May perform with eyes closed if supervised.	Emphasize that balance comes first. Stop activity if balance feels threatened. Lower arm movements will also increase stability.
Level 3: Voluntary trunk movements	Sitting on Dyna-Disc with feet hip-width apart. Arms on thighs when eyes open; arms holding on to chair when eyes closed. Can perform all activities.	Emphasize somatosensory cues. Close supervision on backward lean and smaller movement to foster confidence.
Level 4: Voluntary leg movements	Sitting on Dyna-Disc with feet hip-width apart. Arms on thighs for leg raises and ankle circles (heel on floor); arms holding on to chair during marches and single leg raises.	Emphasize good body alignment. Cue to keep heel on floor during ankle circles. Emphasize erect posture during marches and single leg raises performed at lower height.
Level 5: Perturbations	Sitting on Dyna-Disc with feet hip-width apart. Hands on chair. Provide only small and predictable perturbations to build confidence.	Emphasize good body alignment and good foot contact with floor.
Level 6: Dynamic weight shifts	Sitting on Dyna-Disc with feet hip-width apart. Hands on thighs during all weight shifts except lateral (place on hips). Close supervision when weight shifts are performed with eyes closed.	Emphasize good postural alignment, relaxed shoulders, and feet in firm contact with floor. Emphasize shift of belly button vs. head. Begin with all weight shifts returning to midline.
Level 7: Weight shifts against gravity	Cannot perform these progressions until able to move to balance ball with ball holder.	

Culminating Activities for Seated Balance Activities

The culminating group activities described in this section are intended to provide participants with the opportunity to practice the many different exercise progressions they have been introduced to in each of the seven levels of seated balance activities. By introducing an object to be passed and retrieved, whether with the hands or the feet, you are further increasing the demands of the task by requiring participants to divide their attention between the task of balancing and that of passing the object. Balance must be more subconsciously controlled as attention is diverted to the task of reaching, passing, catching, or throwing. The balance level to which these particular culminating activities best apply is indicated at the start of each activity description. The name of the most appropriate culminating activity or activities is also listed immediately following the discussion of the core exercise progressions associated with the particular set of balance activities. Before introducing any of the culminating activities, be sure to review the safety tips described in the box below.

Important Safety Guidelines to Follow When Introducing Culminating Balance Activities

- Do not introduce group activities until participants can safely perform all of the seated balance exercises on one of the seated support surfaces described earlier *and* with the arms in the most difficult position (folded across the chest).
- Move some participants onto a less challenging seated support surface (e.g., chair with backrest, chair with Dyna-Disc, balance ball with holder) so you can introduce this group activity earlier in the program but still maintain a safe exercise environment.
- Restrict the size of your groups to no more than four to six participants and provide external support (i.e., chairs in close proximity) for participants.
- Bear in mind that older adults are just as competitive in game situations as younger adults. Thus, you should continually remind them that "balance comes first" and they should not attempt to perform a movement during any game if they begin to feel unstable.

■ SEATED BUNNY HOP

This group activity is performed to the song "The Bunny Hop" and is designed to reinforce each of the arm and trunk movements performed in levels 2 and 3. The instructor can vary the combination of arm and trunk movements performed throughout the song. Introducing music also adds an external timing component, thereby increasing the balance challenge. This activity also fosters working memory as the number of movements performed is increased.

■ "PASS THE POTATO, PLEASE"

This is a good culminating activity to introduce after the core exercise progressions associated with levels 2 and 3 have been adequately practiced. This first variation of the activity is self-paced so it does not introduce too high a level of balance challenge too early. Participants are seated on various support surfaces in a circle (no more than four participants in each circle). A ball is passed in a clockwise direction until the instructor calls "Change." The ball is then passed in a counterclockwise direction. As participants become more comfortable performing the activity, the height of the pass can be varied, as well as the weight of the ball. A nice progression of this activity would be to encourage participants to also pass the ball to participants either directly across from them in the circle or on a diagonal. In this way, they can practice the different trunk movements introduced in level 3. The instructor can also move around the outside of the circle and have the participant retrieve and then pass the ball back from different heights and angles to practice other arm and trunk movements (figure 4.19).

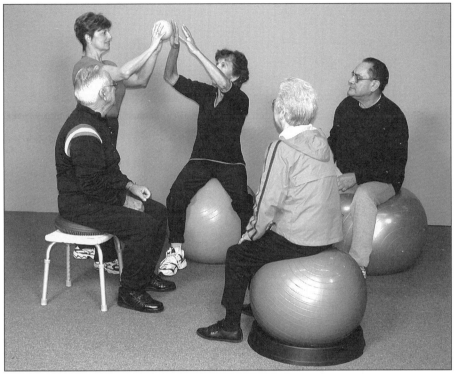

Figure 4.19 Participants playing "Pass the potato, please."

■ "HOT POTATO!"

A slightly more challenging version of the previous passing activity is called "Hot potato!" This culminating activity can also be introduced to reinforce the exercise progressions practiced in levels 2 and 3. The object of this activity is to pass the ball around the circle as quickly as possible. Requiring participants to perform the task more quickly places an added challenge on the postural control system. You can also increase the cognitive demands associated with the activity by periodically calling out the verbal command to change the direction in which they are passing. Adding this cognitive demand will provide you with the opportunity to watch how quickly a participant is able to process and respond to each verbal command. A second ball can also be introduced into the circle to further increase the various physical and cognitive demands associated with the task. Balls of different weights can also be used to add a resistance component to the activity.

■ BALLOON VOLLEYBALL

This is the most challenging culminating activity to introduce after level 2 and 3 exercise progressions have been practiced. What makes this activity more challenging than the two previous activities is that you further increase the task demands by adding a higher-level external timing component. As with the previous two variations of culminating activity, small groups of class participants (four to six) are seated in a circle formation and attempt to tap a balloon to one another as many times as possible before the balloon contacts the floor. Unlike the ball-passing activities, participants must now react more quickly because they do not know when the balloon will reach them. Attention is being further diverted from the task of balancing, requiring that it be controlled at a more subconscious processing level.

■ "SHIFT AROUND THE CLOCK"

"Shift around the clock" is an excellent culminating activity to introduce after participants have practiced all the core progressions described in level 4. Instruct participants to move to various positions on an imaginary clock face (e.g., 3 o'clock, 5 o'clock, 11 o'clock). Begin each weight shift to a position on the clock from a midline position. Return to the midline after each movement. As soon as participants become familiar with moving to each of the positions on the imaginary clock face from a midline position, eliminate the return to this position and have participants move from one clock position to another without pausing at the midline. Increase the speed with which the clock positions are announced to further challenge participants. Both memory and motor coordination will be improved as an outcome of this activity. As the program progresses, you could also manipulate certain task (e.g., alter the base of support, add a secondary task such as counting or reading) or environmental (e.g., alter the support surface beneath the feet, reduce or remove vision) demands described in the box on page 110 to add still more challenge to the activity.

■ SEATED SOCCER

This is an excellent culminating activity to introduce following completion of the core exercise progressions in level 4. This activity is a fun way to (a) improve seated balance control when the base of support is reduced and (b) divide the participant's attention so that the act of balancing becomes less consciously controlled again. Be sure to manipulate each individual's capabilities by selecting a seated support surface that will maximize their safety during this activity. Participants should be seated on various support surfaces in a circle formation (three to four in each group). The object of the activity is to trap and then kick the ball from person to person in the circle. Encourage participants to stop the ball with one foot and then kick it with the other foot. When first introducing this activity to the class, be sure to position chairs between each person in the circle and encourage the less stable participants to hold on to a chair during the trapping and kicking phases of the action.

Important Safety Tips for Seated Soccer

- Do not introduce this culminating activity until participants can safely perform the most difficult seated balance exercise progression in level 4 (i.e., single leg raises) on one of the seated support surfaces described earlier and with the arms in the most difficult position (folded across the chest).
- Move some participants onto a less challenging seated support surface (e.g., chair with backrest, chair with Dyna-Disc, balance ball with holder) so you can introduce this group activity earlier in the program but still maintain a safe exercise environment.
- Remind participants that "balance comes first"—and they should not attempt to perform a movement in the game if they begin to feel unstable.
- Demonstrate the most appropriate way to kick the ball (i.e., instep kick) before starting the activity.
- Encourage participants to stop the ball with one foot and then kick it with the opposite foot.
- Discourage participants from kicking the ball while it is still moving.

Summary

When introducing any of the exercise progressions described in the seven levels of seated balance activities, remember to match the individual's capabilities to the challenge of the task and the environment in which the task must be performed. As each participant becomes more comfortable performing each activity on the selected equipment, consider moving them onto a more challenging surface when performing the lower-level exercise progressions in later classes. For example, if the participant is able to perform exercises in level 2 while seated on a chair and Dyna-Disc with arms folded across the chest and eyes closed, consider moving them onto a balance ball with a ball holder beneath it when these exercise progressions are repeated in a subsequent class. Initially, participants can adopt an easier hand position (on the ball itself) and only perform the exercise progressions with their eyes open until they are ready to accept more challenge. Participants may then need to return to the chair and Dyna-Disc configuration to perform the more challenging and higher-level exercise progressions.

Several ways to progressively increase the challenge associated with each balance exercise in the seven levels of seated balance activities have also been described on page 110. Remember that you are attempting to manipulate the demands imposed by the task or the environment so as to increase the challenge associated with each balance exercise. Given that the manipulation of these two variables will directly affect the individual's ability to perform the task, do so in a way that does not compromise safety or negatively affect a participant's self-confidence. You can further reinforce what has been learned in each level by incorporating culminating activities that allow participants to practice the many balance skills they have acquired in a fun, gamelike atmosphere. Consider what type of support surface you would have Jane and Bill sitting on during the performance of any of the culminating activities described above. For example, would you change the type of support surface they were sitting on for certain games, and if so, why?

Standing Balance Activities

The type of support surface to use for the standing center-of-gravity control activities will again depend on the *individual capabilities* of the participant. Some participants may need to begin each exercise progression while standing on the floor with a wide base of support, whereas other participants may be ready to begin activities standing on an altered support surface (e.g., foam, rocker board) or with an altered support base. The exercise progressions described in the seven levels of standing balance activities are designed to progressively challenge each participant's standing balance.

Once participants are able to perform each of the core exercise progressions associated with the seven levels of standing balance activities described in this section, you can again begin to increase the level of balance challenge by manipulating either the task or environmental demands in ways similar to those described in the previous section. By manipulating just one or two aspects of the task, you will add variety to the practice session and challenge the sensory, motor, and cognitive systems at the same time. A set of culminating activities is also described that will enable your clients to practice several different exercise progressions simultaneously in a fun, gamelike atmosphere.

General Safety Guidelines for Standing Balance Activities

- Alert all assistants to participants who may have difficulty performing standing activities with eyes open or closed so they can be closely supervised. Also alert assistants to participants with medical conditions (e.g., peripheral neuropathy, joint replacements, osteoporosis) that make it difficult to perform standing exercises on compliant surfaces.

- Certain participants may need to perform these exercises with their back to the wall (about 2 feet away), with a chair in front of them, or with very close supervision (or all three).

- Do not ask participants to perform the next exercise progression until they can safely perform the task at hand. For example, do not ask participants to perform an exercise with the eyes closed if they are not able to do it safely with the eyes open.

- Instruct participants to open their eyes immediately if they feel they are about to lose their balance.

- Instruct participants how to safely mount and dismount compliant (foam, half-foam roller, or Dyna-Disc) and moving (rocker board) surfaces.

- Have participants practice how to get safely on and off foam, foam roller, or Dyna-Disc surfaces in the forward, backward, and lateral directions before introducing the exercise progressions.

Level 1: Checking Your Standing Posture

Before introducing any of the standing balance activities described in this section, teach your class participants how to check their standing posture. Demonstrate the correct standing posture to your class and then have them practice while standing with their back against a wall. If you are fortunate enough to have a wall of mirrors in your facility, you could have them practice standing with a correct posture while facing the mirror and then standing sideways to it. Provide the following verbal cues as you observe whether your class participants are standing correctly:

- "Stand with your back against the wall, feet flat on the floor with the heels approximately 6 inches from the wall."

- "Relax your arms and let them hang by your sides." (Observe whether the space between the arm and the body is equal on both sides for each client.)

- "Hold your head erect and direct your eyes forward to focus on a target." (Check whether the chin is parallel to the floor.)

- "Gently move your head straight back until your ears are directly above your shoulders."

- "Your upper back should be erect and your chest slightly elevated."

- "Pull your abdominal muscles in and up so that your stomach flattens." (Check to see that each client's lower back has a slight forward curve and that the hips are level, the kneecaps are facing forward, and the ankles and feet are straight.)

- "Notice that the weight is evenly distributed under your feet."

- "Breathe normally and hold that position for 15 seconds with your eyes open. Now close your eyes and try to concentrate on the feeling of standing correctly."

Your clients can also check their alignment by placing one hand behind their neck with the back of the hand against the wall and the other hand behind their lower back with the palm facing the wall. If they are able to move their hands forward and backward more than an inch, the curves of the spine are not in proper alignment. Another good homework assignment to give your clients is to practice standing posture either against a wall or in front of a full-length mirror at home.

Important Reminders

- Stand tall and imagine that the top of the head is being pulled toward the ceiling by a string.
- Keep the eyes directed forward and focused on a visual target at eye level.
- Try to maintain each standing position for as long as possible (30 seconds maximum).

Level 2: Standing Balance With Altered Base of Support (ABOS)

The exercise progressions described in this level are intended to help participants learn how to control the center of gravity when in a standing position. As the base of support is altered during this set of exercise progressions, subtle shifts of the COG will be necessary so that upright balance can be maintained. For example, as participants move from a Romberg (feet together) to a sharpened Romberg (tandem stance) position, they must recognize that their base of support is now narrower and longer and adjust the position of the COG accordingly. To maintain stable, upright control in a sharpened Romberg position, the COG must be shifted forward to a position directly above the heel of the front foot and toe of the rear foot. The COG is then moved again as the participant adopts a one-legged stance so that it is now directly above the stance leg as the other leg is lifted off the floor. The ultimate goal of the exercise progressions at this level will therefore be to teach the participants the strategy for manipulating the COG as the base of support is altered. Once acquired, this strategy should serve the older adult well in performing daily activities that involve a changing base of support (e.g., walking, stepping into and out of the bathtub, standing in confined spaces).

Exercise Progressions

■ 1. STANDING FLOOR ACTIVITIES

Altered base of support.

a. Stand with feet together (Romberg position). Hold the position for 15 seconds. Repeat with the eyes closed (figure 4.20a).

b. Move the feet into a semitandem position (front foot ahead of the rear foot with a small space between the feet). Hold the position for 15 seconds. Repeat with the eyes closed (figure 4.20b).

c. Stand in sharpened Romberg position (heel-to-toe standing position). Hold the position for 15 seconds. Repeat with the eyes closed (figure 4.20c).

d. Adopt a unilateral stance (participant may rest the raised leg on the foot of or against the stance leg). Hold the position for 15 seconds. Repeat with the eyes closed (figure 4.20d).

An easy way to manipulate the balance challenge associated with this set of exercise progressions is by either (a) altering the position of the arms during the exercise (i.e., at sides, folded across chest) or (b) altering the support surface beneath the feet (e.g., foam, rocker board, Dyna-Disc, half-foam roller). It may be necessary to reduce the balance challenge for some participants by asking them to adopt a less difficult arm position, particularly in the eyes-closed exercises (i.e., at sides), whereas other participants may be ready to perform the exercise progressions with the arms folded across the chest or while standing on a more challenging surface, or both. See page 125 for additional ideas.

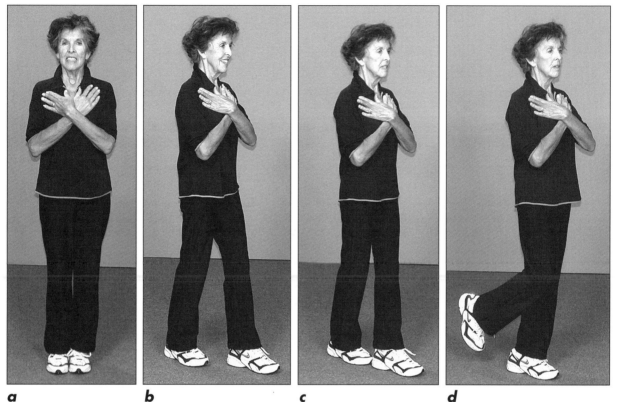

a   b   c   d

Figure 4.20 Four examples of activity progressions with altered base of support: *(a)* feet together (Romberg); *(b)* feet in semi-tandem; *(c)* feet in sharpened Romberg; and *(d)* one-legged stance.

Getting Safely On and Off Altered Support Surfaces

- Instruct participants to always "test" the altered support surface by putting one foot onto the middle of the surface and feeling its (a) level of compliance, in the case of a foam or Dyna-Disc surface, or (b) direction and amount of tilt, in the case of a rocker board.

- When one foot has been placed on the altered surface and positioned in the center, slowly transfer weight onto that foot and bring the other foot up onto the surface (figure 4.21).

- Instruct clients to stand tall with slightly flexed knees (i.e., soft knees) and focus on a visual target directly in front of them at eye level.

- Instruct clients to step off any altered surface in a forward direction, taking a moment to firmly plant the lead foot on the firm surface before lifting the other foot off the altered surface.

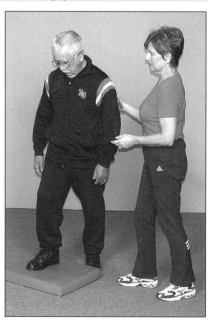

Figure 4.21 Getting safely on and off altered support surfaces.

■ 2. STANDING WHILE PERFORMING A COGNITIVE TASK

a. Repeat all exercises performed successfully in level 1 while performing a secondary cognitive task (e.g., reading aloud, counting backward) (figure 4.22).

b. Repeat the exercises performed successfully in the first progression while standing on a compliant surface and performing a secondary cognitive task.

c. Repeat the exercises performed successfully in the first progression while standing on a rocker board and performing a secondary cognitive task.

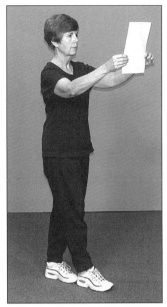

Figure 4.22 Participant standing in sharpened Romberg position while reading aloud.

■ 3. STANDING WHILE PERFORMING AN UPPER BODY MANUAL TASK

a. Repeat all exercises performed satisfactorily at level 1 on a firm surface while reaching for objects placed at different heights. Manipulate the weight and shape of the objects to increase the level of challenge.

b. Repeat all exercises performed successfully at level 1 on a firm surface while catching and throwing objects of different weights and shapes (figure 4.23).

c. Repeat all exercises performed successfully at level 1 on a compliant surface while reaching for objects of different weights placed at different heights.

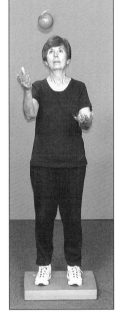

Figure 4.23 Standing on a rocker board (ABOS) while tossing a ball from hand to hand.

■ 4. STANDING WHILE PERFORMING A LOWER BODY MANUAL TASK

a. Foot drawing: Participants use a foot to draw or write on the floor. Effective activities include writing their first name with the right foot and their last name with the left foot, drawing circles, squares, diamonds, and so on.

b. Moving a small towel in different directions with the foot: Have participants push the towel away from and back toward the body in a variety of directions, scrunch and unscrunch the towel with one foot, and then transfer the towel (using the foot) to the opposite foot. Repeat the activities. (This activity is best performed with shoes removed.)

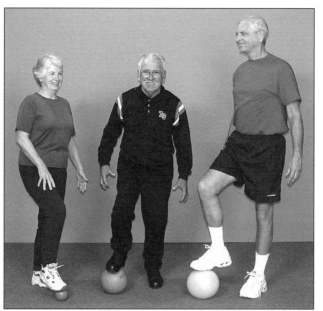

Figure 4.24 Standing with foot on top of ball.

c. Standing with one foot placed on a medium-sized ball (figure 4.24): Move the ball in different directions (forward, backward, diagonally, in a circle, etc.) while maintaining standing balance. Place the ball under the opposite foot and repeat the activity. Position less stable participants close to a chair or wall so they can steady themselves during any portion of the exercise.

d. Replace the ball with a more compliant one that does not allow as much weight to be placed on it for support. Repeat the above activity.

(The most compliant object to place under the foot is a balloon). Do not move to this more advanced progression until the previous progression can be performed without assistance.

Level 3: Multidirectional Weight Shifts

The primary purpose of the exercises described for level 3 is to expand each participant's region of stability so that activities of daily living that require greater ranges of body motion or extreme leaning (i.e., pulling weeds in the garden, leaning into cupboards or the washing machine) can be accomplished. An expanded region of stability will also place an individual at a lower risk for losing balance in case of an unexpected perturbation. These exercises are also intended to teach participants how to move the body more efficiently through space and in a way that is most appropriate for the task demands. Improved joint flexibility and lower body strengthening will also be promoted as the distance through which participants are required to shift and transfer weight increases.

Tactile and Verbal Feedback to Enhance Learning

- Provide verbal cues, and provide tactile feedback by placing chairs a suitable distance in front of and behind participants or positioning participants appropriately between a wall and a chair. Move the chair(s) closer to the participants if you observe that they are bending at the hips before reaching the chairs.

- Watch to see that participants are not rising up onto their toes as they lean forward. Instruct them to reduce the lean distance so their heels remain in contact with the floor.

- Verbally instruct participants to stand tall and keep their eyes focused on a target at eye level in front of them.

- Participants should touch the chair with the hips as they move forward and touch the chair or wall behind with the buttocks as they move in a backward direction.

- During lateral weight shifts, participants should turn to one side so they can continue to use the chairs or wall to provide tactile feedback. The hips should make contact with each chair (or the chair and wall) as they move in a lateral direction.
- Instruct participants to relax the shoulders and "slide their hips along a tray" as they perform the lateral weight shifts.
- On diagonal weight shifts, encourage participants to feel the changing pressures under their feet as they shift weight in the forward diagonal (pressure moves forward under the toes) and backward diagonal (pressure moves back toward the heel) directions.
- Have them perform a quick visual check to see that the knee is directly above the foot at the end of the forward diagonal weight shift.
- Check to see that participants are maintaining slightly flexed knees on the lateral and diagonal weight shift exercise progressions. A good verbal cue to use is "soft knees."

Exercise Progressions

■ 1. FORWARD-BACKWARD WEIGHT SHIFTS

a. Shift weight forward until pressure can be felt under the balls of the feet and the heels begin to lift off the floor. Return to the midline position. Repeat five times, then repeat with the eyes closed for the same number of repetitions. The upper and lower body should be moving in the same direction.

b. Shift weight backward through the hips until the toes begin to rise from the floor. Return to the midline. Repeat five times. Repeat with the eyes closed for the same number of repetitions.

c. Shift weight in the forward and backward directions without pausing at the midline. Repeat the movement sequence 10 times. Repeat with the eyes closed for the same number of repetitions.

■ 2. LATERAL WEIGHT SHIFTS

a. Shift weight through the right hip until the inside edge of the right foot begins to lift from the floor. Return to the midline. Repeat five times before changing sides.

b. Repeat the weight shift to the left side. Return to the midline.

c. Shift weight from left to right without pausing at the midline. The shoulders should remain relaxed and level throughout the exercise.

■ 3. FORWARD DIAGONAL WEIGHT SHIFTS

a. Position the right foot so that the heel of that foot is ahead of the toes of the left foot.

b. Slowly shift weight forward through the right hip until the knee is directly above the toes of the right foot. The right knee should bend as the weight transitions forward. The upper body should remain erect and facing forward throughout the weight shift. The shoulders should remain relaxed and level.

c. Hold for a count of three and return to the midline. Repeat five times.

d. Reverse the position of the feet so that the heel of the left foot is now ahead of the right foot.

e. Repeat the diagonal weight shift forward and to the left.

f. Hold for a count of three and return to the midline. Repeat five times.

g. Repeat each forward and diagonal weight shift with the eyes closed.

■ **4. BACKWARD DIAGONAL WEIGHT SHIFTS**

a. Position the left foot so that the heel is ahead of the toes of the right foot.

b. Shift weight backward and diagonally through the hip until foot pressure is centered over the right heel. Bend the right knee during the backward transition. The upper body should remain erect and facing forward. The shoulders should remain relaxed and level.

c. Hold for three counts and return to a midline position.

d. Repeat five times before changing the position of the feet.

e. Repeat the backward and diagonal weight shifts to the left.

f. Repeat the exercise with the eyes closed.

■ **5. FORWARD AND BACKWARD DIAGONAL WEIGHT SHIFTS**

a. Begin by moving diagonally forward to the right and then diagonally backward to the left without pausing at the midline position.

b. Repeat 10 times before repositioning the feet and performing the exercise on the opposite diagonal.

c. Repeat the exercise with the eyes closed.

■ **6. COMBINATION BACKWARD WEIGHT SHIFTS**

a. Position the feet hip-width apart and focus the eyes on a forward visual target at eye level. The upper body should remain erect with the shoulders relaxed and level.

b. Shift weight backward through the right hip until the pressure increases under the right heel. Return to the midline.

c. Shift weight directly backward through both hips until the pressure increases under both heels. Return to the midline.

d. Shift weight back through the left hip until the pressure increases under the left heel. Return to the midline.

e. Repeat the exercise with the eyes closed.

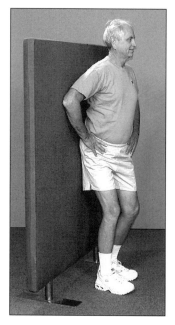

Position participants close to a wall for this last exercise progression so they can use the wall as a tactile cue at the end of each backward movement (figure 4.25). Touching the wall reinforces the need to shift the weight through the hips. A fun set of cues to use during this exercise is "right cheek touches, both cheeks touch, left cheek touches."

Refer to the box on page 125 for other ideas on increasing the balance challenge associated with each of these exercise progressions once the participants have become comfortable performing them on a firm surface with their eyes closed. In addition, a good culminating activity to have your class participants perform at the end of this set of exercise progressions is the "shift around the clock" activity described on page 114 of the seated balance section. The only difference is that the participants will now perform the activity in a standing as opposed to a seated position.

Figure 4.25 Backward weight shifts against a wall.

Level 4: Weight Transfers With Head and Body Movements

The marching progressions described in this section challenge the participants' level of motor coordination (i.e., four-corner marching—head turns first) as well as adaptive postural control, particularly when the client is marching in place and the head is turned to one side during the marching activity. These activities will help improve the client's ability to perform daily activities that might require them to turn their head as they are walking, for example, to check oncoming traffic as they cross the road or in response to a friend's greeting. Because many older adults become unstable when they perform these types of activities, the marching progressions described in this section will be very helpful.

Exercise Progressions

■ 1. MARCHING IN PLACE ON A FIRM SURFACE

Emphasize lifting the knees directly to the ceiling. Perform this exercise for 30 seconds. Keep the upper body and head erect and the eyes directed forward.

■ 2. MARCHING IN PLACE WITH HEAD TURNS

Begin marching in place for eight counts with the head erect and the eyes directed forward. Continue marching for an additional eight counts while turning the head a quarter turn to the right. Turn the head back to a forward position while continuing to march for eight counts. Continue marching, but now turn the head a quarter turn to the left (figure 4.26).

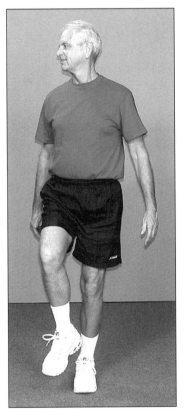

> ### Important Safety Tip
>
> Increase the number of marching counts between turns if the participant experiences any dizziness. Encourage gaze fixation with each quarter turn.

Figure 4.26 Marching in place with the head turned to the left.

■ 3. FOUR-CORNER MARCHING

Begin marching for eight counts with the head and eyes directed forward. Continue to march for eight counts but turn the head and body a quarter turn to the right. Continue marching and turning the head and body a quarter turn for eight counts until four turns have been completed.

■ 4. FOUR-CORNER MARCHING—HEAD TURNS FIRST

Repeat the four-corner marching exercise, but now turn the head before the body on each quarter turn. Continue to encourage gaze fixation on each quarter turn.

Level 5: Dynamic Weight Transfers Through Space

Exercise Progressions

■ 1. FORWARD RIGHT AND LEFT STEP

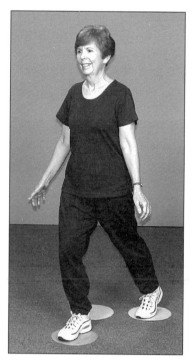

a. Begin with a weight shift through the left hip to unload weight from the right leg. Step forward with the right foot (figure 4.27). Make sure the knee is bent as the right foot contacts the floor and that the knee is directly above the right foot at the completion of the forward step. Hold the position for three counts. Then shift weight backward through the left hip until the weight is centered over the left foot. Step backward with the right foot (use colored spots to indicate the desired stepping distance). Perform each forward step activity multiple times before changing the leading leg.

b. Repeat the exercise with the eyes closed.

Figure 4.27 Colored spots on the floor are used to guide the desired stepping distance during the forward weight shift.

■ 2. FOUR-CORNER STEPPING

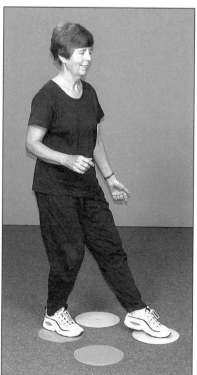

a. Step in a forward direction with the right foot followed by the left foot. Shift weight onto the left foot, and then step back with the right foot followed by the left foot (use colored spots to indicate the desired stepping distance) (figure 4.28).

b. Repeat the exercise with the eyes closed.

Figure 4.28 Backward weight shift on four-corner stepping activity.

There are many fun ways to increase the level of balance challenge associated with each exercise progression. Refer to the box below for ways to manipulate the task or environmental demands to increase the balance challenge. To help participants practice how to manipulate the COG during standing activities, you can introduce culminating activities such as line passing, creek crossing, and rock hopping. Each of these activities requires the class participants to dynamically control the COG while leaning in different directions or transferring weight through space.

Increasing the Standing Balance Challenge by Manipulating the Task and Environmental Demands

Task demands

- Alter pacing of the exercise (i.e., increase or decrease speed of weight shifts, transfers, stepping sequences) using a hand clap, metronome, or music of various tempos.
- Instruct participants to repeat each of the multidirectional weight shift progressions in level 3 but gradually increase the distance the participants must shift their weight. You will notice participants beginning to flex at the hips as the forward-backward lean distance increases. Do not increase the lean distance beyond the point where participants begin to flex the hips.
- Add an external timing component (music, counts).
- Add a secondary task to be performed simultaneously with the balance activity (e.g., count backward, read aloud, reach for objects, catch and throw objects).
- Move participants to the next bench or step height once they are able to perform all exercise progressions in level 7 safely (example: progress from 4-inch to 6-inch bench height).

Environmental constraints

- Have participants perform selected exercise progressions with vision reduced or absent.
- Alter the support surface under the feet during exercise progressions performed in levels 3, 4, and 5 (e.g., foam, rocker board, Dyna-Disc).
- Have participants perform activities while facing a wall with a busy visual pattern taped onto it (e.g., vinyl checkerboard tablecloth, large square of material with complex visual pattern). Alternatively, move a checkerboard through the visual field and instruct participants to follow it with the eyes only.

Level 6: Kicking Stationary Objects

Exercise Progression

■ 1. BALL KICKING

Practice kicking a ball against a wall or to a partner. Encourage participants to alternate the leg used to kick or trap the ball on each repetition.

Important Safety Tips When Kicking Stationary Objects

- Position less accomplished participants so they are kicking against the wall as opposed to another individual.
- Position less stable participants close to a wall or chair so they can hold on during the kicking phase of the action.
- Instruct participants to stop the ball completely with the foot before attempting to kick it back to the wall or a partner.
- Demonstrate and then encourage participants to kick the ball with the instep for better control.
- Increase the amount of supervision and support available to participants during this exercise because it requires greater postural control, particularly during the kicking portion.

Level 7: Weight Shifts and Transfers Against Gravity

When performing each of the exercise progressions described for level 7, be sure to select the bench height that is best suited to the capabilities of each participant. A good way to determine the best height is to start each participant at the 2-inch bench height and observe their overall level of postural stability while performing at least four forward and backward toe touches. Progress them to the 4-inch bench height if they perform the toe touches satisfactorily. If the participant begins to lose balance on the forward toe touches or rotates the trunk on the backward toe touches at either of these two bench heights, then do not progress them to the next bench height (6 inches). Pay close attention to good form during these progressions, particularly when the participant is performing sustained heel raises in a forward or backward direction or step-up, step-down, and swing-through step activities that require the participants to be in a one-legged stance as the leading leg travels up onto and over the bench.

Exercise Progressions

■ **1. ALTERNATING TOE TOUCHES ONTO BENCH**

Alternate touching feet onto 2-, 4-, or 6-inch bench. Be sure that participants only place the forefoot on the bench with each toe touch. The knee should be directly above the lead foot on contact.

■ **2. ALTERNATING AND SUSTAINED FORWARD HEEL RAISES**

Weight is taken onto the foot touching the bench until the stance leg leaves the floor (figure 4.29). Hold for 2 to 5 seconds. Have participants imagine that they have a string tied around their waist that is being pulled forward as their foot contacts the bench and assumes the weight of the body.

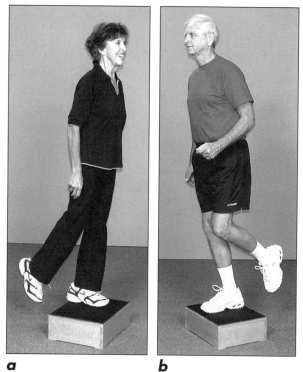

a   *b*

Figure 4.29 Forward (*a*) and backward (*b*) sustained heel raises.

■ 3. BACKWARD TOE TOUCHES

Alternate feet contacting the bench. Be sure that participants only place the forefoot on the bench with each toe touch.

■ 4. SUSTAINED BACKWARD TOE TOUCHES

Weight is shifted onto the foot touching the bench until the stance leg leaves the floor. Increase counts from 2 to 5. Encourage participants to shift weight through the lead hip and keep the head directed forward. Only the forefoot should contact the bench.

■ 5. SIDE TOE TOUCHES

The foot closest to the bench is lifted up onto the bench and toward the center.

■ 6. SUSTAINED SIDE BENCH RAISES

Lift the foot closest to the bench up onto the bench and shift weight until the other foot is no longer in contact with the floor. Hold for 3 seconds and lower the foot to the floor. Emphasize an erect posture with the eyes directed forward at a visual target during the rising portion of each exercise progression. Watch for excessive hip rotation on the rising phase. The leg in contact with bench should remain slightly flexed at the knee. Repeat the exercise using the other leg.

■ 7. FORWARD STEP-UP/STEP-DOWNS

Step forward onto and then off of the bench, ending on same side of the bench as the starting position.

■ 8. FORWARD STEP-UP/STEP-DOWNS, OPPOSITE SIDE

Step forward onto and then off of the bench, ending on the opposite side of the bench from the starting position. Turning choices: (a) return to the original position in front of the bench or (b) turn 180° in place and repeat the exercise. Alternate the lead foot on each repetition.

■ 9. FORWARD SWING-THROUGH STEPS

Step forward onto the bench with the lead leg and swing the other leg through, making contact with only one foot (i.e., up with the right, swing through with the left, step down with the right; see figure 4.30). Turn in place and repeat the exercise with the opposite leg acting as the lead leg (i.e., up with the left, swing through with the right, step down with the left).

■ 10. SIDE STEP-UP/STEP-DOWNS

Step sideways onto and then off of the bench, ending on the same side of the bench as the starting position.

■ 11. SIDE STEP-UP/STEP-DOWNS, OPPOSITE SIDE

Step sideways onto and the off of the bench, ending on the opposite side of the bench from the starting position.

Once your class participants have adequately practiced each of the progressions in level 7, you can begin to combine the various types of stepping activities they have been performing on the appropriate height bench into progressively longer step aerobic routines. This culminating activity will not only improve their

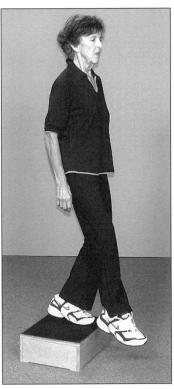

Figure 4.30 Forward swing-through steps on bench.

dynamic COG control, but will also improve their memory and attention skills as you lead them through progressively longer step sequences.

Once again, let's consider the types of standing balance activities that would be most appropriate for Jane to practice during the first or second week of the class. In selecting the recommended exercise progressions that are described in table 4.2, I first considered how each of Jane's identified impairments was likely to affect her ability to perform the various balance activities when in a standing as opposed to a sitting position.

Table 4.2 Sample Set of Standing Center-of-Gravity Control Exercises for Case Study 1: Jane Gain

Balance activity	Level of challenge	Comments
Level 1: Checking standing posture	Stand with back against wall. Place one hand behind neck with back of hand against wall. Place other hand behind lower back, palm to wall.	Emphasize erect posture, eyes focused on a target and chin tucked in. Tighten abdominal muscles and breathe normally.
Level 2: Standing with altered base of support	Stand on firm surface near wall or chair. Practice feet-together (Romberg) and semitandem positions with eyes open and closed. Practice sharpened Romberg and unilateral stance with support (eyes open only).	Emphasize somatosensory cues in eyes-closed progressions. Demonstrate and provide verbal cues relative to movement of COG in semitandem, sharpened Romberg, and unilateral stance positions.
Standing while performing second cognitive task	Stand on firm surface only near wall or chair. Repeat progressions (a) and (b) while counting backward. Practice progressions (c) and (d) while holding onto support.	Observe level of sway during each progression. Encourage change in arm position (folded across chest) if sway is small. Emphasize alignment.
Standing while performing upper body task	Stand on firm surface only near wall or chair. Perform progressions (a) and (b) only with balls of different sizes and weights.	Emphasize good body alignment while performing each activity. Emphasize reaching to various heights and distances from body.
Standing while performing lower body task	Stand on firm surface only near wall or chair. Perform progressions (a), (b), and (c) while periodically holding onto support surface.	Emphasize good postural alignment during all activities. Encourage intermittent release of support on (a) and (b) progressions only.
Level 3: Multidirectional weight shifts	Stand on firm surface near wall or chair. Perform all progressions (1-6), with special emphasis on use of wall for backward weight shift progressions.	Emphasize good postural alignment, relaxed shoulders, and feet in firm contact with floor. Emphasize shift of belly button vs. head and shoulders. Cue pressure change under feet.
Level 4: Weight transfers with head and body movements	Stand on firm surface near wall or chair. Perform all progressions (1-4).	Emphasize erect posture, eyes focused on target, particularly during head turns. Allow self-pacing of activity.
Level 5: Dynamic weight transfers through space	Stand on firm surface near wall or chair. Perform both progressions (with eyes open and closed).	Emphasize good postural alignment, relaxed shoulders, and bent knee on landing. Focus eyes on forward target with each weight shift. Small distance between spots.

Level 6: Kicking stationary objects	Stand on firm surface and hold on to support surface during kicking and trapping movements. Kick against wall, not partner.	Emphasize erect posture. Cue to hold on to chair or wall when trapping and kicking ball. Must stop ball before passing!
Level 7: Weight shifts and transfers against gravity	Stand on firm surface near wall. Use 2- to 4-in. bench for progressions 1 through 4. Do not perform progressions 4 or 6 yet. Perform progression 9 on 2-in. bench only.	Emphasize erect posture and eyes focused on a forward target once foot is positioned on bench. Check whether Jane feels pain on any exercise; if so, discontinue exercise or reduce bench height.
Floor-to-stand transfers	Have Jane perform easiest progression only. Place eggcrate foam on floor to cushion knees.	Emphasize working at own pace. Avoid multiple repetitions. May need medic alert.

Increasing the Level of Balance Challenge

The level of balance challenge can be increased for any of the standing balance activities described in the seven levels by manipulating the task and environmental demands in a variety of ways. Consult the box on page 125 for ideas on how to manipulate the task and environmental demands at each level. As an exercise for yourself, decide which of the balance challenges listed would be appropriate to introduce to Jane after she can safely demonstrate the standing activity.

Culminating Activities for Standing Balance Activities

■ "PASS THE POTATO, PLEASE" IN STANDING POSITION

Participants stand on a firm surface or various support surfaces and facing each other in a circle, a little less than arm's length apart (no more than four participants in each circle). A ball is passed in the clockwise direction until the instructor calls "Change." The ball is then passed in a counterclockwise direction. As participants become more comfortable performing the activity, the height of the pass can be varied (e.g., above the shoulders, below the knees), as well as the weight of the ball.

■ "HOT POTATO!" IN STANDING POSITION

A variation of the first passing activity is called "Hot potato!" The object of this activity is to pass the ball as quickly as possible around the circle. Requiring participants to perform the task more quickly places an added challenge on the postural control system. Add a second ball to further increase the attentional demands associated with the task. Adding balls of different weights will also improve upper body strength. Instruct participants to reverse the direction of their passing on the verbal command of "Change." Because you have now added an external timing component to the task, you must remind participants that balance comes first and they should not try to receive or pass the object if they feel they are about to lose their balance. For more competitive class participants who are not that stable, consider moving them onto a less difficult support surface during this version of the activity.

■ BALLOON VOLLEYBALL IN STANDING POSITION

Participants stand in the same circle formation used in the previous activities (figure 4.31). The goal is to tap a balloon to one another as many times as possible before the balloon contacts the floor. As with the seated version of this activity, attention is

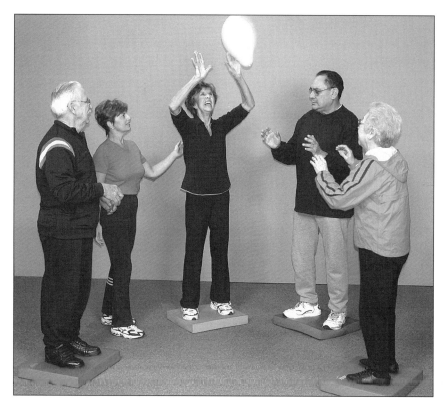

Figure 4.31 Balloon volleyball. This culminating activity can be made more challenging for some participants by altering the type of support surface.

being further diverted from the task of balancing, requiring that it be controlled at a more subconscious processing level. I recommend that you start this activity with everyone standing on a firm surface and note the level of postural control and eye-hand coordination being exhibited by each participant before introducing altered support surfaces in subsequent repetitions. Again, pay close attention to the more competitive class participants, and station an assistant close by to provide a verbal reminder that balance comes first or to provide manual assistance.

■ "SHIFT AROUND THE CLOCK"

While standing with feet flat on the floor and hip-width apart, participants are instructed to lean to various positions on an imaginary clock face (e.g., 5 o'clock, center (midline), 11 o'clock, center). Begin each weight shift to a position on the clock from a midline position. Return to the midline after each movement. Progress the activity by requiring participants to lean from one position on the clock to another without shifting back to the midline (e.g., 1 o'clock, 7 o'clock). Increase the speed at which the clock positions are announced to further challenge participants. Both memory and motor coordination will be improved as an outcome of this activity.

■ FAST FEET

This group activity is designed to encourage class participants to move a little faster when performing weight transfers. Participants stand with their feet flat on the floor and hip-width apart. Begin by asking participants to move either the right or left foot away from and back to the starting position in either a forward, backward, or lateral direction following your command. For example, you might call out the following sequence: "Right forward, left back, right side, left side." Begin at a slow pace and gradually increase the speed of your verbal commands. You can then progress this activity by instructing your participants to transfer their weight more fully by lunging in each direction as it is called.

■ LINE PASSING

This group activity provides participants with an opportunity to practice weight shifting on various surface types while performing a secondary task of passing an object (figure 4.32). Because the participants are standing on altered surfaces, this activity also improves lower body strength. Upper body flexibility is also being enhanced by the different object-passing activities, as is upper body strength when the object being passed is weighted.

Participants (four to six per group) form a line, one behind the other and approximately an arm's length apart. Organize the line so the shortest person is at the front of the line and the tallest is at the rear. The object of the activity is to pass an object down the line beginning with the person at the front. When the object reaches the last person in the line, it is then passed back toward the front. This activity is performed while participants are standing on different surface types (e.g., compliant, moving). When first introducing this activity, have only the odd-numbered people in the line stand on a compliant or moving surface, with the even-numbered participants standing on a firm surface. As the activity becomes familiar to all participants, you can progress to having each participant stand on an altered surface.

Important Safety Tips for Line Passing Activity

- Organize participants in the group according to height so that passing is made easier.
- Make sure that participants remain approximately an arm's length apart when standing in the line.
- Match the difficulty of the surface to the participant's capabilities.
- Organize the line so that participants are standing in proximity to a wall and the last person in line is being well supervised. Have an assistant walk down the line, providing manual assistance where appropriate.

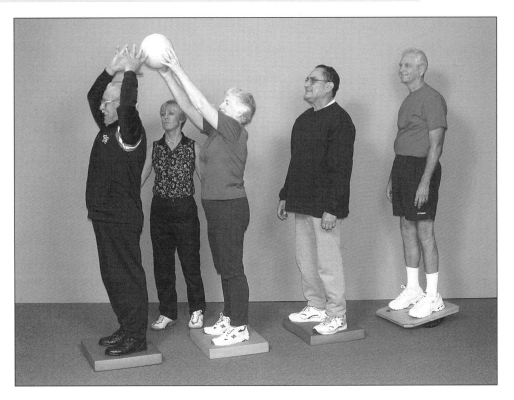

Figure 4.32
Line passing activity.

The following types of passing activities are suggested:

- Left-to-right lateral passing: The first person in line passes the ball by rotating the trunk to the right and passing the ball at waist height to the person immediately behind. The second person then rotates the trunk to the left and passes the ball to the person behind. Alternate passing sides for the return trip to the front. The weight shift should occur to the side opposite the passing side.
- Passing the ball above and behind the head: This activity requires a forward weight shift as the ball is lifted above and behind the head.
- Passing the ball between the legs: Remind participants to keep the head level and eyes directed forward as the ball is passed between the legs.
- Combination of over-the-head and between-the-legs passing.

Increase the challenge of the group activity in any of the following ways:

- Increase the weight of the ball being passed.
- Alter the support surface on which the participant is standing (move from a compliant to a moving surface).
- Add a timing constraint (i.e., maximum number of successful passes in 30 seconds).
- Add a secondary cognitive task such as counting by threes (3, 6, 9, 12, etc.) along the line or calling out the name of an animal beginning with a letter of your choosing.

■ CREEK CROSSING

Lay out two lines of masking tape (approximately 5 to 6 feet in length) of increasing distance apart (approximately 6 to 18 inches) in different areas of the room. The area between the two lines is the "creek" and the areas beyond each line are the "creek banks." The goal for participants is to see how many times they can cross the creek, beginning at its narrowest end, before getting their feet wet (i.e., feet touching the floor in the space between the two lines). A suitable exercise progression is as follows:

1. Instruct participants to step forward across the creek, turn, and step back to the starting side until they are unable to take a long enough step to avoid getting their feet wet.

2. Instruct participants to place only one foot on the opposite bank (i.e., beyond the second tape line) and then return it to the same side of the creek without getting it wet (equates to a forward lunge activity of increasing distance). Have them alternate the lead leg on each repetition.

3. Place objects in the creek (i.e., on the floor between the two lines) for participants to pick up as they cross it. On the return trip, they place the objects back in the creek.

4. Instruct participants to step forward across the creek and then backward when returning to the starting side. (This is an advanced activity and is only suitable for your more accomplished clients.)

■ ROCK HOPPING

Place colored spots at different intervals between the two tape lines representing the creek bed. The goal is to reach the other end of the creek by stepping on the "rocks" (i.e., colored spots) and banks of the creek without getting the feet wet. Increase the balance challenge in the following ways:

- Substitute Dyna-Discs for some of the colored spots so that the surfaces of certain "rocks" are more unstable as participants move down the creek.
- Place objects in the creek that participants must bend down to retrieve on their way down the creek (figure 4.33).

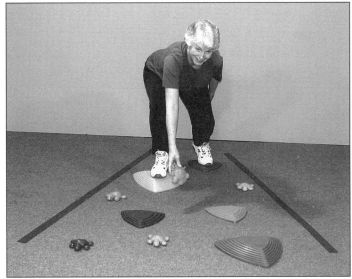

Figure 4.33 Rock-hopping activity. The activity can be made more challenging by requiring participants to pick up objects from the creek bed.

■ CIRCLE SOCCER

Organize groups of four to five participants in a circle at a comfortable distance from one another. The object is for the participants to kick a soccer ball to one another, keeping the ball within the circle as it is passed among the group (figure 4.34). Have participants call a person's name before kicking the ball to them. One point is scored for every successful trap and kick within the circle. Encourage less stable participants to hold onto a chair as they trap and kick the ball.

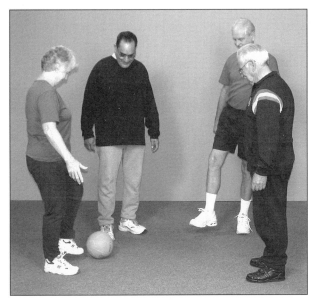

Figure 4.34 Group soccer activity.

Floor-to-Standing Transfers

All participants must practice floor-to-standing transfers many times throughout the program (figure 4.35). Many older adults are unaware of the procedures for rising safely from the floor. This is an important skill to teach your participants in case they experience a fall when alone at home. It has been well documented that morbidity and mortality rates associated with falls increase the longer the person lies after falling to the ground. The floor-to-standing progression has been divided into levels of difficulty from easiest to most difficult. You will also notice that two different floor-to-standing transfer strategies are described under the more difficult category. The first strategy emphasizes upper body strength, whereas the second strategy emphasizes lower body strength and hip flexibility. The most difficult transfer strategy is described but not illustrated because it is very difficult for most older adults to use successfully unless they are well conditioned and free of injury.

Floor-to-Standing Transfer Progressions

■ EASIEST PROGRESSION

Supine/prone to side-lying position to side sitting to kneeling with hands on the floor, then crawling to an external support to pull up to standing

■ MORE DIFFICULT (EMPHASIZES UPPER BODY STRENGTH)

Supine/prone to side-lying position to side sitting to kneeling with hands on the floor, then hand-walking to standing

■ STILL MORE DIFFICULT (EMPHASIZES LOWER BODY STRENGTH)

Supine/prone to side-lying position to side sitting to kneeling to half-kneeling to standing

■ MOST DIFFICULT

Supine/prone to symmetrical sit-up to squat to leg reliance to standing (not shown)

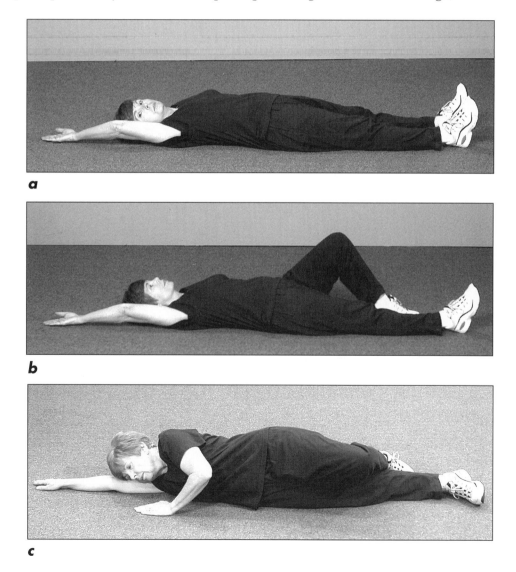

a

b

c

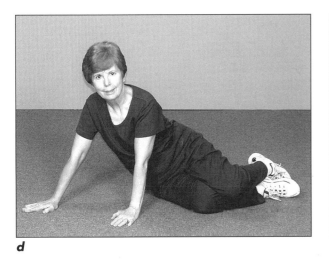
d

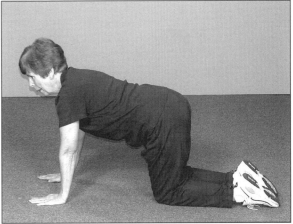
e

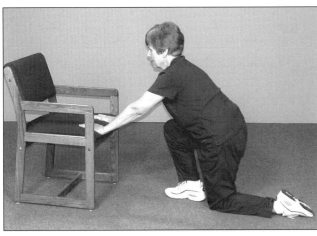
f

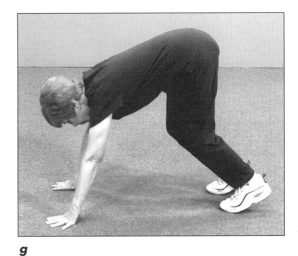
g

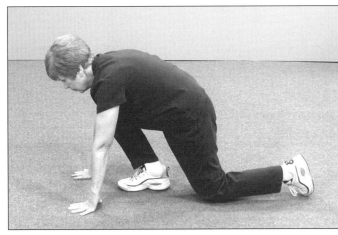
h

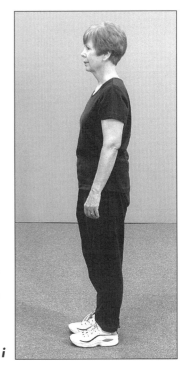
i

Figure 4.35 Floor-to-standing transfer progressions: *(a)* supine or prone position, one arm extended; *(b)* flex opposite knee; *(c)* roll toward extended arm until side-lying position is reached; *(d)* push up into a side-sitting position; *(e)* rotate the body until kneeling with hands on floor; *(f)* hand walk to external support (easiest transition to standing); *(g)* hand walk to standing (requires good upper body strength); *(h)* half-kneel to standing (requires good hip ROM and lower body strength; *(i)* standing position.

Summary

The primary emphasis throughout this chapter has been on describing a set of progressive balance activities in seated, standing, and moving environments that will help the older adult clients in your program better understand how to control the COG when they are required to stand steadily in space, lean through their limits of stability, or perform a variety of weight transfer activities. Not only are they learning how to consciously control the COG in static and dynamic balance environments, but also how to control it subconsciously when they are unexpectedly perturbed or performing a second task that forces them to divide their attention between the new task and the task of balancing. Many of the exercise progressions presented, particularly the bench activities in level 7, also help foster improved anticipatory postural control skills as the participants negotiate the bench in a variety of ways.

Once each of the core exercise progressions has been adequately practiced, you can begin to increase the balance challenge by altering the task or environmental demands associated with the various exercises. Several ideas for increasing the level of balance challenge were presented on pages 110 and 125. As important as it is to maximize the balance challenge associated with a set of exercise progressions, it is equally important that you do so while minimizing the risk of injury. Throughout the chapter, I have incorporated safety tips and exercise precautions that you should carefully review and follow whenever you are presenting a set of exercise progressions. Also remember that the FallProof program is designed to be taught in group activity settings, so not all class participants will be ready for the same level of balance challenge when performing a set of activities. Here is where your knowledge of the client and your interpretation of their preprogram test results will help you determine what types of COG activities each client requires and the level at which they should begin practicing those activities.

TEST YOUR UNDERSTANDING

1. To achieve a stable standing posture, the center of gravity should be positioned such that
   a. the COG is outside of the base of support
   b. the COG is contained within the base of support
   c. the COG is close to the anterior border of the base of support
   d. the COG is close to the posterior border of the base of support
   e. the base of support is contained within the COG

2. How can you modify the task or environmental demands to accommodate an individual who has difficulty performing dynamic weight shifts in the backward direction while sitting on a balance ball? Have the individual perform the activity
   a. while sitting on a chair with a Dyna-Disc
   b. while sitting on the balance ball with a ball holder
   c. only in the forward and lateral directions
   d. because the goal is to challenge the individual's capabilities
   e. while sitting on the balance ball with hands resting on the ball

3. During seated center-of-gravity control training, task difficulty can be manipulated by altering hand placement. The order of difficulty, from easiest to most difficult, is as follows:

   a. hands on ball, hands held above head, hands folded across chest

   b. hands folded across chest, hands on thighs, hands on ball

   c. hands holding on to assistant, hands on ball, hands folded across chest

   d. hands on ball, hands on thighs, hands folded across chest

   e. hands on thighs, hands on ball, hands folded across chest

4. Which of the following culminating activities is not an effective way to practice various seated activities that require dynamic center-of-gravity control?

   a. seated bunny hop

   b. "Hot potato!"

   c. seated soccer

   d. balloon volleyball

   e. "walk the gauntlet"

5. Which of the following is an example of changing the environment to increase the level of difficulty?

   a. performing a continuous sequence of movements

   b. altering the type of support surface beneath the feet during an activity

   c. performing the selected movement while holding a weighted object

   d. changing the starting arm position from holding the seated surface to hands resting on thighs

   e. changing the seated support surface from a balance ball to a chair with a Dyna-Disc

6. Which of the following is not an appropriate example of an exercise involving dynamic weight transfers through space?

   a. marching in place

   b. rock hopping

   c. forward right and left stepping

   d. four-corner stepping

   e. creek crossing

7. Which of the following is an example of changing the task demands to increase the balance challenge?

   a. reducing the amount of vision available

   b. altering the support surface beneath the feet

   c. performing the activity with a reduced base of support

   d. altering the seated support surface

   e. performing the activity in front of a busy background (e.g., a checkerboard)

8. Which of the following is an appropriate example of a culminating activity for standing center-of-gravity control training with weight shifts?

   a. shift around the clock

   b. line passing

   c. seated soccer

   d. "walk the gauntlet"

   e. rock hopping

9. Which of the following is an example of a way to increase the task demands of a seated balance activity with voluntary leg movements?
    a. changing the seated support surface
    b. changing the starting arm position
    c. reducing the amount of vision available
    d. altering the support surface beneath the feet
    e. performing a secondary task at the same time

PRACTICAL PROBLEMS

1. Experiment with performing the various exercise progressions at different levels of balance challenge so you can begin to better understand how the difficulty of an exercise changes with each variable (i.e., task or environmental demand) that you manipulate. To an outside observer, many of these exercise progressions look very simple; however, until you try them yourself, you may not appreciate just how challenging many of them can be, even for a younger adult.

2. Develop a set of exercise progressions for each level of seated and standing balance activities for Bill Divine based on the recommended exercises that were described for Jane Gain. Assume it is the first week of class and you are preparing your COG training component to be presented during the skills section of the class. Indicate the level of initial balance challenge you would establish for Bill and identify the exercise progressions you would present in the 20-minute skills section you have planned during the first two or three classes scheduled for the first week. Also indicate whether you would manipulate the balance challenge in any way during or between the various exercise levels. Finally, indicate what type of support surface you would have Bill working on during the culminating activities you select for each class. Be sure to review the possible underlying impairments you identified after reviewing Bill's test results (presented in chapter 3) so that you can establish the appropriate initial level of balance challenge for each of the selected exercise progressions.

Multisensory Training

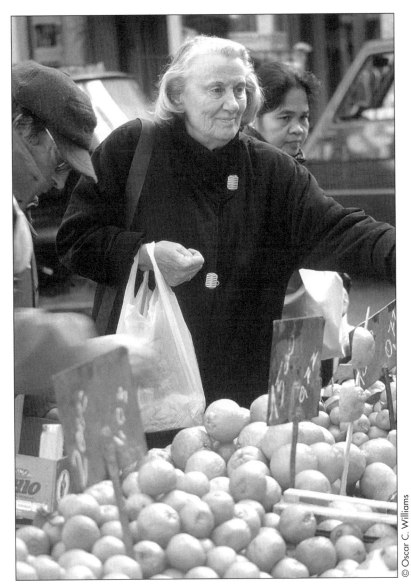

© Oscar C. Williams

Objectives

After completing this chapter, you will be able to

- describe how each of the three sensory systems (i.e., visual, somatosensory, vestibular) contribute to postural control in different sensory environments,
- understand how the type of sensory system impairment will affect exercise selection and progression,
- develop a set of exercise progressions designed to improve the use of each of the three sensory systems to control balance, and
- structure a safe practice environment.

Our ability to perceive where we are in space and how we should respond to changing sensory conditions during our daily lives is heavily dependent on (a) the amount and quality of information we receive from our peripheral sensory receptors and (b) how we organize and integrate the information from the different sensory sources once it has reached the central nervous system. It has been well documented that each of the three sensory systems (i.e., visual, vestibular, and somatosensory) that contribute to balance and mobility experience significant changes as a function of the aging process. Visual acuity, contrast sensitivity, and depth perception decline; the threshold for detecting vibration and joint movement increases; and the number of sensory receptors (hair cells) within the vestibular apparatus also declines (Rose, 2001a). A reduction in the gain of the vestibulo-ocular reflex with advancing age has also been documented (Wolfson et al., 1997).

Although older adults are generally able to compensate for small changes occurring in each of these systems with age, impairments associated with particular medical diagnoses (e.g., macular degeneration, peripheral neuropathy, Ménière's disease) and severe deconditioning will adversely affect their postural control system and limit both the types of activities they can successfully perform and the environments in which they can safely function. The activities in this component of the program are intended to optimize the functioning of the sensory systems that are not impaired while compensating for the system or systems that are known to be permanently impaired. The effectiveness of sensory training programs on selected measures of balance have already been demonstrated for healthy older adult groups in previous research studies (i.e., Hu & Woollacott, 1994a, 1994b), providing a strong rationale for their inclusion in a multidimensional fall risk reduction program targeting older adults who are at increased risk for falls.

The use of vision is optimized by teaching gaze-stabilization strategies during seated, standing, and locomotor activities. Performing balance activities on a compliant or moving support surface will also promote the use of vision for controlling balance by compromising the somatosensory system, thereby making it more difficult to obtain accurate sensory information from the surface. Conversely, to optimize the use of the somatosensory system as the primary source of sensory information for controlling balance, it is necessary to compromise vision and maximize the quality and quantity of somatosensory information obtained by having clients perform balance activities with the feet in contact with a firm, broad surface. Lowering the room lights, having the participant wear dark glasses, or engaging vision by introducing a second task that requires vision (e.g., reading, tracking, reaching for, or catching objects) represent effective ways to reduce the older adult's reliance on vision to control balance. Vision can also be removed by having participants perform activities with the eyes closed once they reach a higher level of performance and feel comfortable performing activities in the absence of vision.

Finally, an increased reliance on vestibular inputs for balance can be achieved by compromising both the visual *and* somatosensory systems. Performing a variety of balance activities on surfaces that are compliant or moving, or both, while vision is distracted (by introducing movement in the field of view), engaged in performing a second task, or the eyes are closed will encourage greater reliance on vestibular information for balance. Of course, knowing which multisensory activities are most appropriate for each participant requires a careful review of the medical history completed at the outset of the program (to ascertain whether certain sensory systems are permanently impaired due to an existing pathology) and the results of the M-CTSIB performed during the prescreening and assessment described in chapter 3.

In addition to exercises for improving each of the three sensory systems that contribute to balance and mobility, several exercises are introduced in this chapter that are intended to improve the older adult's ability to coordinate head and eye movements. These exercises involve the visual system alone or the visual and vestibular systems working together. For example, when the head is stationary and only the eyes are moving as they track an object through the visual field (i.e., smooth pursuit movements), the visual system is being exercised. Once the head begins to move, however, the vestibular system is also activated. As described in chapter 1, the vestibulo-ocular reflex becomes important when we turn our head quickly to focus on a target or acknowledge a friend who has called our name. In these situations, the VOR is activated to prevent retinal slip (i.e., occurs when the speed of eye movements is not equal to the speed of the head movement) by moving the eyes at the same velocity as the head but in the opposite direction (Herdman, 1999). This reflex helps us perceive that the world is stable as we move through space. Older adults who have abnormalities of the VOR will often experience vertigo (i.e., an illusion of oneself or the environment moving). In other situations, when the head and eyes are tracking an object, the VOR must be canceled so that the head and eyes now move in the same rather than opposite directions. Individuals who are unable to effectively cancel the VOR in these situations will not exhibit smooth eye movements as they track objects. The eyes may periodically jump in order to catch up with the moving object and bring it back into focus.

The exercises presented in this chapter are designed to train each of the three sensory systems to function more efficiently as well as improve the older adult's ability to coordinate eye and head movements. More specifically, the goals of this component of the program are as follows:

- Improve the functioning of the somatosensory system by compromising or removing vision
- Improve the use of visual inputs for balance by compromising the somatosensory system
- Improve vestibular system function by compromising both the somatosensory and visual systems
- Enhance the interaction between the visual and vestibular systems

Finally, as an instructor, you should follow two guiding principles when selecting exercises intended to force the use of each of the three sensory systems that contribute to balance: (1) force the use of systems when the impairments are temporary or changeable and (2) compensate or substitute for system impairments that are permanent or progressive.

Important Safety Reminders

- It is important to review the health history of each participant prior to introducing *any* multisensory training activities to ensure that you are not asking participants to perform any activities that would compromise their safety. Be sure to review the test results and interpretation sheet associated with the M-CTSIB before choosing any of the multisensory activities described in this first section of the chapter that are intended to force the use of particular sensory systems.

- Ask participants to cease performing any activity if they become dizzy or disoriented. If certain clients regularly experience dizziness during a class, recommend that they pay a visit to their primary care physician to discuss the problem.

- Remember that for sensory systems with temporary impairments, the goal is to introduce activities designed to force their use, whereas in the case of permanent sensory system impairments, the goal is to compensate for the loss by introducing activities designed to improve function in the remaining system(s).

- Do not introduce the next exercise progression in any level until the previous one can be performed without imbalance.

- Be aware that some participants may be able to perform the more advanced activities associated with one set of sensory exercises but not those associated with another set of exercises due to an impairment in a different sensory system.

Forcing the Use of the Somatosensory System to Control Balance

Participants who do not have a medical diagnosis indicating that the somatosensory system is permanently or progressively impaired (i.e., peripheral sensory neuropathy or loss of sensation in the feet or lower limbs) should derive considerable benefit from engaging in balance activities that force them to select somatosensory (i.e., touch and proprioception) inputs instead of other sensory systems to control balance. Before you decide whether forcing the use of the somatosensory system is desirable, however, you must first review the health/activity questionnaire completed by each participant in conjunction with the results of the M-CTSIB test conducted. Take a moment to review the health/activity questionnaires completed by our two case study participants to determine if any impairments are indicated that are likely to affect their use of this system.

After checking whether any medical diagnosis or self-report of sensation loss in the feet and ankles appears on the questionnaires, review the results obtained for condition 2 of the M-CTSIB (eyes closed, stable surface). Recall that participants who perform poorly (i.e., demonstrate a large amount of sway or prematurely open their eyes) in this condition are not using somatosensory inputs effectively to control their balance—they are visually dependent. In the absence of any information on the questionnaires that suggests they are experiencing a loss of sensation, you can be reasonably sure that introducing activities designed to force the use of the somatosensory system will be helpful, albeit challenging, during the early stages of practice. Here, again, take a quick look at the scores obtained by Jane and Bill on condition 2 of the M-CTSIB to determine if they are using somatosensory inputs appropriately.

Improving the older adults' use of the somatosensory system for controlling balance will be particularly important when they must perform daily activities in situations of reduced or absent lighting (i.e., walking in the community at night, entering a dark room, or getting up to go to the bathroom at night). The older adult who is experiencing significant changes in vision as a function of age or pathology will also benefit significantly from engaging in this type of sensory training. As a result of operating balance and mobility training programs at Braille Institute facilities, we have found that older adults, even those who have lived with serious visual impairments for many years, do not use somatosensory inputs for balance as well as one might think. Despite their serious visual impairments, they do not automatically switch to using somatosensory inputs as their primary information source.

You must follow two important guidelines when presenting balance activities designed to force the use of the somatosensory system. First, all balance activities must be performed on a broad, firm surface; and second, vision must be compromised in some way. Four simple ways to compromise vision are as follows:

- Reduce the amount of vision by lowering the lights in the room or have the participants wear dark glasses during an activity.
- Remove vision by turning off all the lights in the room or ask participants to close their eyes during the activities.
- Engage vision by asking participants to read aloud or reach for or catch objects while performing an activity.
- Distract vision by having participants perform activities in front of a busy visual pattern or while an object with such a pattern (i.e., checkerboard) is being moved through their visual field.

Level 1: Seated Balance Activities

Exercise Progressions

a. Participants are seated on a chair with no backrest, with the arms in one of four positions—holding onto a support surface, resting on the thighs, folded across the chest, or extended out at sides—and the feet are hip-width apart and in contact with a firm surface. Have them maintain balance with vision reduced (i.e., dark glasses) or absent for 30 seconds (figure 5.1). Focus the participants' attention on pressure experienced below the buttocks and feet.

b. With vision reduced or the eyes closed, have participants lean the trunk in the forward, backward, lateral, and diagonal directions as directed by the instructor. Focus their attention on feeling the pressure as it shifts under the buttocks and from one region of the foot to another. Progressively increase the angle of trunk lean so that the pressure under the buttocks and feet progresses from light to moderate to heavy.

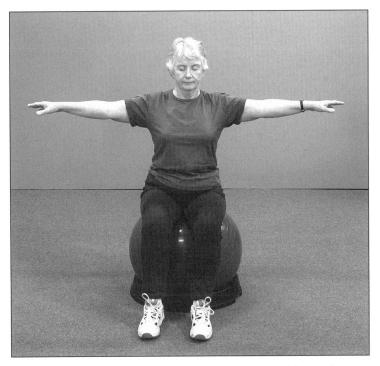

Figure 5.1 Performing activities with the eyes closed forces the participant to rely on somatosensory inputs for balance.

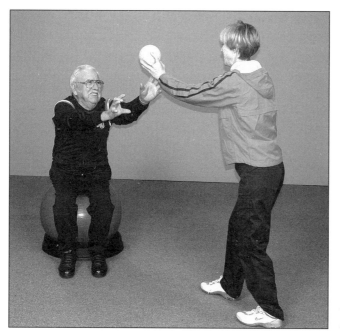

Figure 5.2 Engaging vision forces the participant to rely on somatosensory inputs for controlling balance.

c. Have participants reach for objects (i.e., of different sizes, weights, shapes) placed at various distances and heights relative to the body (figure 5.2). Encourage trunk movement in a variety of directions. Progress to throwing objects to participants, varying the throwing heights and weights of the objects according to the participants' individual capabilities.

d. Practice shifting weight in the forward, backward, lateral, and diagonal directions with vision reduced (i.e., wear dark glasses) or the eyes closed.

e. While participants are seated on a firm support surface with feet hip-width apart, move an object with a busy surface pattern (e.g., a checkerboard) quickly through their visual field (figure 5.3). Participants are to remain seated in a stable, upright position, keeping their head stationary, and try to ignore the object moving through their field of view. This activity is intended to distract vision and make it impossible to focus on a stationary target in space.

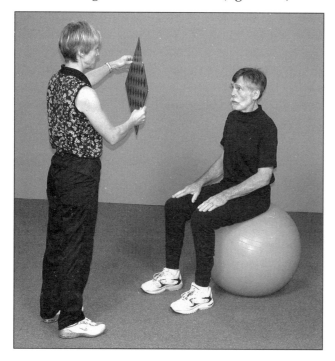

Figure 5.3 The participant must rely on somatosensory inputs to control balance when vision is distracted by moving an object with a busy surface pattern through the visual field.

f. Practice each of the seated exercise progressions described in (a) through (e) with the feet in an altered base of support (e.g., Romberg, semitandem, sharpened Romberg, one-legged stance) with vision reduced, absent, engaged in the performance of a second task, or distracted by a busy visual pattern. Altering and or reducing the base of support in any of these ways will further challenge the somatosensory system by reducing the amount of information now available from this system.

Many of the seated center-of-gravity training activities described in chapter 4 can be reintroduced during this component of the program. You only need to remember that vision must be manipulated so that the client is forced to rely on the somatosensory system for balance-related information and the feet must always be in contact with a firm, broad surface so that surface information is maximized. You can also increase the level of balance challenge associated with a set of exercise progressions by manipulating several different task demands (see table 5.1 on page 152). You have already learned how the environmental demands must be manipulated in this section.

An easy way to increase the balance challenge in this section is to move the client to a more difficult seated support surface. Although performing exercises while seated on a Dyna-Disc™ or balance ball reduces the amount and quality of the somatosensory information received at the level of the buttocks, the goal of the exercise will not be compromised as long as the participant's feet are in contact with a firm, broad surface.

Level 2: Standing Balance Exercises

Exercise Progressions

a. Repeat all the exercise progressions performed satisfactorily in level 1, except the trunk lean exercise progressions in (c), while standing.

b. Introduce any of the weight shift/transfer activities described in chapter 4 on a firm, broad surface while manipulating the amount of vision available. Appropriate exercise progressions include those described in levels 3, 4, and 5 of the standing COG balance training section in chapter 4.

Level 3: Moving Exercises

Exercise Progressions

■ 1. WALKING ACROSS THE ROOM

a. Walk across the room on a firm surface while reading a poem or story out loud (figure 5.4).

b. Walk across the room on a firm surface while reaching for objects passed by a partner.

c. Walk across the room on a firm surface while throwing and catching an object to oneself or a partner.

d. Walk across the room on a firm surface while wearing dark glasses or with the eyes closed.

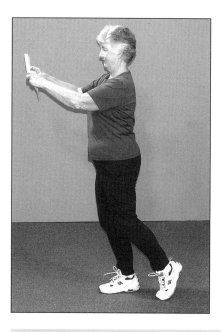

Figure 5.4 Walking while reading aloud.

Do not progress participants to a higher-level exercise progression until they are able to perform the lower-level progression satisfactorily.

Important Safety Tip

Be sure to position participants close to a wall when walking with eyes closed. Allow more fearful participants to open their eyes or lightly contact the wall with a finger periodically to enhance somatosensory input. To reduce fear during early repetitions, you can also walk beside participants and verbally indicate their progress.

As with the seated and standing exercise progressions, you can increase the balance challenge during the moving activities by manipulating the demands of the task (see table 5.1). Good ways to increase the balance challenge during the performance of moving activities are (a) introduce an external timing component (hand clap or metronome to pace the exercise) or (b) alter the arm position (i.e., folded across chest).

In summary, the most important things to remember when selecting any exercise intended to make the somatosensory system the primary source of sensory information for maintaining balance, whether in a seated, standing, or moving environment, is to ensure that (a) the surface beneath the feet is always firm and broad *and* (b) vision is compromised in some way.

Forcing the Use of the Visual System to Control Balance

In the previous set of exercises, when you were trying to create a practice environment that would force your clients to rely more on the somatosensory system for controlling balance, you learned that it was important to provide a firm, broad surface for all activities and compromise vision in some way. Well, the goal in this section is just the reverse. To teach participants how to use their visual system more effectively to maintain balance, you must now alter the type of surface on which they are standing to make it more difficult to use surface information. Three easy ways to force participants to use vision for maintaining balance are as follows:

- Perform exercises on a compliant surface (i.e., foam) with the eyes open and focused on a forward visual target that is at eye level. Many of the exercise progressions described in the center-of-gravity control training chapter are appropriate to include here.

- Perform exercises on an unstable or moving surface (i.e., rocker boards, treadmill) with the eyes open and focused on a forward visual target that is at eye level. Maintaining a balanced posture or weight shifting in different directions are examples of appropriate activities.
- Reduce the base of support (i.e., Romberg, one-legged stance).
- Review the health/activity questionnaires completed by Jane and Bill and the results of condition 3 of the M-CTSIB to determine whether either participant has any diseases of the eye that would make it difficult to use vision to maintain balance and how well they use vision, in the absence of any visual impairment, for maintaining upright balance. A review of their test results for this condition will help you determine whether these exercises are appropriate for them and, if they are, the appropriate starting level.

Level 1: Seated Exercises

Exercise Progressions

a. Participants are seated on a compliant surface (i.e., Dyna-Disc or balance ball) with their feet on a foam pad or rocker board. The goal is to maintain upright balance while focusing on a visual target placed immediately in front of them and at eye level (figure 5.5).

b. Repeat the previous exercise with the feet in a reduced or altered BOS position (i.e., Romberg, semitandem, sharpened Romberg, one-legged stance).

c. Participants perform a variety of arm, trunk, or leg movements (see levels 2, 3, and 4 in the seated balance section of chapter 4). Vision remains fixed on a forward visual target at eye level.

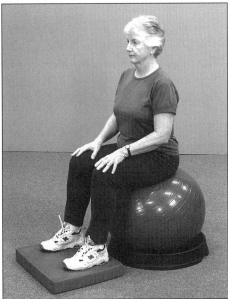

Figure 5.5 Altering the support surface beneath the feet and encouraging participants to focus on a visual target will improve their use of vision to control balance.

Level 2: Standing Exercises

Exercise Progressions

a. Repeat all exercise progressions performed satisfactorily in a seated position while standing on a compliant or moving surface.

b. Introduce selected weight shift and transfer activities while participants stand on a compliant or moving surface and focus on a visual target placed directly

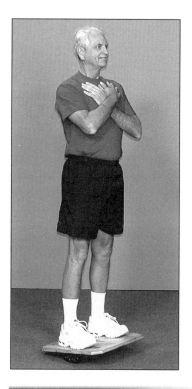

in front of them and at eye level (figure 5.6) (refer to the exercises in levels 3, 4, and 5 of the standing balance section in chapter 4).

c. Repeat weight shift and transfer activities while participant adopts a reduced base of support.

Figure 5.6 Standing on a rocker board while focusing on a visual target.

Level 3: Moving Exercises

Exercise Progressions

a. Participants walk across a compliant surface (i.e., eggcrate foam) while focusing on a visual target immediately in front of them.

b. Participants walk across a compliant surface with an altered base of support (e.g., toes only, heels only, tandem) (figure 5.7). Encourage participants to focus on a target directly in front of them as they move across the room.

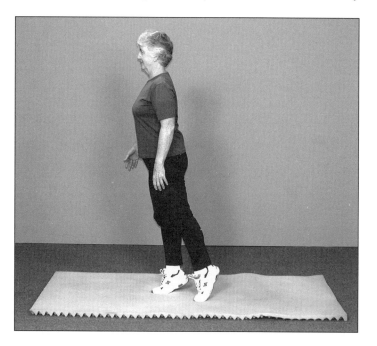

Figure 5.7 Walking across eggcrate foam on toes while focusing on a visual target.

Forcing the Use of the Vestibular System to Control Balance

To encourage participants to use the vestibular system as the primary system for maintaining balance, it will be necessary to compromise the use of both the visual *and* somatosensory systems for balance. This can be accomplished by varying the task demands or environmental constraints in one of two ways:

- Perform exercises on an unstable or compliant surface with reduced or absent vision.

- Perform exercises on an unstable or compliant surface while vision is engaged in the performance of a second task (e.g., reading, tracking objects with the eyes only). The support surface must be compliant or moving to make it more difficult to use somatosensory information for balance. Although somatosensory information is still available, it is now distorted and therefore not as useful to the client for controlling balance.

Before proceeding, take a moment to briefly review the health/activity questionnaires completed by Jane and Bill, our two case studies, to determine whether any permanent impairments have been identified in the vestibular system that would contraindicate presenting activities designed to force the use of the vestibular system. Once you have done that, review their respective test results on condition 4 of the M-CTSIB to see if they experienced any difficulties maintaining balance in a sensory environment that requires using the vestibular system more to maintain upright balance.

Level 1: Seated Exercises

Exercise Progressions

a. Maintain an upright, stable posture while seated on a compliant surface (e.g., Dyna-Disc on chair, balance ball) with the feet also placed on a compliant or moving surface. Close the eyes and maintain balance for 30 seconds. (The exercise can be made less difficult by lowering the room lights or asking the more unsteady participants to wear dark glasses).

b. Repeat the exercise with the feet in a reduced base of support (e.g., feet together, tandem, one-legged stance).

c. Maintain seated balance while performing voluntary arm or leg movements. Vision is removed or compromised and the feet are in contact with a compliant or moving surface during this exercise progression also.

d. While seated on a compliant surface with an altered surface beneath the feet (e.g., foam pad, Dyna-Disc, rocker board), toss an object from one hand to the other while visually tracking its movement (figure 5.8). Gradually increase the height of the toss between the hands until the head begins to move.

e. While seated on a compliant surface with an altered surface beneath the feet (e.g., foam pad, Dyna-Disc, rocker board), reach for objects placed at different heights and distances from the body. Use multicolored objects, if available.

f. While seated on a compliant surface with an altered surface beneath the feet (e.g., foam pad, Dyna-Disc, rocker board), use only the eyes to follow

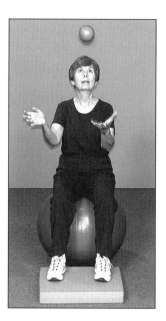

Figure 5.8 The vestibular system becomes an important source of balance information when the eyes are engaged in performing a secondary task and the support surface beneath the feet is altered.

the movement of a checkerboard (held by an assistant) through the visual field. The checkerboard should be moved in vertical, horizontal, and diagonal directions.

Level 2: Standing Exercises

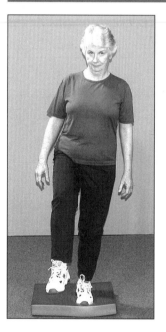

Exercise Progressions

a. Repeat each of the seated exercise progressions in a standing position.

b. While standing on a compliant surface (e.g., foam balance pad), begin marching in place with vision reduced or absent. Practice marching for no more than 5 to 10 steps with the eyes closed, followed by 5 to 10 steps with the eyes open, until good stability is observed (figure 5.9).

Figure 5.9 The vestibular system provides important information for balance when the surface beneath the feet is altered.

Important Safety Tips

- Position the foam pad on a surface that will prevent it from sliding during the marching activities (i.e., on a nonslip or carpeted surface).
- Because postural instability increases when this activity is performed with the eyes closed, it is important that you position clients close to a wall with a chair directly in front of them that they can touch lightly when performing the eyes-closed portion of the activity.
- To increase safety, ensure that there is adequate space between clients during this activity.
- Instruct participants to lightly hold on to the chair in front of them during the early eyes-closed repetitions of this exercise. This will give you an opportunity to observe the level

of postural stability of individual clients when support is provided and decide whether certain clients are ready to perform the marching activity without holding on to the chair or should continue lightly holding on to the chair in subsequent repetitions.

- Check to see that clients are not experiencing high levels of dizziness during this activity. If dizziness is a problem, instruct participants to reduce the height of the marching step, close their eyes for a shorter time, or hold on to the chair until they are able to perform the activity without experiencing dizziness. If none of these strategies work, ask the participant to stop performing the activity with the eyes closed.

Level 3: Moving Exercises

Before you introduce these higher-level activities to your clients, you must determine how to organize the practice environment to ensure the safety of the group. When working with a group on moving activities, particularly when vision is being manipulated, one of two strategies will maximize the safety of the group:

- Set up the compliant surfaces along a wall in your facility and have participants perform the activities sequentially as you verbally cue them to lightly touch the wall if they become unstable. You should also follow the more unstable clients in a close supervisory position.

- A second strategy that is often effective is to divide the group and position half of the participants at one end of the room and the other half at the other end, with the groups facing each other. Then have a row of participants (two to three) begin by performing the moving activity until they reach the opposite end of the room and take a position as the last row of the group on that end. The first row of that group then begins the exercise in the opposite direction. You can follow behind each row of performers to monitor their safety. Make sure that you distribute your more unstable participants in different rows to make supervising them easier.

Exercise Progressions

a. Walk across a compliant surface (i.e., eggcrate foam, floor mats) with vision reduced or absent (figure 5.10).

b. Walk forward across a compliant surface with vision reduced or absent using an altered base of support (e.g., toes, heels, tandem).

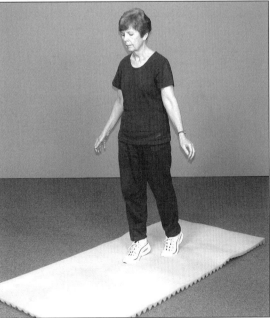

Figure 5.10 Walking across foam with eyes closed is a challenging vestibular activity for some older adults.

Table 5.1 Multisensory Training at a Glance

Core program components	Additional task demands	Environmental manipulations
Stimulate use of somatosensory system: Reduce, remove, or engage vision while performing exercise progressions. Have feet in contact with a firm, broad surface.		

Seated on firm surface
  Trunk leans in different directions
  Reaching for objects
  Catching and throwing objects
  Resisting perturbations
	Altered base of support (e.g., Romberg, semitandem, tandem)
	Altered hand position (e.g., hands on object, thighs, across chest)
	Add external timing demand
	Add second task to engage vision
		Reduce or remove vision
		Add compliant surface under buttocks (e.g., Dyna-Disc, gym ball)

Standing on firm surface
  Dynamic weight shifts
  Marching in place
	Altered base of support
	Altered hand position (folded across chest)
	Add head movements (e.g., lateral, up-down)
	Add a second task to engage vision (e.g., ball toss, target search)
		Reduce or remove vision

Moving on firm surface Altered gait patterns	Altered base of support Add external timing demand	Reduce or remove vision
Stimulate use of visual system: Perform exercise progressions on compliant or moving surfaces.		
Seated on compliant surface with altered surface beneath feet	Altered base of support (e.g., Romberg, tandem, one leg)	Alter type of support surface beneath feet (e.g., foam to Dyna-Disc)
Standing on altered surface	Altered base of support March in place	Alter type of support surface (e.g., Dyna-Disc to rocker board)
Walking across compliant surface	Altered base of support (e.g., toes, heels) Vary gait pattern (e.g., backward, long steps)	Alter type and/or thickness of support surface
Stimulate use of vestibular stystem: Reduce, remove, engage, or distract vision. Have feet in contact with compliant, moving support surface while performing exercise progressions.		
Seated on compliant surface with reduced vision and altered surface beneath feet	Add secondary task to engage vision Reduce base of support	Remove vision Alter type and/or thickness of support surface
Standing on altered surface with reduced vision	Add secondary task to engage vision March in place	Remove vision Alter type of support surface (e.g., Dyna-Disc to rocker board)
Walking on altered surface with reduced vision	Add secondary task to engage vision Reduce base of support Vary gait pattern	Remove vision Alter type of support surface (i.e., increase thickness of compliant surface)

Culminating Activities

When you have practiced each of the individual exercise progressions associated with forcing the use of the somatosensory, visual, or vestibular systems, you can introduce culminating activities so that the participants can practice what they have learned in a fun, gamelike atmosphere. Several of the culminating activities described in the previous chapter can be introduced again in this component of the program. For example, games such as "Pass the potato, please," "Hot potato!" and balloon volleyball can be used to force the use of the somatosensory system, if played while clients are standing on a firm surface, or the vestibular system, if played while clients are standing on a compliant surface. In both variations of the game, vision is the system being manipulated because the client must track the moving object during the game. "Shift around the clock" is a good culminating activity for reinforcing what the clients have learned earlier in the visual training section as long as their feet are in contact with a compliant or moving surface so that the somotosensory system is compromised. Although you may have involved clients in these games in earlier classes to reinforce various aspects of center-of-gravity control, reintroducing them here will reinforce the many skills that have been learned during the multisensory training component. The game remains the same; only the reason for playing it has changed.

Eye-Head Coordination Exercises

The exercises presented in this section are designed to improve a participant's ability to (a) move the eyes smoothly through space while focusing on a moving target, (b) move the head and eyes smoothly through space while focusing on a moving target, and (c) quickly move the head and eyes from one target to another without losing visual focus. These are excellent exercises to incorporate into the cool-down section of the class or as a station activity. As you read through the exercise progressions that require participants to perform the exercises in seated, standing, and finally moving situations, be thinking of the two case studies, Jane and Bill, and the results of their M-CTSIB tests, as well as some of the individual test items from the FAB Scale that tested their ability to use the various sensory systems for balance. Based on those results, identify any exercises in this section that are likely to be more difficult for either Jane or Bill and how you might modify the difficulty of the balance activity to ensure their safety and success.

Level 1: Eye Movements With Stationary Head While Seated

Exercise Progressions

■ 1. SMOOTH PURSUIT (SLOW) EYE MOVEMENTS

The eyes move slowly through space while the head remains stationary. Hold a single target directly in front of the eyes and at arm's length from the face. Visually follow the target with the eyes as it is slowly moved (a) from side to side, (b) up and down, or (c) diagonally while keeping the head still (figure 5.11). Perform the exercise in a seated position and continue for 30 seconds before resting.

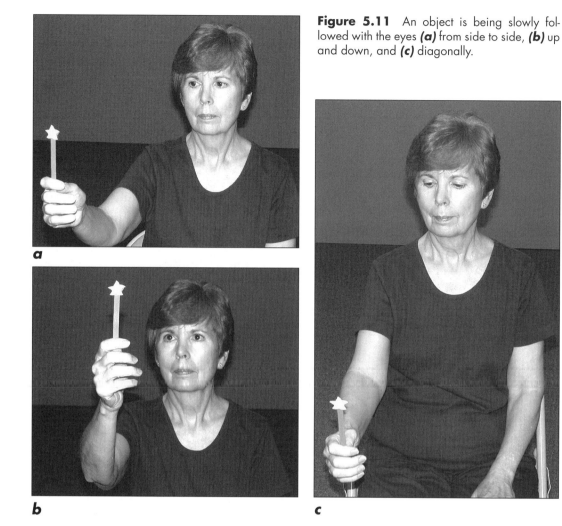

Figure 5.11 An object is being slowly followed with the eyes *(a)* from side to side, *(b)* up and down, and *(c)* diagonally.

■ 2. SACCADIC (QUICK) EYE MOVEMENTS

    a.   Hold or focus on two targets held in front of the face (at eye level) and approximately 4 to 6 inches apart. Move the eyes *quickly* from target to target while the head remains still (figure 5.12).

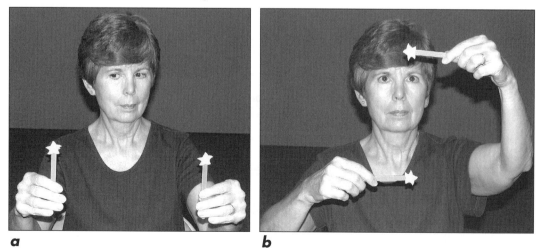

Figure 5.12 Activities requiring quick eye movements in different directions such as *(a)* side to side and *(b)* up and down are an important part of the multisensory training component.

b. Repeat the previous exercise with targets positioned vertically and 4 to 6 inches apart. The eyes now move up and down between the targets.

c. Repeat the exercise with targets positioned diagonally and 4 to 6 inches apart. The eyes now move diagonally.

d. Participants quickly move their eyes from one visual target to another visual target (e.g., numbers, letters) placed on a blank wall directly in front of them. You may verbally cue them as to which target to move to or allow them to do it at their own pace.

e. Seat participants directly in front of a busy background (e.g., checkerboard pattern, floral pattern) with targets placed at different points on the background. Instruct participants to move their eyes from one target to the next on your command. Place targets at positions of the clock face (e.g., 12 o'clock, 3 o'clock, 8 o'clock) and then call out random positions. You can also ask participants to spell out words by finding letters against the busy background.

Once participants have adequately practiced each of these exercise progressions in a seated position, you can repeat the same set of progressions in a standing position. This will add a balance component to the activities. You can further increase the level of balance challenge by altering certain task or environmental demands associated with each progression. For example, you can have your class participants repeat each of the eye movement exercises introduced in level 1 while standing in different altered BOS positions or on an altered surface. Because each of the eye exercises in level 1 engages vision in the performance of a task, standing balance must be controlled at a more subconscious level and the participant must now rely on the other sensory systems (somatosensory and vestibular) to control upright balance.

Level 2: Combination Head and Eye Movements in a Seated Position

The exercises presented in this level are designed to improve the ability to visually focus on targets when the head is also moving in space. Good gaze-stabilization skills are needed when shopping for groceries or walking in busy malls. We are constantly moving our head and eyes in different directions as we scan the shelves for various food items or look at window displays as we move through a shopping mall. The fact that we are usually walking and perhaps dodging people as we perform these different head and eye movements adds to the difficulty of the task. The exercise progressions presented in this section are intended to simulate these types of sensory environments.

Although these exercises are primarily designed to teach participants how to coordinate the movements of the head and eyes when performing tasks in a variety of situations, you should be aware that many of the activities requiring head turns will also activate the vestibular system. For participants who have a diagnosed vestibular impairment or performed poorly on condition 4 of the M-CTSIB during the preprogram assessment, many of the standing and walking activities, in particular, will be difficult if not impossible to perform. You will need to identify those participants who are likely to experience difficulty and make the necessary adjustments to the exercise progressions. Remember that the faster the head turns, the more the vestibular system is activated. Reducing the speed or number of head turns will reduce the difficulty of the task. It will also be important to reinforce the need for participants to focus their eyes on a target during the various head-turn activities to minimize instability.

Do not allow participants who are experiencing instability during the seated exercises to progress to the standing or moving activities until they are ready.

If any participants report that they are feeling dizzy while performing an activity or shortly afterward, ask them how dizzy they are feeling using the 0 to 10 dizziness scale described in chapter 2. Do not ask any client to repeat the exercise until the dizziness has subsided, and if the dizziness increases on the next repetition, have them stop performing the activity altogether. If participants experience repeated bouts of dizziness during any class, encourage them to pay a visit to their primary care physician to discuss the matter. Many older adults experience repeated bouts of dizziness that are often dismissed as an inevitable part of the aging process when they are actually the result of an underlying vestibular impairment or, in some cases, a cardiovascular problem. Certain medications can also cause dizziness, so be sure to check the participant's medication list.

Exercise Progressions

a. Participants slowly move the head in a lateral or vertical direction while focusing the eyes on a stationary visual target held directly in front of them and at eye level in space. Gradually increase the speed of the head turns while maintaining a clear visual focus on the target. Instruct participants to stop increasing the head speed once the visual target becomes blurred.

b. With the participant in a seated position with eyes fixed on a visual target, begin moving another visual target (e.g., checkerboard) through the field of vision (see figure 5.3). Both the head and eyes follow the moving target up and down, side to side, and diagonally for 60 seconds before resting.

c. Move the eyes between two horizontal targets that are held at arm's length and at eye level. The targets should be placed close enough together that when one target is being focused on, the other can be seen in the periphery. Align the head and eyes with one of the targets, move the eyes to focus on the second target, and then move the head to that target (figure 5.13). Repeat in the opposite direction. Vary the speed of the head movement while maintaining a clear focus on the target at all times. Perform at least 10 to 20 head and eye excursions before resting.

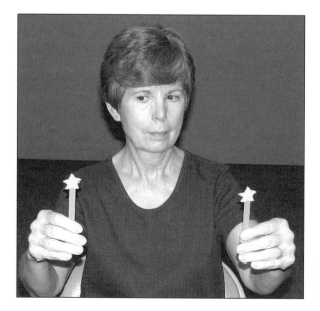

Figure 5.13 The goal of this activity is to move the eyes to a new visual target before the head is lowered to the target.

This is a difficult head-eye coordination pattern for many older adults, so start slowly. You may have to cue the movements verbally early in the repetitions until your clients learn to coordinate the head and eye movements.

d. Repeat the previous exercise but with the two targets positioned vertically. One target should be at approximately the height of the forehead and the other at chin height.

e. Move the eyes quickly between targets set against busy backgrounds (i.e., numbers or letters affixed to a busy background that fills the visual field). The task can be made more challenging by having participants search for numbers in sequential order or create a word by searching the letters sequentially. The word is announced once completed.

After your clients have adequately practiced each of the exercise progressions in this level, you can repeat the progressions with the clients in a standing position. You can also increase the level of balance challenge by altering the BOS position or the support surface beneath the feet once your clients are able to do the exercises well.

Level 3: Head and Eye Movements While Weight Shifting in a Standing Position

Exercise Progressions

a. Lateral weight shifting with head turns. Begin with head turns in the same direction as the weight shift. Progress to head movements in a direction opposite to the weight shift.

b. Repeat the activity with weight shifts in the forward-backward and diagonal forward-backward directions combined with head movements that are up and down (weight shift forward, head tilted up, weight shift backward, head tilted down, or reverse the directions for each).

Level 4: Head and Eye Movements While Walking

Progress each of the walking exercises described in this level by starting with a higher number of steps per head turn. Some participants will experience more difficulty with certain directional head movements than with others. If you observe large gait deviations during any of these exercises, increase the number of steps before the head turns until little or no deviation in gait is observed. Reduce the number of steps as dynamic balance improves. Encourage rapid eye fixation with each head turn.

Exercise Progressions

■ 1. WALKING WITH HEAD TURNS TO RIGHT, CENTER, AND LEFT POSITIONS

a. Begin walking on a firm surface with the head and eyes directed forward. After a set number of steps (one to four), turn the head to the right for the same number of steps and then return the head to center with the eyes directed forward (figure 5.14). Repeat the walking activity, but this time direct the head to the left and then back to center.

b. Repeat the previous exercise, but this time have participants turn the head to the right for a certain number of steps (one to four) and then to the left for the

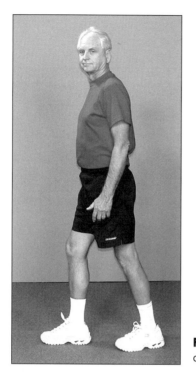

same number of steps. During this exercise, the head does not stop in the center position at any time.

c. Repeat the previous exercise, but this time have participants call out the number or word that is posted at regular intervals along the wall on either side. Their ability to read off the numbers or words successfully tells you whether they are stabilizing their gaze with each head turn.

d. Have participants walk across the room while turning to catch and then throw a ball on command. Alter the walking pattern to increase the challenge of the activity (e.g., toes, heels, tandem).

Figure 5.14 Walking while turning the head requires good adaptive postural control.

■ 2. WALKING WITH VERTICAL HEAD MOVEMENTS

a. Repeat exercise 1, but this time tilt the head up to the ceiling and back to a centered position with the eyes directed forward for a set number of steps. Repeat with the head and eyes moving down to the floor and then back to a vertically centered position for the same number of steps.

b. Repeat exercise 2 with the head and eyes moving up to the ceiling and then down to the floor for a set number of steps. The head does not stop in a centered position on this exercise.

■ 3. WALKING WITH DIAGONAL HEAD MOVEMENTS

Repeat exercises 1 and 2, but this time the eyes and head move diagonally up to the right and down to the left, then up to the left and down to the right.

Although many of the exercise progressions described in level 4 are sufficiently challenging in and of themselves, you can increase the level of balance challenge for your more accomplished class participants. These exercises, especially when performed on altered support surfaces, at faster speeds, and with an altered base of support, are challenging even for very healthy older adults who have no apparent balance problems.

Culminating Activity

"Walk the Gauntlet"

This activity is an excellent way to introduce sensory conflict into the practice situation and reinforce several of the exercise progressions introduced during the first section of this chapter, as well as the eye-head coordination section. The participants are confronted with a complex and moving visual scene as they try to move quickly but safely in a forward direction. Prior to starting this culminating activity, have your class participants form two lines approximately 6 to 8 feet apart. Participants then

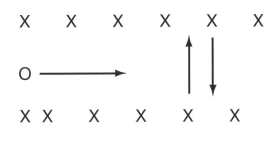

Figure 5.15 "Walking the gauntlet" formation.

turn to face the person directly opposite them in a staggered fashion (see figure 5.15). One participant is positioned at the end between the two lines.

On the instruction to "Go," the participant at the end begins walking quickly and safely down the middle as each person on the two outer lines attempts to cross to the other side before the participant reaches them (figure 5.16). If the participants on the two outer lines time their movements appropriately, it will force the participant walking the gauntlet to change speed or direction repeatedly to avoid body contact. This activity attempts to simulate the type of sensory conflict that arises when walking through a crowded shopping mall or along a busy sidewalk.

When playing this game, you need to establish the "no touching" rule. Be sure to emphasize the need for body control at all times during this activity. It is also a good idea to follow closely behind the more unstable participants as they walk the gauntlet so you can provide a manual assist if they are inadvertently bumped or simply become disoriented while moving through the complex and moving visual scene. This is perhaps the most often requested culminating activity during a class and one that promotes good cooperation and socialization among class members.

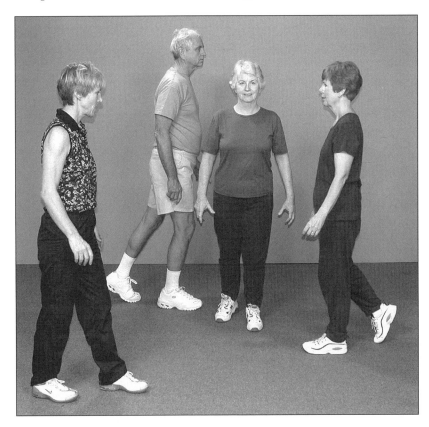

Figure 5.16
"Walking the Guantlet" simulates the type of sensory conflict encountered in crowded malls and on busy sidewalks.

Summary

The exercise progressions in this component of the program are intended to improve the older adult's ability to select the appropriate source(s) of sensory information to control balance in a given situation, as well as to organize the sensory inputs derived from each sensory system so that the motor response generated is appropriate. Several of these exercise progressions are also intended to help the older adult select the most appropriate sensory inputs when the information provided by certain sensory systems is inaccurate. In these sensory conflict situations, the older adult must be able to ignore the inaccurate sensory inputs (usually provided by vision) in preference to other sensory systems that are providing more accurate sensory information (i.e., somatosensory and/or vestibular systems).

Once you have carefully reviewed each client's health/activity questionnaire and the results of the M-CTSIB, which is the only test included in the initial evaluation that specifically assesses whether the use of sensory information is normal or abnormal in different sensory conditions, you can determine whether you should choose exercises that focus on forcing the use of a sensory system that is only temporarily impaired or exercises that improve function in the intact sensory systems to compensate for a permanent impairment of a sensory system. A review of the test items on the FAB Scale that also emphasized the use or activation of sensory inputs for balance (e.g., walking with head turns, standing on foam with eyes closed, turning 360° in a circle) will also help you make wise decisions about setting the initial level of difficulty associated with a balance exercise.

Finally, keep in mind that even if your older adult participants perform well on the M-CTSIB and selected FAB Scale items, they will still benefit from practicing the multisensory activities presented in this chapter. That is because the aging process itself leads to an overall decline in the quality of information provided by each of the three sensory systems. This is particularly true for the vestibular system, which is not subjected to the same level of activation as when the older adult was much younger. The reason for this is that the older adult tends to stop engaging in the types of high-velocity head movements they enjoyed as a young person (e.g., twirling in circles, jumping, hopping, skipping, certain sporting activities such as skiing, roller skating, or surfing). Given the plasticity of the sensory systems that has been demonstrated in a number of research studies, all older adults will benefit from regularly engaging in activities designed to "tune up" the sensory systems.

TEST YOUR UNDERSTANDING

1. The primary purpose of multisensory training is to improve
   a. the ability to maintain a better upright position in space
   b. use of the ankle, hip, and step strategies to maintain balance
   c. gait pattern and stability in gait
   d. the use of visual, somatosensory, and vestibular information for maintenance of upright posture
   e. the use of both motor and sensory systems for maintenance of balance

2. The major goals of multisensory training include all of the following except
   a. identifying permanent sensory loss and compensating for it

    b. identifying temporary sensory loss and stimulating its use

    c. stimulating sensory systems in an intentional, systematic way

    d. manipulating the environment to encourage the use of the targeted system

    e. altering task demands to facilitate improved motor coordination

3. The assessment tool that provides the most information about sensory organization and integration is the

    a. Berg Balance Scale

    b. Fullerton Advanced Balance Scale

    c. Modified Clinical Test of Sensory Interaction in Balance

    d. "walkie-talkie" test

    e. Senior Fitness Test

4. Which of the following is an example of an activity to stimulate the use of somatosensory cues?

    a. walking on grass while focusing on a target

    b. standing on a firm surface while tossing a ball

    c. standing on foam while tossing a ball

    d. standing on a rocker board with eyes closed

    e. walking on a firm surface while focusing on a target

5. When attempting to alter the information provided by the somatosensory system, a task can be made more difficult by manipulating the base of support. Which of the following is an appropriate progression from easiest to most difficult? Standing with eyes closed and

    a. feet shoulder-width apart, feet together, feet in split stance, feet in tandem stance

    b. feet together, feet in tandem stance, feet in split stance, feet shoulder-width apart

    c. feet shoulder-width apart, feet in tandem stance, feet in split stance, feet on foam

    d. feet shoulder-width apart, feet together, feet in tandem stance, feet in split stance

    e. feet shoulder-width apart, feet together, single-legged stance, feet on foam

6. Which of the following is an appropriate activity to stimulate the use of vision for upright balance?

    a. walking on a firm surface while turning the head

    b. walking on grass while turning the head

    c. standing on foam and looking at a target on the wall

    d. standing on foam and tossing a ball

    e. playing balloon volleyball while standing on foam

7. Which of the following tasks is the least effective for stimulating use of the vestibular system?

    a. walking on grass while turning the head

    b. standing on a firm surface while tossing a ball

    c. standing on foam while tossing a ball

    d. standing on a rocker board with eyes closed

    e. walking on a treadmill while reading

8. Which of the following would be an appropriate verbal cue for gaze stabilization during a task?

   a. "Direct your eyes forward and focus on a visual target."

   b. "Can you feel that your head is directly above your shoulders?"

   c. "Close your eyes and feel where your body is in space."

   d. "Try to turn your head and scan the environment with your eyes as you are walking."

   e. "Feel your feet in contact with the floor."

9. If a client loses balance immediately on condition 4 (eyes closed, foam surface) of the M-CTSIB, an inappropriate activity to start with would be

   a. walking on a firm surface while turning the head

   b. walking on grass while turning the head

   c. standing on foam and looking at a target on the wall

   d. standing on a firm surface and tossing a ball

   e. standing on a firm surface with the eyes closed

10. Which of the following activities would be the most appropriate if a client is unable to keep the eyes closed during condition 2 (eyes closed, stable surface) on the M-CTSIB?

   a. walking on eggcrate foam while turning the head

   b. standing on a firm surface while reading

   c. standing on a firm surface in tandem stance with the eyes closed

   d. standing on a rocker board while counting backward by threes

   e. marching in place while standing on foam

PRACTICAL PROBLEMS

1. Familiarize yourself with the activities presented in each section of this chapter so you can better understand how the use of each sensory system is forced during a particular activity. Actually practicing each of the activities with additional balance challenges will help you better appreciate how difficult many of these activities will be for your older adult clients.

2. Develop a set of multisensory activities for Bill or Jane that reflect the sensory systems you consider most in need of being exercised. Provide a rationale for the exercises you selected based on your review of their completed health/activity questionnaires, their results on each of the four conditions of the M-CTSIB, as well as selected items on the FAB Scale.

3. Develop a brief 10-minute presentation that you would deliver to a group of instructors who work with healthy older adults in physical activity settings to justify the need for including multisensory training activities into their activity classes for seniors. What precautions would you add during this presentation?

6

Postural Strategy Training

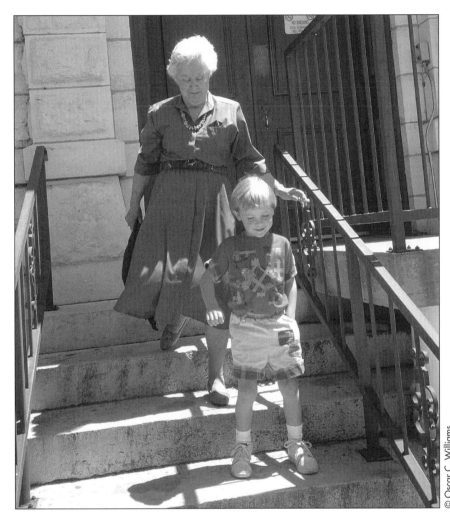

© Oscar C. Williams

Objectives

After completing this chapter, you will be able to

- understand how the task demands and environmental context influence the type of postural strategy used to maintain or restore balance,
- manipulate the challenge of a balance activity by altering the task demands or environmental constraints (or both),
- develop a set of exercise progressions designed to improve the voluntary and involuntary use of the ankle, hip, and step strategies, and
- manipulate the task or environmental demands (or both) to ensure a safe practice environment.

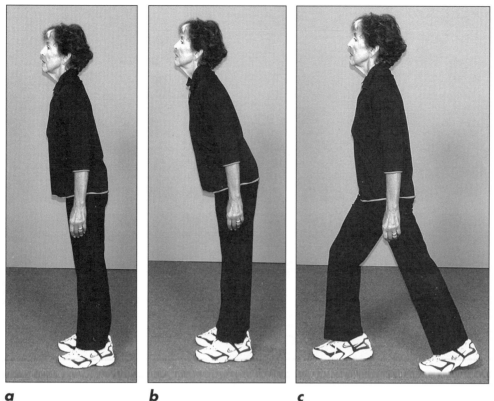

Figure 6.1 Three major postural control strategies have been identified: the **(a)** ankle, **(b)** hip, and **(c)** step strategies.

a   b   c

The progressive balance activities presented in this chapter are designed to improve each of the three postural control strategies (i.e., ankle, hip, and step) discussed at length in chapter 1. These postural control strategies (figure 6.1) are most commonly used to assist us in maintaining and controlling our balance while performing daily tasks in and around the home or while moving about the community. Not only will the demands associated with the task influence the type of postural strategy selected, but so too will the environment in which the task is being performed. Helping the older adult become more efficient in selecting and implementing the most appropriate postural strategy for the task demands and environmental situation is the primary reason for incorporating this set of exercise progressions into the program.

Each of the postural strategies required for maintaining and controlling balance can be practiced by manipulating the task or the environment (table 6.1) in at least three different ways: (a) setting the goal of maintaining balance while standing on different support surfaces, (b) instructing participants to voluntarily sway through an increasingly larger distance in multiple directions while standing on different support surfaces, and (c) instructing participants to minimize or control the amount of sway in response to progressively greater applications of external force.

Just manipulating the type of support surface on which the individual is standing can often trigger the use of a particular postural strategy. For example, when standing quietly on a firm, broad surface, we can control sway by using an ankle strategy. Performing the same task on a narrow or unstable surface, however, necessitates use of a hip strategy to maintain balance. This change in strategy is necessary because the surface against which we are pushing is now narrower than the length of our feet or the surface "gives" or moves as we push, making it more difficult to maintain balance using the smaller muscle groups of the ankle. In people who are experiencing balance and mobility problems, standing on these more difficult surfaces may often result in the immediate use of a stepping strategy rather than a hip strategy. The use

Table 6.1 Postural Strategy Training at a Glance

Core program components	Additional task demands	Environmental manipulations
Ankle strategy		
Standing position (involuntary)	Increase distance of anterior-posterior excursion	Reduced or absent vision
Standing position (involuntary)	Apply small perturbation at hips (push or pull)	
Hip strategy		
Standing position (voluntary)	Increase distance of anterior-posterior excursion Increase speed of sway (i.e., metronome, clap)	Alter support surface (i.e., narrow, compliant) by using a half-foam roller, foam pad, or rocker board
Standing position (involuntary)	Apply perturbation of moderate force at hips Introduce a second task (e.g., cognitive, manual)	
Step strategy		
Forward step (voluntary)	Increase forward lean beyond limits of stability Alter direction of step—backward, lateral	Alter support surface (i.e., foam)
Forward step (involuntary)	Transition from step off low bench to floor Require step up onto or over obstacle Increase lean angle prior to release	Alter support surface (i.e., foam)

of a stepping strategy may be prompted by a heightened sense of fear as the amount of sway increases or by the absence of a hip strategy.

Presenting balance activities that require progressively larger movements of the COG through space will also facilitate practicing of the ankle, hip, or step strategies. The ankle joints will generally be able to control sway only through a small sway envelope in a forward or backward direction. As the sway distance increases, however, the control moves up to the hip joints, as the larger and stronger hip muscles are required to prevent a loss of balance. Increasing the sway distance still farther results in the need to take one or more steps, thereby establishing a new base of support. The speed at which the individual sways will also determine which type of postural strategy is selected. Swaying at a slow speed will trigger one type of strategy (i.e., ankle), whereas swaying at a higher speed will, in most cases, spontaneously lead to the use of a hip strategy.

The external application of different amounts of force, particularly when unexpected, requires a more automatic postural adjustment and is therefore the most advanced set of progressions presented in this chapter. What one observes in a person with good balance is the selection of the postural strategy that best matches the amount of force applied. For example, a person usually responds to a small application of force (i.e., light push or pull) with rotation about the ankle joints. As the amount of force increases, the larger muscles in the hip region are recruited because the ankle joints can no longer generate enough torque to counter the destabilizing force adequately. Finally, a large application of force (i.e., strong push or pull) results in a stepping action to quickly re-establish a good, stable base of support. Activities also will be presented in this chapter that require participants to make subtle and not-so-subtle adjustments in body position in anticipation of a destabilizing limb movement.

The types of daily activities that require the use of postural strategies include stepping onto and off of curbs, climbing and descending stairs, avoiding obstacles, stepping onto and off of escalators or moving walkways, and recovering from an unexpected loss of balance. As you can see from these examples, learning how to select and efficiently execute the most appropriate postural strategy for the task or environmental context is a requirement for successful community ambulation. Knowing what to do in any situation, whether it be consciously or unconsciously, will also decrease an older adult's risk of falling.

Level 1: Voluntary Postural Strategies—Ankle, Hip, Step

The activities described in level 1 are intended to help the participant learn when to use a particular postural strategy. You will see that through simple manipulation of certain task variables such as distance and speed, different strategies will spontaneously emerge. For example, if you ask an individual to begin swaying in a forward and backward direction while you clap your hands slowly (i.e., one clap per second), you will generally see that the sway is controlled by the ankle joints. As you increase the speed of the clap (i.e., two to three claps per second), however, you will begin to see a spontaneous switch from ankle to hip control as the larger hip muscles become active. Involvement of the hip muscles is necessary because the speed of the sway now exceeds the capabilities of the ankle joints to generate enough force to control the sway. The movement of the body will also change from an in-phase (upper and lower body move in the same direction) to an out-of-phase (upper and lower body move in opposite directions) pattern. Finally, if you ask the individual to increase the distance of the sway while keeping time with the faster clapping speed, you will see the step strategy come into play as the stability limits are exceeded. What is interesting about this scenario is that you never had to tell the individual which strategy to use at any given time—it simply emerged as a function of how you manipulated the demands of the task.

General Safety Tips

- Instruct assistants to closely supervise participants when standing on narrow support surfaces. Where possible, set apparatus close to a wall or behind a sturdy chair to maximize participant safety.
- When using resistance bands during step strategy activities, be sure to wrap the band around the hips so that it is flat against the body and hold onto it firmly. Do not release your grip on the band after you release the tension to force the step.

Exercise Progressions

■ 1. ANKLE STRATEGY

a. Have the participant stand on the floor and sway between closely spaced objects (i.e., wall, chairs; see figure 6.2). Use a metronome or slow hand clap (i.e., one per second) to produce a slow pace. Look to see that the ankle muscles are controlling the amount of sway and that the upper and lower body move in the same direction (in-phase pattern). Move the objects closer together if you begin to see sway being controlled with the hip. Recognize, however, that participants with weak ankle muscles or other ankle and foot abnormalities, such as sensory peripheral neuropathy or severe rheumatoid arthritis in the toes, will find this activity difficult to perform.

b. Instruct the participant to practice the previous exercise with the eyes closed so that they can focus more on how the movement "feels."

c. Have the participant practice swaying in a forward and backward direction without external supports providing tactile cues.

d. Have the participant repeat the previous exercise with the eyes closed.

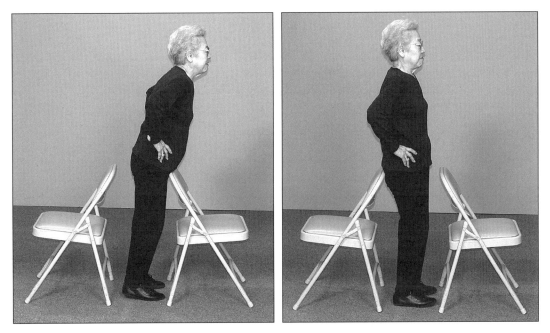

Figure 6.2 Practicing the ankle strategy between two chairs. The upper and lower body move in the same direction, or "in phase."

■ 2. HIP STRATEGY

a. Instruct the participant to sway forward and backward while increasing the distance and speed of the sway. As the distance and speed increase, the participant will spontaneously move into the use of a hip strategy to control the sway. Encourage the participant to feel the pressure increase under the toes as they lean forward and then increase under the heels as they lean backward. Also encourage them to be aware of the changing angle of the hips as they lean forward and backward.

b. Have the participant stand on a surface that is narrower than the length of the feet (i.e., sideways on a beam or half-foam roller)(figure 6.3). In some cases, you will notice that the more unstable participants immediately begin to control their sway using the larger hip muscles as opposed to the ankle muscles. To trigger the hip strategy in more stable participants, instruct them to begin

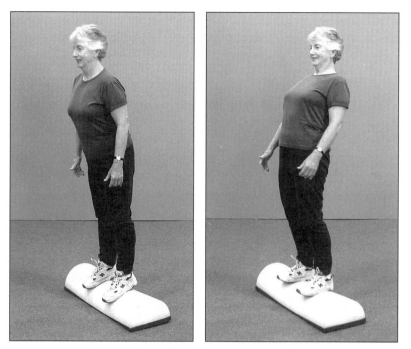

Figure 6.3 Practicing the hip strategy on a half-foam roller. The upper and lower body now move in opposite directions, or "out-of-phase."

swaying back and forth. The participant will step off the narrow surface if the hip strategy is either not currently part of their repertoire or is not well developed. Having the participant reach for objects held in front of their body at a distance that forces them to reach can also lead to spontaneous use of a hip strategy.

c. Repeat the previous exercise while the participant stands on a rocker board oriented in a forward and backward direction. This exercise can often be used to elicit a stepping strategy if participants exceed their maximum limits of stability.

■ 3. STEP STRATEGY

a. Instruct participants to lean forward until they think they have reached their stability limits and then take a step. Have them practice initiating the step first with the right leg and then with the left leg. Notice the angle of lean at which the individual chooses to initiate the step and the length of the step taken. To increase safety and reduce participant anxiety, position an assistant or a more stable participant in front of the participant performing the exercise. Encourage longer steps by placing a line on the floor at a progressively greater distance in front of the participant (distance should not exceed 40% of the participant's total height). Instruct the participant to look straight ahead as they step, not at the line they are attempting to cross. The assistant who is spotting during the exercise can monitor how successful the participant is in stepping beyond the line.

b. Repeat the voluntary step activity in a backward direction. Position yourself or an assistant behind and slightly to the side of the participant to increase safety. Observe whether the participant leans back through the hip (not from the head) before initiating the step. If you do not have an assistant available to help, move down the line, asking each participant in the group to initiate the backward step while you are in a position to spot each person adequately. The other participants in the group can be watching and providing feedback as to whether the step was initiated correctly. (The value of having participants engage in observational learning of this type is discussed further in chapter 10.)

c. Repeat the voluntary step activity in a lateral direction. Observe the type of step pattern selected (side step or crossover step). Observe whether the participant shifts weight through the hip before initiating the step. Practice this stepping activity in both lateral directions.

Important Reminder

Do not progress participants to level 2 activities until they are able to initiate a voluntary step confidently and efficiently in each direction. A sign that participants are ready to progress to level 2 activities is when they are consistently shifting weight through the hip on the backward and lateral step activities before step initiation. It may take several sessions before performance consistency in certain directions (e.g., backward) is evident, so participants may need to continue practicing certain level 1 activities in combination with level 2 activities.

Level 2: Involuntary Postural Strategy Training

The exercise progressions described in level 2 are considered advanced progressions and should not be introduced until your class participants are able to initiate a voluntary step consistently and effectively in each direction. You and your assistants also must practice the release maneuver with the resistance band many times before working with participants. The activities described in this level are best suited to individual as opposed to group practice and may not be appropriate for all participants (e.g., very unstable or fearful participants).

Although the activities described have been found to be extremely effective exercise progressions for retraining the step strategy, they should not be performed unless you and your assistants are competent in releasing the tension on the resistance band during the step activity. Remember that the safety of all participants is your number-one concern; so if you do not think you have the ability to perform this technique efficiently and safely, then skip all level 2 activities.

Instructions for Resistance Band Release Maneuver

- Wrap a 6- to 8-foot length of resistance band (medium to heavy resistance level) around the hips. Ensure that the full width of the band is flat against the body and both ends are of equal length once you grasp the band in your hands.

- When performing either the forward or backward resistance band release maneuver, position yourself to the side of the client, as shown in figure 6.4. Hold onto both ends of the band with your dominant hand and position the other arm (a) in a guarding position directly in front of the client and at chest level during the forward release or (b) in a guarding position directly behind the upper back during the backward release.

- Position yourself slightly behind and to the side of the client when performing the lateral step activities. Hold both ends of the resistance band firmly in your dominant hand and position the other hand in a guarding position behind the upper back on the side to which the client will execute the lateral step.

- Increase the tension on the band as the client begins to lean into it by slowly pulling it in a direction opposite to the one in which the client is leaning.

- When the client reaches the desired lean angle, quickly release the tension on the band by quickly reversing the direction in which you were originally pulling it so that the hand holding the band is now moving in the same direction as the client is leaning. *Note:* Do not release the band itself.

- As the step is initiated, move with the client so you can provide a manual assist if needed. The arm that is guarding the client should remain in the original position until the client has stopped moving.

- For your own safety, do *not* perform this release maneuver with any client whose height or weight would make it difficult for you to provide a manual assist.

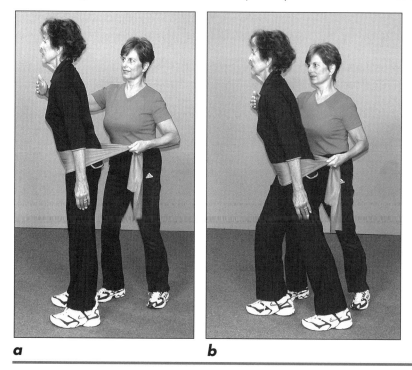

a　　　　　　　　　　　*b*

Figure 6.4 Correct release maneuver using resistance band on forward step, from the start position *(a)* to the end position *(b).*

Improvement in the use of each of these subconsciously invoked strategies is often not observed until a sufficient amount of strength and flexibility has been achieved. Therefore, you must include activities designed to increase lower body strength and flexibility during the class and as assigned homework between class sessions. Several upper and lower body strength activities are described in chapter 8.

Exercise Progressions

■ 1. MANUAL PERTURBATIONS OF INCREASING FORCE

a. Introduce manual perturbations of progressively greater forces. A small perturbation should cause the participant to make a countermovement using the ankle muscles, a medium perturbation should lead the participant to initiate a countermovement with the hip muscles, and a large perturbation should cause the participant to take a step to reestablish balance. In many cases, you will see the participant take a step even when the amount of force applied is small. This should be considered less problematic than a failure to make any response at all to the perturbation.

b. Stand behind the participant and introduce the perturbation at the hips. Pull the hips back quickly and watch for a countermovement in the forward direction. Alternatively, quickly push the hips forward and see whether the participant begins to move in a backward direction to counter the pushing action.

■ 2. FORWARD STEP STRATEGY FROM A LEANING POSITION

a. The forward step strategy can be practiced with different tensions of resistance band or sport cord attached to a waist belt. The participant stands on a 2- to 4-inch-high bench and leans forward against the length of resistance band or sport cord. The head and eyes are directed forward (see figure 6.5a). Release the tension on the band unexpectedly using the release maneuver described earlier in this section. Release the tension on the band when the participant reaches different lean angles so that you can observe how early in the lean the individual initiates a step. Step forward with the participant to further decrease the tension on the band and control the participant's amount of sway after the step (figure 6.5b). Look to see that the participant takes a step that is appropriate for their height and that they step with each foot on different attempts.

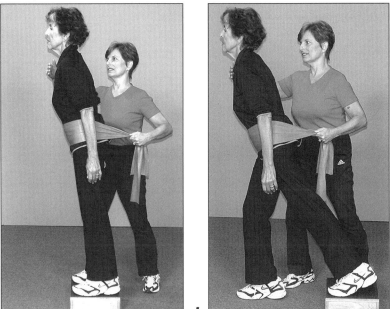

Figure 6.5 Forward step strategy. Start position **(a)** and end position **(b).**   *a*   *b*

b. Once the participant is able to step down from the bench consistently, repeat the exercise with the person standing on the floor. Ask the participant to lean forward against a resistance band that is wrapped around the hips. Once again, release the tension on the band unexpectedly using the correct resistance band release maneuver. Step forward with the participant to further decrease the tension on the band and control the participant's amount of sway following the step.

c. Once the participant is able to step forward safely on a level surface with consistency, repeat the exercise with the participant standing on a foam surface (2 to 4 inches thick). Initiating a step on a foam surface emphasizes the need for more dorsiflexion at the ankle joint and greater knee and hip flexion during the swing phase of the step.

d. Step strategy while walking: The participant attempts to walk against the resistance of the band wrapped around the hips. The instructor releases the tension on the band unexpectedly during the walking exercise.

> ### Making the Initiation of the Step Strategy Easier
>
> Using a 2- to 4-inch-high bench in the early repetitions of this progression makes it easier for participants to step safely because the height of the swing phase during the step is minimized as a result of them stepping down as opposed to forward on a firm surface. Before presenting this activity, ensure that the bench does not slide on the floor surface.

■ 3. BACKWARD STEP STRATEGY FROM A LEANING POSITION

Repeat the stepping exercise on a firm, level surface only. The instructor or assistant stands in front of the participant while holding onto a length of resistance band or sport cord wrapped low around the hips (see figure 6.6a). Encourage participants to lean backward through the hips until they feel tension across the buttocks. The instructor unexpectedly releases the tension on the band or cord at different angles of lean to elicit a backward step (6.6b). The safest way to perform the release is to hold both ends of the band with one hand while gently resting your other hand on the participant's shoulder. This additional tactile cue will remind the participant to initiate the backward lean from the hips instead of the head. Cue participants to "feel the resistance increase as the hips move backward into the band." Do not release the tension on the band until the participant is clearly initiating the backward lean from the hips.

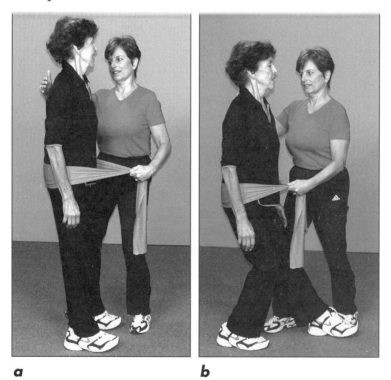

a   b

Figure 6.6 Start *(a)* and end *(b)* positions for backward step strategy. Instruct the participant to lean backward through the hips during this exercise progression.

■ 4. SIDE STEP STRATEGY FROM A LEANING POSITION

Repeat the stepping exercise against resistance on a firm, level surface only. The instructor or assistant stands to the side of the participant holding a length of resistance band wrapped around the participant's hips. The participant leans to the side, feeling tension from the band at the level of the hips (figure 6.7a). The instructor unexpectedly releases the tension on the band at different angles of lean. Two types of side step strategies may be observed during this exercise, as illustrated in figure

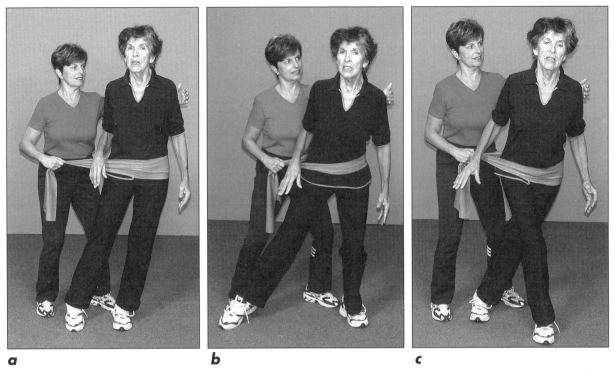

a   *b*   *c*

Figure 6.7 From an initial leaning position **(a)**, a loss of balance in a lateral direction may result in **(b)** a same-leg step strategy or **(c)** a crossover strategy.

6.7b and c. The same-leg step strategy requires a quick weight shift back onto the other leg before the leading leg is lifted (figure 6.7b), whereas the crossover strategy involves crossing the weighted leg over the midline and a subsequent step with the initially weighted leg to reestablish a wide base of support (figure 6.7c).

Important Verbal Cues

- "Lean over your ankles as you lean forward; keep your head erect and eyes focused on a target at eye level in front of you."
- "For backward and lateral step directions, lean from your hips, not your head."
- "Feel the tension of the resistance band increase as your hips lean into it."
- "Take additional steps after the band is released if you do not feel stable enough after a single step."

Summary

The exercise progressions presented in this chapter are designed to improve your older adult clients' ability to select the appropriate movement strategy when the task or environment demands it. As you learned in reading this chapter, manipulating the task or environment in at least three different ways will enable your older adult clients to practice each of the ankle, hip, and step movement strategies. Manipulating the task demands by increasing the speed and distance through which you ask an older adult to sway in a forward and backward direction will determine whether an ankle or hip strategy is used to control sway. Changing the support surface a client is standing on from one that is firm and broad to one that is narrower than the length of the feet or unstable will often be sufficient to trigger the hip strategy to control balance. Finally, the step strategy will be the movement strategy of choice when the task requires older adults to lean beyond their maximum limits of stability. Each of these strategies can also be activated at a subconscious level simply by progressively increasing the amount of force applied during a perturbation activity from small (ankle strategy) to medium (hip strategy) to large (step strategy).

Practicing each of the progressions described in the ankle, hip, and step strategy sections of the chapter will also help the older adult learn how to perform each strategy efficiently so it can be reproduced consistently when needed. Although it will take much longer for many older adults to learn to reproduce the correct strategy subconsciously when they are unexpectedly perturbed with different amounts of force, repeated practice of the three strategies at a conscious level will certainly be helpful. In addition to constructing the appropriate practice environment and manipulating the demands of a task so that a particular strategy is more likely to be selected, you also will need to have your clients practice the various lower body strength activities described in chapter 8 on a regular basis. Even though the older adult may have the ability to produce the correct movement strategy, adequate levels of strength are still required to ensure that it is scaled appropriately and executed effectively.

TEST YOUR UNDERSTANDING

1. When standing quietly on a firm, broad surface, a person controls postural sway by using
   a. an ankle strategy
   b. a hip strategy
   c. a step strategy
   d. a suspensory strategy
   e. a standing steady strategy

2. If you want to encourage participants to use a hip strategy to control postural sway, you would ask them to
   a. sway slowly and over a short distance
   b. step over obstacles of different heights
   c. reach for objects while standing sideways on a narrow beam
   d. attempt to remain standing while you perturbed them using a large amount of force
   e. march in place while throwing objects from hand to hand

3. The primary goal of postural strategy training is to improve an individual's ability to
   a. move the center of gravity efficiently and confidently through space
   b. perform each of the four identified movement strategies with efficiency
   c. select and execute each of the three movement strategies required to maintain or restore upright balance
   d. alter the gait pattern to meet the goals of the task being performed
   e. maintain upright balance when the base of support is altered

4. To elicit a stepping strategy,
   a. the COG must be within the base of support
   b. the COG must move beyond the individual's limits of stability
   c. the base of support must be reduced

    d.   an external force must be applied to the body

    e.   the participant must first be able to demonstrate a hip strategy

5.   A common age-related change that has been demonstrated in the research literature is

    a.   the absence of an ankle strategy among older adults with poor range of motion at the hip

    b.   the disappearance or ineffective use of the ankle and step strategies

    c.   the disappearance of the step strategy

    d.   the ineffective use or disappearance of the hip and step strategies

    e.   the more frequent use of the step strategy when the base of support is exceeded

6.   Which of the following movement strategies appears to require the greatest allocation of attention?

    a.   the ankle strategy

    b.   the hip strategy

    c.   the step strategy

    d.   the suspensory strategy

    e.   the feet-in-place strategy

7.   When asked to sway over a greater distance and at a faster speed, an individual is most likely to use a _____ strategy to prevent a loss of balance.

    a.   hip

    b.   stepping

    c.   ankle

    d.   suspensory

    e.   mixed

8.   An effective way to promote the use of either leg to initiate the stepping strategy is to

    a.   "fix" the swing leg in order to force the use of the opposite leg

    b.   ask the participant to practice stepping up onto and over a bench with alternate legs leading

    c.   prevent the individual from moving the stance leg in order to force the use of the opposite leg

    d.   gently tap the leg that you would like the individual to use just prior to the start of the exercise

    e.   stand on the same side as the leg you would like the participant to use

9.   When eliciting a step strategy using a resistance band, the instructor should

    a.   tell the participant when tension on the band is about to be released

    b.   completely release the band as the participant steps

    c.   increase the tension on the band by pulling it away from the participant as the step is initiated

    d.   increase the tension on the band by pulling it away from the participant as the lean is initiated and then quickly release the tension at a lean angle likely to lead to a step

    e.   not release the tension on the band until the participant reaches a lean angle of at least 45°

PRACTICAL PROBLEMS

1. Practice the resistance band release maneuver with fellow instructors or able-bodied friends of different heights and weights so that you can learn to perform the release maneuver safely and effectively. Solicit feedback from your helpers to determine whether the amount of tension you applied was sufficient as they initiated the lean and whether they felt safe during the release phase of the maneuver. I cannot stress enough the need to practice this technique many times before you even consider trying it with your older adult clients.

2. Practice perturbing the same group of able-bodied friends by applying quick pushes or pulls at the level of the hips while they are seated on a balance ball or standing on an altered support surface. Observe the type of response they initiate at the different levels of force. Now solicit help from two or three of your most accomplished older adult fitness class members and practice applying force at different levels. You will certainly not be able to apply the same level of force when perturbing your older, albeit very healthy, adult clients, but practicing with your colleagues will help you understand different force levels from a relative perspective.

3. Develop an appropriate set of postural control strategy activities for Bill and Jane. Based on your knowledge of these individuals, which of the postural control strategies do you think Jane and Bill are likely to find the most difficult to acquire? Provide a rationale for your response.

Gait Pattern Enhancement and Variation Training

7

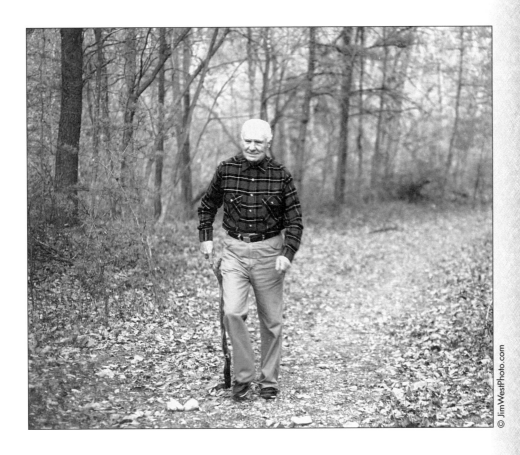

© JimWestPhoto.com

Objectives

After completing this chapter, you will be able to

- describe the important phases of the gait cycle and the neural mechanisms that control gait,

- identify the changes in the gait cycle that are due to age or pathology,

- describe the characteristics of gait in persons with various medical conditions, and

- develop a set of progressive gait activities designed to help older adults develop a more flexible and efficient gait pattern.

The ability to move about successfully in a variety of environmental contexts that impose different timing (e.g., stepping onto and off of escalators, crossing busy streets) or spatial demands (e.g., stepping over obstacles, walking in crowded malls) requires a gait pattern that is both flexible and adaptable. At its most fundamental level, successful locomotion is contingent on the ability to integrate the control of posture with upper and lower body limb movements. For example, initiating gait, walking, stopping, and turning are all movements that also require a change in our postural orientation.

Successful locomotion is contingent on the ability to integrate postural control with upper and lower body movements.

Overview of the Gait Cycle

gait cycle—The time between the first contact of the heel of one foot with the ground and the next heel-ground contact with the same foot.

Because the act of walking is cyclical in nature, the **gait cycle** is arbitrarily defined as the time between the first contact with the ground by the heel of one foot and the next heel-ground contact with the same foot. The gait cycle is measured in seconds. One single-limb cycle usually requires approximately 1 second to complete and is composed of two phases: stance and swing. The stance phase begins when the foot first contacts the ground, and the swing phase begins as the foot leaves the ground. When walking at a preferred speed, adults usually spend as much as 60% of the gait cycle in the stance phase and 40% in the swing phase. (See figure 7.1 for an illustration of the complete gait cycle.) As you can see in the illustration, both feet are in contact with the ground from the time the right heel contacts the ground until the left toe leaves the ground (approximately 10% of the gait cycle) and then again from when the left heel contacts the ground until the right toe leaves the ground (approximately 10% of the gait cycle). The time during the gait cycle when both feet are in contact with the ground is referred to as **double-support time.**

double-support time— The time during the gait cycle when both feet are in contact with the ground.

During the gait cycle, three major tasks must be achieved: weight acceptance, single-limb support, and limb advancement. Weight acceptance (initial contact and loading) is perhaps the most demanding task that must be accomplished during walking. Successful completion of this task requires adequate knee flexion (approximately 15°) so that the shock associated with accepting the body's full weight on impact is absorbed, good limb stability as the foot contacts the ground, and the ability to keep the COG moving forward in preparation for the swing phase of gait. The key muscle groups involved in completing this task are the hip extensors (to provide limb stability), quadriceps (to constrain knee flexion), and dorsiflexors (during the heel strike, foot contact with the ground, and preparation for limb loading).

During the single-limb support task that occurs during midstance and terminal stance, one limb must assume the responsibility for supporting total body weight, which must also be simultaneously progressed forward in preparation for the swing phase. The key muscle groups activated during this task include the hip abductors (to stabilize the hip), trunk muscles (to maintain an upright position), quadriceps (to assist forward progression of the COG), and plantar flexors (to control the forward movement of the tibia during mid- and terminal stance).

The final task that must be completed during each gait cycle is that of advancing the limb (preswing and swing). This task begins during preswing as the knee begins to flex (approximately 35°) in preparation for the limb being lifted off the floor. During the swing phase, the limb will be advanced. The knee will continue to flex

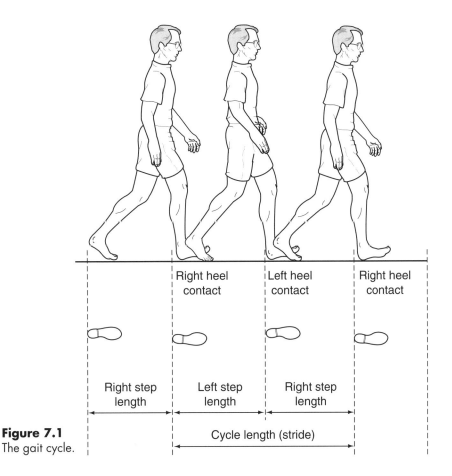

Figure 7.1
The gait cycle.

Labels in figure: Right heel contact · Left heel contact · Right heel contact · Right step length · Left step length · Right step length · Cycle length (stride)

to approximately 60° to allow for toe clearance (approximately 1 centimeter above the floor) before reaching full extension in preparation for heel contact. How far the limb is advanced during this phase will determine step length. The key muscle groups involved in the completion of this final task are the hip flexors, knee flexors, dorsiflexors, quadriceps, and hamstrings (during terminal stance). All of the muscle groups involved in completing each of these tasks must remain strong to preserve the quality of the gait pattern and minimize the risk of falls in your older adult clients. In chapter 8 you will find strength and endurance exercises that specifically target each of these major muscle groups.

Three major tasks must be achieved during the gait cycle:

• Weight acceptance
• Single-limb support
• Limb advancement

To achieve a normal gait pattern, an individual must have four major attributes: an adequate range of joint mobility; appropriate timing of muscle activation across the gait cycle; sufficient muscle strength to meet the demands involved in each phase of the gait cycle; and unimpaired sensory input from the visual, somatosensory, and vestibular systems. Particularly important muscles for gait include the hip extensors, knee extensors, plantar flexors, and dorsiflexors. A significant weakness in any of these muscle groups will adversely affect the quality of the gait pattern. For lateral stability during walking, the hip abductor muscle groups also must remain strong.

Four major attributes are needed for normal gait:
- Adequate range of joint mobility
- Appropriate timing of muscle activation
- Sufficient muscle strength
- Unimpaired sensory input

Although many aspects of gait can be measured using sophisticated instrumentation (e.g., force plates, electromyography, high-speed videotaping), the variables that are probably of greatest interest to you as a balance and mobility instructor involve the temporal and distance factors associated with gait. Two variables that you are already familiar with as a result of administering the 50-foot walk test are **stride length** (the distance covered from one heel strike to the next heel strike by the same foot) and **cadence** (the number of steps per unit of time). Not only do these two variables determine walking speed, but they also influence how much we swing our arms; how far we rotate the hip, knee, and ankle joints; and how long we remain in double-limb support during each gait cycle. You can also conduct a qualitative analysis of gait as each older adult client completes the 8-foot up-and-go test and the 50-foot walk test at preferred and fast speeds. Pay particular attention to how your older adults swing their arms while walking, the degree of dorsiflexion at the ankle joint as the heel strikes the floor, the degree of knee flexion before and during the swing phase, the position of the trunk and head during the gait cycle, and the overall symmetry of the gait pattern across limbs.

stride length—The distance covered from one heel strike to the next heel strike by the same foot.

cadence—The number of steps per unit of time.

Mechanisms Controlling Gait

The act of walking constitutes one of the most complex activities we engage in as humans. Although higher brain centers (e.g., cerebral cortex, basal ganglia, cerebellum, brainstem) play an important role in the overall control, variation, and adaptation of the locomotor pattern, complex networks of neurons (often referred to as **central pattern generators**) located in the spinal cord are responsible for the rhythmic and subconscious coordination of the major muscle groups involved in walking. Each of the three sensory systems described in chapter 2 also plays a critical role in locomotion. Vision, in particular, plays an important role in the control and modulation of gait because it can help us anticipate changes occurring in the visual environment, not just react to them.

Patla (1997) has identified two strategies associated with the proactive visual control of locomotion: avoidance and accommodation. An **avoidance strategy** is one that involves the momentary modification of the gait pattern to avoid a barrier within the environment. For example, vision assists us in placing the foot during gait, avoiding obstacles by signaling the need to lift the limb higher so that we can successfully step over them, or changing the direction of the walking pattern if the obstacle is perceived to be too high to clear successfully (figure 7.2). Vision is also used to help us stop. On the other hand, an **accommodation strategy** is defined as the adaptation of the gait pattern in response to a change in the physical environment (e.g., slope of the ground, type of walking terrain). Characteristics of the gait pattern will be altered in this latter scenario. For example, vision helps us accommodate changes in the physical environment by signaling the need to alter stride length (e.g., decrease stride length when walking across an icy surface) or increase the contractile power of certain muscle groups as the task demands change (i.e., climbing stairs).

central pattern generators—Complex sets of neurons located in the spinal cord that are believed to control the rhythmic and subconscious coordination of the major muscle groups involved in walking.

avoidance strategy—The momentary modification of the gait cycle to avoid a barrier in the environment.

accommodation strategy—Adaptation of the gait pattern in response to a change in the physical environment.

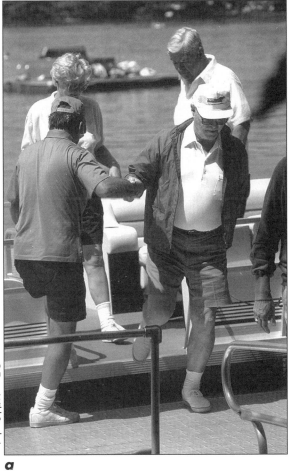

a

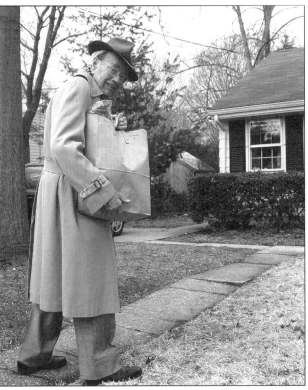

b

Figure 7.2 Vision helps us avoid barriers in the environment *(a)* or adapt our walking pattern when we step onto a different surface *(b).*

© Terry Wild Stock, Inc.

© Susan Siegrist

Just as the somatosensory system is critical for controlling standing balance, it also plays an important reactive role during locomotion. Sensory input received from proprioceptors in the muscles and joints and from cutaneous receptors has been shown to contribute to the reflexive control and modulation of gait by providing limb position information during critical phases of the gait cycle. The proprioceptors also inform us about the position of the limb in space during the various phases of the gait cycle. Finally, the vestibular system, in conjunction with vision, plays an important role in stabilizing the head during walking through the vestibulo-ocular reflex. This important reflex allows us to stabilize vision even though the head is moving during locomotion. Specific impairments within the vestibular system lead to increased instability during gait because it becomes more difficult to stabilize the head (Berthoz & Pozzo, 1994).

The proprioceptors inform us about limb position during the gait cycle, whereas the visual and vestibular systems help us stabilize the head during walking.

The musculoskeletal system also plays an important role in locomotion by providing the muscular force necessary to support the body during the stance phase of gait and move it forward during the swing phase. Because gravity is acting against the body, adequate levels of muscle strength will be necessary to minimize the energy expended during gait while maximizing biomechanical efficiency. Adequate range of motion is also necessary in the joints of the trunk and lower limbs.

Age-Associated Changes in Gait

Although it is difficult to know whether the changes we observe in the gait pattern of healthy older adults are due to the aging process alone or some underlying disease process, clear differences exist when healthy older adults are compared to younger adults. The most evident change is in the variables of gait speed. Even healthy older adults with no history of falling walk at a preferred speed that is, on average, 20% slower than the speed exhibited by younger adults. Conversely, when walking at a fast speed, a 17% difference in gait speed between the two groups has been noted (Elble, Thomas, Higgins & Colliver, 1991). What is most interesting is that the slowing in gait speed that accompanies age is largely due to a decrease in stride length as opposed to cadence. Unfortunately, this reduction in stride length also has negative consequences for other aspects of gait, including reduced arm swing; reduced rotation of the hips, knees, and ankles; increased double-support time; and a more flat-footed contact with the ground during the stance phase before toe-off (Elble, 1997).

> The age-associated decrease in gait speed is largely due to a decrease in stride length rather than cadence.

Common adaptations you are likely to observe among your older adult clients are the tendency to load the limb more cautiously during the weight acceptance task, a flatter foot-to-floor contact pattern, less forward progression of the limb during single-limb support, and reduced knee flexion during the preswing and swing phases of gait. A summary of the changes commonly observed in the temporal and distance variables in the gait pattern of older adults is presented in the box below.

Summary of Gait Changes Observed in Older Adults

Temporal and distance factors

- Decreased velocity
- Decreased step frequency
- Increased stride width
- Increased time in double support
- Decreased step length
- Decreased stride length
- Increased stance phase
- Decreased time in swing phase

It has also been demonstrated that when approaching obstacles, older adults further reduce their gait speed and clear the obstacle using a slower, shorter step. This reduction in step length decreases the likelihood of tripping, but it often causes the heel or sole of the foot to contact the obstacle before it returns to the ground on the other side (Chen, Ashton-Miller, Alexander & Schultz, 1991).

Age-related changes in each of the sensory systems are also likely to adversely affect gait speed. In addition to providing continuous feedback that is essential for adapting the gait pattern to changes in terrain and a changing visual display, vision serves an important **feedforward** role by helping us anticipate changes in the environment and thereby preserve a smooth and continuous walking pattern (Rose, 1997). Age-related decreases that occur in the visual perception of motion are also likely to adversely affect the gait pattern, leading to inaccurate responses in some situations or slower movement responses in others. Although some of the changes

feedforward—Vision is used to anticipate changes in the environment and prepare the motor system in advance of action.

in gait are inevitable with age, much can be done to prevent or slow those declines through the careful selection of gait pattern enhancement and variation exercises.

Effect of Pathology on the Gait Pattern

Unfortunately, not all changes in the gait patterns observed among older adults can be attributed to the aging process. Certain medical conditions, particularly those of neurological origin, can also adversely affect different aspects of gait. Let's briefly consider five neurological conditions that will produce abnormal or pathological changes in the gait pattern: stroke, Parkinson's disease, peripheral neuropathy, cerebellar ataxia, and Alzheimer's disease. Although typical gait patterns are associated with each medical condition, both the type and severity of the problems observed during gait will vary within the medical condition and among persons who have been diagnosed with the same disorder.

> The type and severity of problems observed during gait will vary depending on the medical condition and among persons diagnosed with the same disorder.

Stroke

The problems commonly observed in the gait pattern of an older adult who has sustained a stroke are the result of muscle weakness and **spasticity** (increased muscle tone due to hyperexcitability of the stretch reflex) that often accompany a stroke. Because a stroke usually affects one side of the body more than the other, the gait pattern typically will be asymmetrical. The inability to appropriately time the onset and offset of the muscle groups involved in gait will result in an uncoordinated gait pattern—the toe instead of the heel may contact the floor at initial foot contact, the knee may be hyperextended during stance, and the toe may drag on the floor during the swing phase. A "step-to" gait pattern is often observed wherein the unimpaired limb steps forward and the impaired limb catches up to it on the next swing phase but does not pass it, as would be observed in a normal gait pattern. Older adults who sustain more serious strokes may also need to use an assistive device (e.g., single-point or three-point cane) on their unimpaired side to help them maintain dynamic balance while walking.

spasticity—Increased muscle tone due to hyperexcitability of the stretch reflex.

Parkinson's Disease

In contrast to the gait pattern observed in an older adult who has sustained a stroke, the older adult with Parkinson's disease (PD) will exhibit a shuffling gait pattern. The foot is often flat at initial contact, the muscles are rigid, trunk rotation is limited, and the posture is stooped, particularly in the later stages of the disease. Older adults with PD will experience difficulty initiating the gait pattern and, once started, will also have difficulty regulating the length of the step or stopping the gait cycle. These commonly observed impairments are due to the disease affecting primarily the basal ganglia, which plays an important role in both the initiation and scaling (changing the amplitude of a movement) of the gait pattern. Older adults with PD also have difficulty adapting their gait pattern and thus will experience greater difficulty during turning movements or stepping over an obstacle. PD also markedly affects older adults' ability to adapt their posture. In particular, older adults with PD have difficulty shifting their COG forward when attempting to stand up from a chair and tend to fall backward as a result. Because of the shuffling gait pattern, they do not adequately clear the floor with the toe and are thus at risk for tripping during the swing phase of gait.

Peripheral Neuropathy

Because the continuous flow of somatosensory information is critical to knowing where the limbs are in space during the gait cycle, as well as to our ability to adapt the gait cycle to the changing demands of the environment, any disruption in this input will result in abnormal gait patterns. In particular, a wider base of support, slower velocity, and decreased floor clearance often occur during walking. In more severe cases, a foot slap will be evident during initial contact. Older adults experiencing peripheral neuropathy (loss of sensation in the feet or lower limbs) will no longer be able to sense where the feet and lower limbs are in space, leading to delays in the initiation of certain phases of the gait cycle (i.e., swing). The ability to adapt the gait pattern will also be compromised, particularly when vision is not available to anticipate changes occurring in the environment (e.g., visual impairment, low lighting).

Cerebellar Ataxia

ataxia—General term used to describe uncoordinated movement.

Any damage to the cerebellum also produces an abnormal gait pattern that is often referred to as **ataxia.** Recall that the cerebellum plays an extremely important role in the maintenance of equilibrium or balance during the gait cycle because of its ability to provide continuous error detection and correction information. What you are most likely to observe in an older adult with cerebellar dysfunction is a poorly coordinated gait pattern characterized by a wide base of support and irregular or unpredictable step length. Individuals with cerebellar dysfunction may also veer to the right or left when walking and have difficulty stopping, starting, and turning.

Alzheimer's Disease

Finally, Alzheimer's disease (AD) also results in adverse changes in the gait pattern. Generally, the individual with AD adopts a shuffling gait pattern that is nonpurposeful and significantly slower because of the shorter step cycle. The knees are often in excessive flexion throughout the gait cycle, and the individual frequently requires verbal cuing to maintain a walking pattern. Individuals with dementia are at particularly high risk for falls and should not be included in a group training program unless adequate supervision is available and their judgment skills are good. Although the FallProof program currently operates in facilities that serve older adults in the early stages of AD, the program has been significantly modified to ensure the safety and success of the clients involved.

Orthopedic Conditions

contractures—Loss of passive joint range of motion.

Certain orthopedic conditions may also produce abnormal gait patterns. Individuals with soft tissue **contractures** (loss of passive joint range of motion) are unable to move the joints through the required range of motion at certain phases of the gait cycle and exhibit restricted movement patterns as a result. Pain in the joints caused by arthritis will also lead to abnormal gait patterns as the older adult seeks to limit movement in an effort to reduce pain. Fractures and total joint replacement surgery have also been associated with the development of abnormal gait patterns.

Cardiovascular Disease

A variety of cardiovascular conditions also result in the development of an abnormal or pathological gait pattern. Individuals experiencing **orthostatic (postural) hypo-**

tension, for example, often experience a fluctuation in blood pressure on rising that causes dizziness and disequilibrium during the gait cycle. Chronic pain in the calf muscles due to **intermittent claudication** also leads to abnormal adjustments in the gait pattern. Gait speed is also generally much slower in older adults with cardiovascular problems as a result of poor aerobic conditioning.

In summary, certain medical conditions produce specific impairments that are likely to result in an abnormal or pathological gait pattern. The major impairments that contribute to the development of these patterns include the following:

- Joint deformity (e.g., contractures)
- Pain (e.g., joint, heel)
- Impaired motor control (e.g., spasticity)
- Muscle weakness (e.g., stroke, cardiovascular disease)
- Sensory system deficits (e.g., peripheral neuropathy)
- Central processing dysfunction (e.g., Parkinson's disease, Alzheimer's disease, stroke)

orthostatic (postural) hypotension—A drop in systolic and/or diastolic blood pressure leading to dizziness, light-headedness, or loss of consciousness.

intermittent claudication—Severe pain in the lower extremities that occurs with activity. It results from inadequate arterial blood supply to the exercising muscles. The pain subsides with rest.

Check Your Walking Pattern

Here is a quick and easy way to check the quality of your walking pattern. All you need is a full-length mirror.

Walk directly toward the mirror and observe the following:

- Your knees are pointing forward.
- Your hips are level.
- Your arms swing rhythmically as you walk.
- Both sides of your body are symmetrical (arm swing, step length, etc).
- You are walking tall (e.g., your head is erect and your ears are directly above your shoulders).

Walk alongside a wall mirror (a full-length mirror is helpful for this activity) and observe the following:

- Your heel makes contact with the floor first on each step.
- You can feel the pressure roll up to the toes as you push off from the floor.
- Your knee is almost fully extended before your heel contacts the floor.
- Your steps are of equal length.
- Your ears are directly above your shoulders and your body is upright.

Gait Pattern Enhancement and Variation Training

The activities in this component of the program are designed to build on the balance activities already described in earlier chapters and help the older adult achieve a gait pattern that is efficient, flexible, and adaptable to changing task and environmental demands. For example, requiring older adults to start and stop quickly; walk with longer, shorter, or wider stride patterns; and turn in different directions will require them to vary the spatial and temporal characteristics of the gait pattern, making it more flexible in the long term. Other activities designed to enhance or vary the gait pattern include walking on the toes or heels; stopping, starting, and turning on command; and stepping over obstacles, onto and off different surface types, and up and down inclines.

As the older adult becomes more confident in their balance abilities and demonstrates better overall performance, secondary tasks can be added to force a more subconscious control of balance due to the need to divide attention between multiple tasks. To accomplish this goal, activities that require the older adult to count backward by threes, reach for or catch objects, or turn the head while walking should be incorporated into the training program. These activities will further challenge each individual's abilities while rendering the practice environment more like the everyday performance environment.

Level 1: Walking With Directional Changes and Abrupt Starts and Stops

a. Instruct participants to make abrupt starts and stops on command (e.g., verbal, whistle, music) while walking. (Provides participants with the opportunity to practice their gaze-stabilization techniques while moving. Use the following verbal cue: "Focus your eyes on a target directly in front of you and walk directly toward it.")

b. Have participants change direction on verbal command or when the music is paused. Ask them to make a quarter turn followed by a half turn and, finally, a full turn on command.

c. Repeat the activity while walking using different gait patterns (e.g., backward, side step, marching with high knees). Periodically pause the music and announce a new walking pattern.

Level 2: Walking With Altered Base of Support

a. Have participants walk forward using a narrow step width (mark floor with lines spaced 2 inches apart).

b. Have participants walk forward using a wide step width (mark floor with lines spaced 8 to 12 inches apart).

c. Combine narrow and wide stepping exercises by having participants complete a certain number of narrow steps followed by the same number of wide steps. Increase or decrease the number of steps completed using each gait pattern to match the coordination abilities of the participants.

d. "Step-to" walking: Have participants walk forward while taking a long step with one leg and bringing the other leg back even with it on the next step. Repeat the exercise with the opposite leg leading the action.

e. Repeat the previous exercise but instruct participants to change the leg that is stepping long after a set number of steps.

f. Have participants walk forward on their heels across a firm surface.

g. Have participants walk forward on their toes across a firm surface (figure 7.3).

h. Combine heel and toe walking exercises by having participants complete a certain number of steps while walking on the heels followed by the same number of steps while walking on the toes. Increase or decrease the number of steps completed using each gait pattern to match the coordination abilities of the participants.

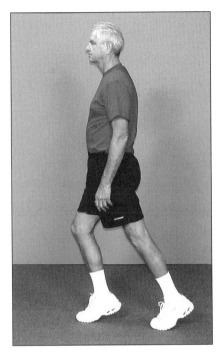

Figure 7.3 Walking with an altered base of support (on toes) is designed to help the older adult develop a more flexible gait pattern.

Level 3: Gait Pattern Variations—Braiding and Tandem Walking

a. Crossover steps (e.g., braiding): Have participants begin the exercise by only crossing the trailing foot behind the leading leg. Then have them repeat the exercise in the opposite direction, crossing the trailing leg in front of the leading leg. Participants should not rotate the hips as the lead foot is placed on the floor behind or in front of the body. A helpful cue to use during all braiding progressions is "Keep your hips (headlights) facing forward."

b. Repeat crossover stepping using a full braiding technique if the participant is able to perform the first progression without instability or excessive hip rotation. The trailing leg crosses forward and in front of the leading leg, then behind the leading leg, on alternate steps (figure 7.4).

c. Repeat the previous exercise in the opposite direction.

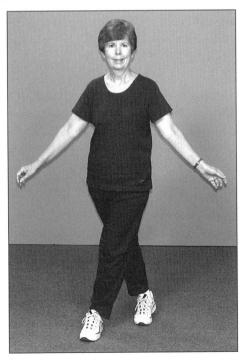

Figure 7.4 Braiding activities can be used to help older adults vary their gait patterns.

d. Perform semitandem walking (make heel contact when the right foot is forward of the toe of the opposite foot) in the forward and backward directions.

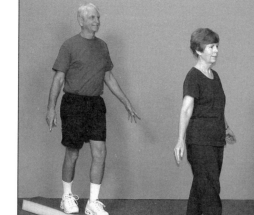

Figure 7.5 Walking along a narrow beam requires altering the gait pattern to remain stable.

Use a length of wood (10-foot-long two-by four) or two lines of masking or vinyl tape (spaced 2 inches apart) to provide a visual path.

e. Repeat the previous exercise while semitandem walking on a narrow beam elevated above the floor or on a half-foam roller (6 to 12 inches wide).

f. Repeat the previous exercise while walking in a full tandem (sharpened Romberg) position (e.g., right foot contacts the floor when directly in front of the toes of the left foot).

g. Repeat the previous exercise while tandem walking on a raised narrow beam or half-foam roller (figure 7.5).

Important Reminder

- The braiding activity is not appropriate for all participants because it requires crossing the midline on each step, and the risk of falling is increased if the technique is not performed correctly. The full braiding technique should not be performed if participants with a hip or knee joint prosthesis or a diagnosis of osteoporosis are unable to satisfactorily perform the lead-up braiding activity described in the first exercise progression.

- The braiding technique can also be modified so that the foot does not cross the midline during the activity. Braiding should be discontinued if the participant complains of discomfort in the hip region.

Level 4: Gait Pattern Enhancement/Variation Obstacle Course

One of the best ways to practice the gait patterns introduced in levels 1 through 3 is to set up an obstacle course. The level of balance challenge can be progressively increased by manipulating the task or environmental demands. Some ways you can increase the task or environmental demands when designing obstacle courses include the following:

Task Demands

- Increase the number of obstacle types that must be negotiated along the course.

- Introduce an object to be carried through the course (e.g., laundry basket) (figure 7.6).

- Introduce a cognitive task while the course is being negotiated (e.g., counting by threes).

• Require each participant to perform an activity after stepping onto each piece of equipment in the obstacle course (i.e., march in place 10 times on foam pad, perform swing-through steps on bench, balance for 10 seconds on half-foam roller with eyes closed, step onto and off of Dyna-Disc™).

• Require that different-shaped objects be retrieved from the floor as each participant moves through the course.

• Introduce an external timing demand. For example, require that the course be completed in a given amount of time. Indicate that time will be added if the activities are not performed correctly or with control. This added constraint tends to minimize unsafe behavior.

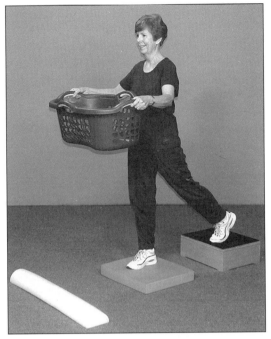

Figure 7.6 Requiring participants to carry an object along an obstacle course divides their attention between the walking and carrying tasks. It also prevents them from looking at their feet.

Environmental Demands

• Have participants negotiate the obstacle course while wearing dark glasses.

• Vary the type of support surfaces placed along the course. For example, intersperse foam of different densities with Dyna-Discs, half-foam rollers, and wedges.

• Introduce a busy background or floor surface (length of material with busy visual pattern) from which participants are required to retrieve various objects.

• Have two to four class participants negotiating the same obstacle course at the same time. Have two participants start the course at one end and two other participants begin at the opposite end. Start the second participant at each end after the first participant has gone about a third of the way through the course. This activity is intended to create a more complex visual environment as participants pass each other on the course.

Summary

The gait pattern enhancement and variation activities presented in this chapter are intended to help the older adult develop a gait pattern that is more efficient, flexible, and adaptable. As you learned earlier in the chapter, the aging process results in a number of changes in the walking pattern. The most observable change is a decrease in gait velocity caused by a reduction in stride length. This change also negatively affects other aspects of gait, including the arm swing; hip, knee, and ankle rotation; and the quality of foot-floor contact. A reduction in stride length also results in longer double-support times during the gait cycle. When required to negotiate obstacles, older adults further reduce their gait speed and take slower, shorter steps as they approach the obstacles. Having your class participants negotiate several different obstacle courses that include obstacles of various heights and varying support surfaces will do much to improve their confidence and their ability to adapt their gait pattern to changing environmental demands. Although you can expect to see much smaller changes in the gait patterns of older adults who are experiencing medical conditions that have affected different areas of the neurological system (e.g., stroke, Parkinson's disease, dementia), it is nevertheless important to have them practice many of the lower-level progressions described in this chapter so they can maintain their functional independence for as long as possible.

TEST YOUR UNDERSTANDING

1. The stance phase
    a. occupies 20% of the gait cycle
    b. occupies 40% of the gait cycle
    c. occupies 50% of the gait cycle
    d. occupies 60% of the gait cycle
    e. occupies 70% of the gait cycle

2. The gait cycle is arbitrarily defined as
    a. the distance between the heel strike of one foot and the next heel strike with the same foot
    b. the time between the heel strike of the right foot and the heel strike of the left foot
    c. the time between the heel strike of one foot on first contact and the subsequent heel-floor contact with the same foot
    d. the distance between the heel strike of one foot and the heel strike of the other foot
    e. any point you wish to start timing from within the gait cycle

3. Which of the following is a common problem observed in the walking pattern of someone who has experienced a stroke?
    a. stooped posture
    b. reduced foot clearance
    c. shuffling
    d. asymmetrical gait pattern
    e. lateral veering

4. All of the following are changes that adversely affect the gait pattern during normal aging except
    a. muscle weakness
    b. poor depth perception
    c. impaired ankle proprioception
    d. spasticity
    e. decreased stride length

5. Which of the following key muscle groups are activated during the single-limb support phase of gait?
    a. trunk muscles, quadriceps, and dorsiflexors
    b. quadriceps, abductors, plantarflexors, and trunk muscles

c. hip extensors, quadriceps, and dorsiflexors

d. hip flexors, hamstrings, and plantarflexors

e. hip flexors, knee flexors, dorsiflexors, quadriceps, and hamstrings

6. A person with Parkinson's disease would most commonly demonstrate the following type of gait pattern:

a. shuffling with decreased step length, forward trunk, decreased trunk movement with lack of arm swing

b. wide base; unsteadiness, lateral veering; difficulty turning, starting, stopping

c. knee hyperextension with foot slap

d. excessive knee flexion, lateral veering, wide base, foot slap

e. retracted pelvis, toe drag, step-to gait pattern

7. The purpose of gait variation and enhancement training is to improve all of the following except

a. the strength of the lower limbs for walking

b. dynamic balance for walking

c. flexibility of the gait pattern

d. gait in different environmental contexts

e. speed of walking

8. Which of the following culminating activities is *not* an effective way to challenge an individual's ability to adapt the gait pattern?

a. walking within a crowded room

b. obstacle course

c. line dancing

d. marching in place

e. braiding activities

9. Which of the following is an example of multiple tasking during gait pattern variation and enhancement training?

a. walking while counting backward

b. walking on heels followed by walking on toes followed by walking on heels

c. going up and down stairs

d. stepping over obstacles at various heights

e. walking backward

10. A person who becomes unsteady during the turn of the 8-foot up-and-go test would benefit from

a. marching in place

b. stepping over obstacles

c. walking with head turns

d. going up and down stairs

e. walking backward

PRACTICAL PROBLEMS

1. Review the health/activity questionnaires completed by Jane and Bill and the results of their 50-foot walk tests at preferred and fast speeds. What can you glean from a review of their questionnaires and test results that might lead you to believe they have an abnormal or pathological gait pattern? If you conclude that either Bill or Jane does have an abnormal gait pattern, list each of the impairments you believe are contributing to it.

2. Design three obstacle courses for Bill or Jane that progress from (a) easy to (b) more difficult and then to (c) most difficult to negotiate. Describe what you have changed about each course that makes it more difficult to negotiate and why the types of obstacles you included in one person's course might differ from the other person's course. Be sure to review either Jane or Bill's test results once more to ensure that the types of surfaces or the activities you have selected challenge their balance abilities appropriately but do not exceed their individual capabilities.

8

Strength and Endurance Training

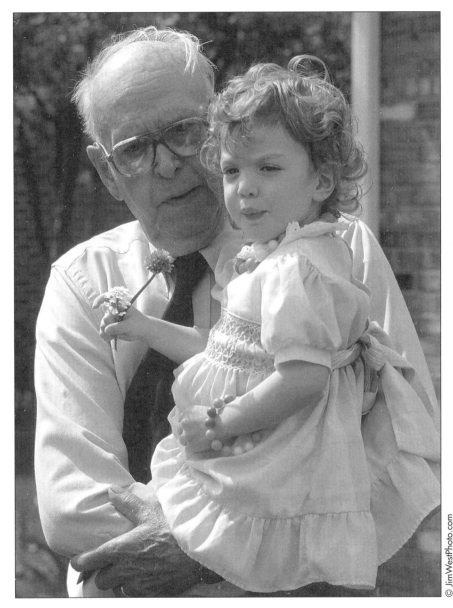

© JimWestPhoto.com

Objectives

After completing this chapter, you will be able to

- understand the contribution of muscle strength to the multiple dimensions of balance and mobility,
- develop a set of exercise progressions designed to improve upper and lower body muscle strength, and
- incorporate strength exercises into a balance environment.

Age-associated declines in muscle mass and strength have been well documented in the literature (Landers, Hunter, Wetzstein Bamman & Wiensier, 2001; Akima et al., 2001). Men and women over the age of 60 have been shown to lose muscle mass at a rate of 0.5% to 1.0% per year, whereas muscle strength declines as much as 20% to 40% between the third and eighth decades of life (Aloia et al., 1991). In the United States, it has been reported that 28% of men and 66% of women above the age of 74 years cannot lift objects that weigh more than 10 pounds, equal to the weight of an average bag of groceries (Rhodes et al., 2000). More recently, researchers have also begun to study age-related changes in muscle power, or the velocity with which a muscle can generate force, so as to better understand its impact on the older adult's level of functional independence (American College of Sports Medicine, 2002; Foldvari et al., 2000).

Given that many activities of daily living (e.g., stair climbing, rising from a chair, walking) require different levels of leg muscle power and that declines in power are much greater than the declines observed in absolute strength, activities designed to increase both absolute strength *and* power should be included in a balance and mobility training program.

> Muscle strength declines as much as 20% to 40% between the third and eighth decades of life.

This chapter describes numerous upper and lower body strength training activities. Some of the strength activities, particularly those that include a balance component, are recommended for inclusion in the class, whereas others should be assigned for homework. Both upper and lower body strength activities have been included that are intended to exercise the key muscle groups involved in balance and gait, described in chapters 1 and 7, respectively (e.g., hip flexors and extensors, hip abductors, knee flexors and extensors, dorsiflexors and plantarflexors). Activities designed to strengthen the musculature of the feet, an often underexercised area of the body, have also been included.

Many of the strength activities described can be performed seated or standing (with or without support). In some cases, alternative methods of performing the strength activity are described to accommodate the greatest number of older adults in your class. Once a participant is able to demonstrate correct form consistently while performing an exercise and performance improves, be sure to add a balance component by first having participants perform the strength activity while seated on a compliant surface (i.e., Dyna-Disc™, balance ball) and then while standing on a compliant or moving surface (i.e., foam pad, rocker board).

Before introducing strength activities into your program, consider the following guidelines related to intensity, progression, and safety:

- Always complete the warm-up and dynamic flexibility exercises prior to having participants engage in any strength exercises.
- Have participants select a hand or ankle weight or resistance band that allows them to perform between 8 and 15 repetitions before fatiguing. (Review the results of the two strength-related test items on the Senior Fitness Test to help you make these decisions.)
- Once participants can complete 15 repetitions of an exercise, encourage them to increase the amount of weight or level of resistance.

- Encourage participants to perform at least one upper and one lower body strength exercise while waiting to perform a balance activity.
- Recommend exercises that target the muscles identified as weak during your initial assessment. A review of each individual's performance on the 30-second chair stand (measure of lower body strength) and arm curl (upper body strength) test items of the Senior Fitness Test will inform you as to whether individuals are below average, average, or above average in terms of their upper and lower body muscle strength.
- More unstable or weak participants should perform the exercises in a seated position to minimize the stability requirements.
- If participants are fatigued, do not ask them to perform any strength or power exercises.
- Remind participants to avoid or stop performing any exercise that they feel is unsafe or causes pain.
- Remind participants never to hold their breath during an exercise. In fact, encourage them to exhale during the exertion phase of the exercise.
- Correct form is important, so take the time to teach the appropriate form to participants. Also instruct program assistants to carefully monitor participants during the performance of each exercise.

Choosing the Appropriate Amount of Resistance

The amount of resistance provided by elastic tubing or resistance band is color-coded. Although manufacturers do not all use the same color-coding system, below is an example of the color coding system used by Theraband®:

- Yellow – light
- Red – medium
- Green – heavy
- Blue – extra heavy
- Black – special heavy

Handles and extremity straps are also available. These accessories will be useful for class participants with weak hand muscles or arthritis.

Selected Upper Body Strength Exercises

The strength exercises described in this section address the muscle groups of the upper body and are organized from the head to the hand, with the exercises involving the larger muscle groups described before those that involve the smaller muscle groups.

■ SHOULDER SHRUGS WITH HAND WEIGHTS

Muscles Targeted

Muscles in the upper back and neck.

a. Sit tall with the lower back pressed firmly against the backrest of a sturdy chair.

b. Relax the shoulders and keep the arms down at the sides while holding the hand weights.

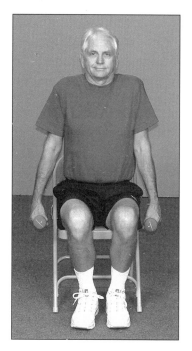

c. Keep the head erect and the chin tucked in so that the ears are directly above the shoulders and the eyes are directed forward. Inhale.

d. Raise both shoulders simultaneously in a shrugging action during the exhale (figure 8.1).

e. Inhale and lower the shoulders to the original starting position.

f. Perform two sets of 10 to 15 repetitions with the appropriate hand weight.

Figure 8.1 Shoulder shrugs with hand weights.

■ BACK EXTENSIONS

Muscles Targeted

Muscles in the upper back and shoulders.

a. Sit tall with the lower back pressed firmly against the backrest of a sturdy chair.

b. Keep the shoulders relaxed and level, the chin tucked in so that the ears are directly above the shoulders, head erect, and eyes focused on a target directly in front and at eye level. Keep the abdomen tucked in.

c. Position the hands behind the head; the fingers should be interlocked and the elbows pointing out (figure 8.2). Inhale.

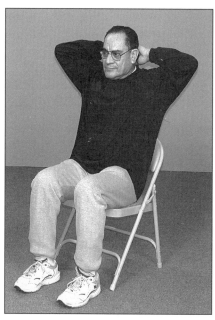

d. Push the elbows back and pinch the shoulder blades together, exhaling as you do so. Hold the position for 10 seconds before returning the arms to the starting position. Breathe evenly during the hold phase.

e. Repeat the exercise 5 to 10 times.

f. Stand behind participants as they perform the exercise to see that they are actually pinching the shoulder blades together.

Figure 8.2 Back extensions.

■ BACK AND ARM EXTENSIONS

Muscles Targeted

Muscles in the upper back and shoulders.

a. Stand with the knees slightly flexed and the feet hip-width apart. Raise the arms to shoulder level with the palms facing up toward the ceiling (figure 8.3).

b. Check postural alignment, position of head, and eyes. Inhale.

c. Pull both arms back with the thumbs leading; pinch the shoulder blades together, exhaling as you do so. Hold the position for 10 seconds while breathing evenly.

d. Return the arms slowly to the starting position.

e. Repeat the exercise 5 to 10 times.

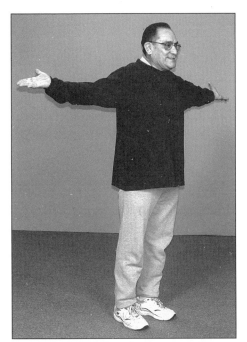

Figure 8.3 Back and arm extensions.

■ SIDE BEND WITH HAND WEIGHTS

Muscles Targeted

Muscles in the upper and middle back, shoulders, and arms.

a. Stand with feet hip-width apart, knees slightly flexed, and weights held in the hands at hip level.

b. Stand tall, tuck in the abdomen and chin, and look directly ahead. Inhale.

c. Slowly bend the trunk to one side as the weight on the other side is raised to armpit level (figure 8.4). Exhale during the side bend. Inhale during the return to starting position.

d. Repeat the exercise on the opposite side.

e. Repeat on both sides 5 to 10 times.

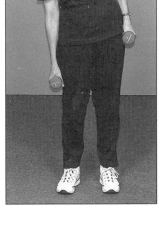

Figure 8.4 Side bend with hand weights.

■ STANDING CHEST PRESS (RESISTANCE BAND)

Muscles Targeted

Muscles in the chest, shoulders, and arms.

a. Stand tall with feet hip-width apart, abdomen and chin tucked in, and eyes focused on a target directly in front and at eye level.

b. Place the resistance band around the back and under the armpits. Make sure the band is flat against the back (figure 8.5).

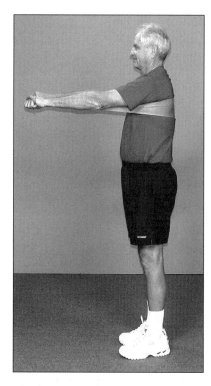

c. Hold onto the ends of the band, adjusting the length by wrapping the band around the hands to increase tension. Inhale.

d. Push the arms directly forward and press the chest muscles together. Exhale during the pushing phase.

e. Pause, then slowly return to the starting position, releasing the tension on the band. Inhale during this phase of the movement.

Figure 8.5 Standing chest press with resistance band.

■ HORIZONTAL PULLS (RESISTANCE BAND)

Muscles Targeted

Muscles in the upper and middle back, shoulders, and arms.

a. Stand in an upright position, feet hip-width apart, abdomen and chin tucked in, eyes directed forward.

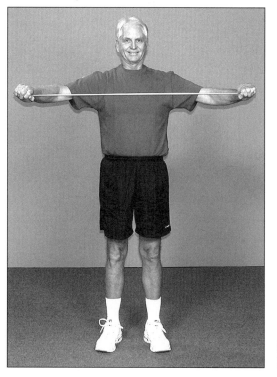

b. Wrap the excess portion of the band around the hands for shoulder-width positioning (figure 8.6).

c. Keep the arms at chest level and the elbows slightly bent.

d. Pull the arms out horizontally to the sides of the body while squeezing the shoulder blades together, exhaling as you do so.

e. Pause, then slowly return to the starting position.

f. Repeat the exercise 5 to 10 times.

Figure 8.6 Horizontal pulls with resistance band.

■ BALL LIFTS WITH ADDED BALANCE CHALLENGE

Muscles Targeted

Muscles in the upper, middle, and lower back; shoulders; arms; and abdominals.

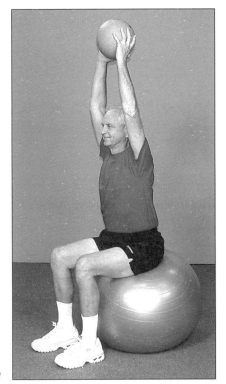

a. Sit tall and in the middle of a balance ball with feet positioned shoulder-width apart.

b. Hold a weighted ball (1-2 kg) directly in front of the body at waist height. Inhale.

c. Extend the arms and raise the ball directly above the head (figure 8.7a). Exhale as you raise the ball.

d. Bend forward at the hips and lower the ball toward the floor (figure 8.7b). Bring the ball back up to the waist.

e. Continue moving the ball in various directions, but always bring it back to the waist.

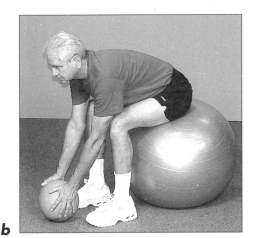

Figure 8.7 Ball lifts on balance ball. Start position *(a);* end position *(b).*

■ DIAGONAL ARM EXTENSIONS (RESISTANCE BAND)

Muscles Targeted

Muscles in the shoulders and upper and middle back and the abdominals.

a. Tie a loop knot at one end of the band and place left foot inside.

b. Hold the other end of the band with the right hand.

c. Sit tall and in the middle of a balance ball with both feet flat on the floor and hip-width apart.

d. Slowly extend the arm across the body, forming a diagonal line from the left foot to the outstretched right hand, head and eyes following the movement of the resistance band.

e. Pause, then slowly return the band to the starting position.

f.   Repeat the exercise 5 to 10 times.

g.   Repeat using the opposite foot and arm.

■ PARTNER PUSH-PULLS (RESISTANCE BAND)

Muscles Targeted

Muscles in the shoulders, upper and middle back, and chest and abdominals.

a.   Position two individuals on balance balls and facing each other at a distance of approximately 4 feet (figure 8.8).

b.   Use two lengths of resistance band, with each partner holding onto one end of each band.

c.   Partners should sit tall and in the middle of the balance ball with the feet hip-width apart and flat on the floor. Inhale

d.   Each partner pulls on one length of band while the other partner pulls on the other length of band in a push-pull motion. Each partner exhales on each pulling motion.

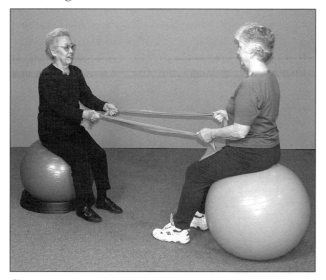

a

e.   The body should remain erect during each phase of the push-pull movement.

f   Repeat the exercise 10 times.

g.   Make sure that partners are of similar height and strength for this activity.

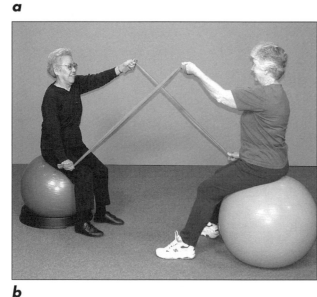

b

Figure 8.8   Partner push-pull with resistance bands: *(a)* horizontal and *(b)* diagonal.

■ STANDING TRICEPS EXTENSIONS (HAND WEIGHT)

Muscles Targeted

Muscles in the elbows, arms, and back.

a. Stand with one knee resting on a sturdy chair with no armrests. The other leg should be to the side of the chair with the knee slightly flexed.

b. Bend the body slightly forward and support the body by resting the forearm on the same side as the flexed knee on the back of the chair.

c. Hold the weight in the other hand at waist level and point the elbow backward at or above shoulder height and toward the ceiling. Inhale.

d. Slowly straighten the arm holding the weight while keeping the elbow, as well as the knee on that side, slightly flexed. Exhale as the arm is extended. Maintain a stable trunk position throughout the extension phase of the movement. The trunk should not sway or arch during the exercise. (Reduce the weight if the trunk cannot be maintained in a stable position throughout the exercise.)

e. Pause, then inhale and slowly bend the arm holding the weight back to the starting position.

f. Complete five repetitions on the same side before moving the weight to the other hand and repeating the exercise.

■ SEATED OR STANDING TRICEPS EXTENSIONS WITH RESISTANCE BAND

Muscles Targeted

Muscles in the back of the upper arms.

a. Wrap the resistance band around each hand until the length of the band is equal to width of shoulders.

b. Raise one arm to shoulder level, bending it at the elbow and palm facing inwards (figure 8.9).

c. Slowly extend the other arm, keeping the elbow close to the side of the body. Exhale as the arm is extended.

d. Pause, then slowly bend the upper arm at the elbow until the hans is just below the hand remaining at shoulder height. Inhale as the arm returns to the starting position.

e. Complete 5 to 10 repetitions with each arm.

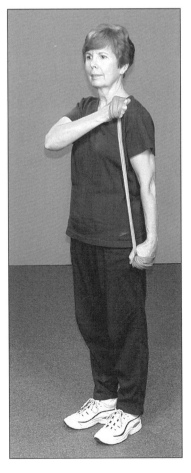

Figure 8.9 Standing triceps extension with resistance band.

Manipulating the Level of Challenge

You can manipulate the level of challenge associated with any of the strength and endurance exercises by manipulating any of the following variables:

- Performance position (seated or standing)
- Level of resistance or amount of weight used
- Plane of motion (e.g., below or above shoulder)
- Number of repetitions or sets performed

■ SEATED BICEPS CURLS WITH HAND WEIGHT

Muscles Targeted

Muscles in the front of the upper arms (biceps) and wrists.

a. Sit tall with the lower back pressed firmly against the backrest of a sturdy chair. Position the side of the body on which the exercise will begin close to the edge of the side of the chair. Tuck in the abdomen and chin, and direct the eyes forward.

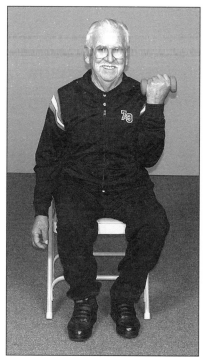

b. Position the feet flat on the floor and hip-width apart. Hold the weight in one hand, with the arm hanging down beside the thigh and the palm facing inward. Inhale.

c. Slowly lift the weight by bending the lower arm up toward the chest, turning the palm of the hand toward the chest as the weight is raised (figure 8.10). Exhale during the lifting phase.

d. Slowly lower the weight to the starting position with the palm facing inward again. Inhale during the lowering phase.

e. Complete 5 to 10 repetitions and repeat the exercise with the opposite arm.

Figure 8.10 Seated biceps curls with hand weight.

■ DOUBLE BICEPS CURLS WITH ADDED BALANCE COMPONENT

Muscles Targeted

Biceps and abdominals.

a. Sit tall and in the middle of a balance ball with the feet flat on the floor and hip-width apart. The resistance band should be positioned beneath the feet with equal lengths of the band wrapped around each hand or grip handles (figure 8.11).

b. Begin with the arms in an extended position. Inhale.

c. Slowly bend the forearms toward the shoulders, turning the palms upward without bending the wrists. Keep the elbows tight against the body throughout the lifting phase. Exhale as the band is lifted.

d. Pause, then slowly return the band to the starting position. Inhale as the band is lowered.

e. Complete 5 to 10 repetitions.

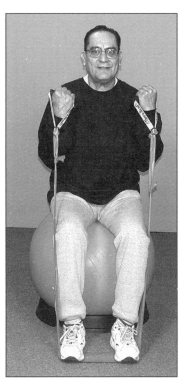

Figure 8.11 Seated double biceps curls with resistance band.

■ STANDING BICEPS CURLS WITH RESISTANCE BAND

Muscles Targeted

Muscles in the front of the arms and wrists.

a. Loop one end of the resistance band around the foot (figure 8.12).

b. Wrap the other end of the band around the hand or grip handles and let the arm hang loosely at the side. Inhale.

c. Slowly bend the forearm toward the shoulder, turning the palm upward without bending the wrist. Keep the elbow tucked against the body as the band is raised. Exhale during this phase.

d. Pause, then slowly return the band to the starting position.

e. Complete 5 to 10 repetitions and then repeat the exercise with the opposite arm.

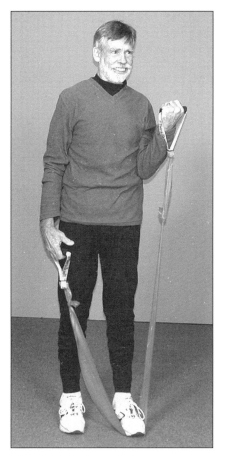

Figure 8.12 Standing biceps curls with resistance band.

■ SEATED PRESS-UPS

Muscles Targeted

Muscles in the elbows, arms, chest, and back.

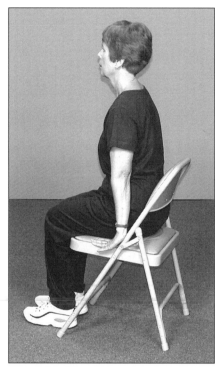

a.   Sit tall with the lower back pressed firmly against the backrest of a sturdy chair (figure 8.13). The shoulders should be relaxed and level.

b.   Tuck in the abdomen and chin and focus the eyes on a target directly in front and at eye level.

c.   Grasp the sides of the chair next to the hips. Inhale.

d.   Slowly lift the body while keeping the back straight. Exhale as the body is lifted.

e.   Hold the position for 5 to 10 seconds, breathing evenly.

f.   Slowly return to a seated position. Repeat the exercise 5 to 10 times.

Figure 8.13   Seated press-ups.

■ PALM SQUEEZES

Muscles Targeted

Muscles in the hands and wrists.

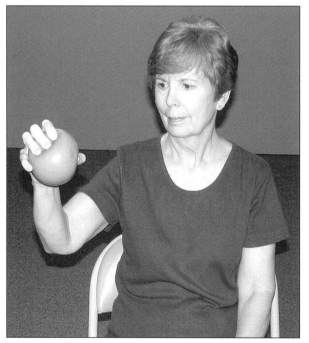

a.   This exercise can be performed in a seated or standing position. The elbows should be at the sides and flexed to 90°.

b.   Grasp a soft ball or object with the hand (figure 8.14). Inhale. Begin squeezing the object firmly. Exhale during the squeezing motion.

c.   Maintain the squeeze for 5 seconds. Complete 5 to 10 repetitions with the same hand before repeating the exercise with the other hand.

Figure 8.14   Palm squeezes.

Table 8.1 Upper Body Strength and Endurance Exercises at a Glance

Exercise	Muscles targeted	Position	Accessories
1. Shoulder shrugs	Upper back and neck	Seated/standing	Hand weights
2. Back extensions	Upper back and shoulders	Seated/standing	
3. Back and arm extensions	Upper back and shoulders	Seated/standing	Wrist weights
4. Side bends	Upper and middle back, shoulders, arms	Seated/standing	Hand weights
5. Chest presses	Chest, shoulders, arms	Seated/standing	Resistance band
6. Horizontal pulls	Upper and middle back, shoulders, arms	Seated/standing	Resistance band
7. Ball lifts	Upper, middle, lower back, shoulders, arms, abdominals	Seated	Weighted ball (1-2 kg), Dyna-Disc, balance ball
8. Diagonal arm extensions	Shoulders, upper and middle back, abdominals	Seated/standing	Resistance band
9. Partner push-pulls	Shoulders, upper and middle back, chest, abdominals	Seated	Resistance bands (2)
10. Standing triceps extensions	Elbows, arms, upper back	Standing	Chair, hand weight
11. Triceps extensions	Elbows, arms	Seated/standing	Chair, resistance band
12. Biceps curls	Front of upper arms, wrists	Seated/standing	Hand weight(s), chair
13. Double biceps curls	Front of upper arms, abdominals	Seated/standing	Resistance band, chair
14. Seated press-ups	Elbows, arms, chest, back	Seated	Chair
15. Palm squeezes	Hand and wrist	Seated/standing	Soft ball/object, chair

Note: Many of the above strength and endurance exercises can be performed with an added balance component: seated—Dyna-Disc or stability ball (with or without holder); standing—foam balance pad, rocker board.

Selected Lower Body Strength Exercises

■ WALL SQUATS

Muscles Targeted

Quadriceps and muscles in the hips, back, and abdomen.

    a.   Start in a standing position with the back against a wall and the feet at a distance of 12 to 24 inches from the wall and hip-width apart. Make sure the floor beneath has a nonslip surface.

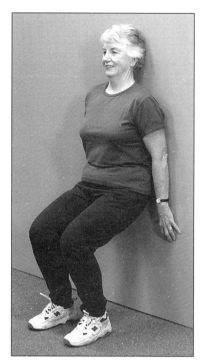

b. Stand with the hips and buttocks slightly tucked and the shoulders relaxed.

c. Slowly slide the back down the wall almost to a sitting position (figure 8.15). The knees should be behind or directly above the ankles. Exhale as the body is lowered.

d. Hold the position for 5 to 10 seconds while breathing evenly, then slowly return to the starting position.

e. Repeat the exercise 5 to 10 times.

Caution: Keep the knee angle of the squat greater than 90° if the participant has particularly weak quadriceps or pain in the knees.

Figure 8.15 Wall squats.

■ SIT-TO-STANDING SQUATS

Muscles Targeted

Quadriceps and muscles in the hips, back, and abdomen.

a. Sit tall while pressing the lower back firmly against the backrest of a chair. Tuck in the abdomen and chin and hold the head erect with the eyes directed forward. The feet should be flat on the floor and hip-width apart. Inhale.

b. Stand up from the chair, lifting the body about two-thirds of the way up (figure 8.16). Exhale as the body is lifted.

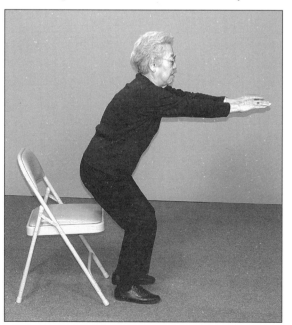

c. Keep the back straight and the knees slightly behind or directly above the ankles.

d. Hold the position for 3 to 5 seconds and then slowly return to the original seated position.

e. Repeat the exercise 5 to 10 times.

Figure 8.16 Sit-to-standing squat.

■ DYNA-DISC THIGH SQUEEZES

Muscles Targeted

Quadriceps, adductor muscles in the hips, back, and abdomen.

a. Perform the sit-to-standing squat exercise described earlier but place a Dyna-Disc between the knees.

b. Rise from the chair while squeezing the Dyna-Disc between the knees (figure 8.17). Exhale during the rising phase of the squat. Hold the position for 3 to 5 seconds.

c. Return to a seated position while keeping the Dyna-Disc between the knees. Inhale.

d. Repeat the exercise 5 to 10 times.

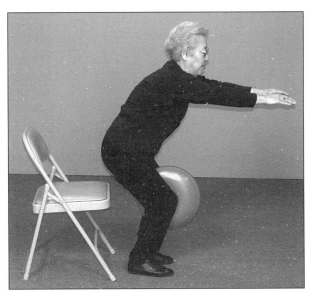

Figure 8.17 Dyna-Disc thigh squeezes.

■ STANDING LEG CURLS WITH ANKLE WEIGHTS

Muscles Targeted

Hamstrings and calf muscles.

a. Stand with the feet shoulder-width apart. Hold onto the back of a chair and stand tall. Inhale.

b. Slowly bend one knee, raising the lower leg behind you to form a 90° angle (figure 8.18). Do not allow the thigh of the leg with the knee being flexed to move behind the other thigh. Exhale as the knee is flexed.

c. Return the leg slowly to the starting position. Repeat the exercise 5 to 10 times with each leg.

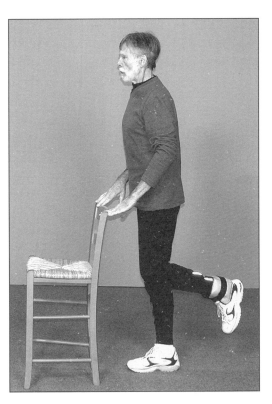

Figure 8.18 Standing leg curls.

■ SEATED LEG EXTENSIONS

Muscles Targeted

Muscles in the abdomen, hips, and legs.

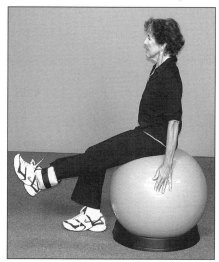

Figure 8.19 Seated leg extensions with ankle weight.

a. Sit tall on a ball or chair, and press the lower back firmly against the backrest of a chair. The abdomen and chin should be tucked in, the head erect, and the eyes directed forward. Inhale.

b. Hold onto the side of the ball and tighten the muscles in the leg.

c. Extend one leg and raise it to an angle of approximately 90° to the floor (figure 8.19). Flex the ankle and point the toes toward the ceiling as the leg is raised. Exhale during the lifting phase.

d. Slowly lower the leg to the starting position. Exhale as the leg is lowered.

e. Complete 5 to 10 repetitions before repeating the exercise with the opposite leg.

f. Add an ankle weight to increase resistance once the movement can be performed correctly and 10 repetitions successfully completed with each leg.

■ STANDING FLEXION AND EXTENSION

Muscles Targeted

Muscles in the hips and legs.

a. Stand upright with the feet together and hold onto the side of a chair or a wall for support. Inhale.

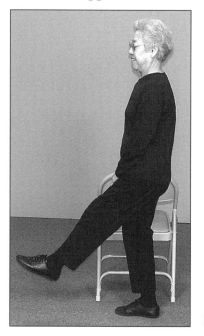

b. Slowly raise and extend one leg in a forward direction (figure 8.20). Exhale as the leg is raised.

c. Inhale and lower the leg back to the floor; pause momentarily before extending the leg in a backward direction. Exhale as the leg is moved backward.

d. Return the leg to the starting position. Inhale as the leg is lowered.

e. Avoid bending at the hips by not raising the leg too high in either direction.

f. Complete five repetitions with the same leg before repeating the exercise with the other leg.

g. Add ankle weights to increase resistance if correct form is being used during the exercise.

Figure 8.20 Standing flexion.

■ LATERAL LEG LIFTS

Muscles Targeted

Hip abductors and adductors, leg muscles.

a. Stand with the feet together and hold onto a wall or chair for support. Shift weight onto one leg. Inhale.

b. Slowly raise the other leg out to the side, leading with the heel (figure 8.21). Exhale as the leg is raised.

c. Slowly return the leg to a centered position. Inhale as the leg is lowered.

d. Complete five repetitions with the same leg before repeating the exercise with the opposite leg.

e. Add ankle weights to increase resistance if correct form is being used during the exercise.

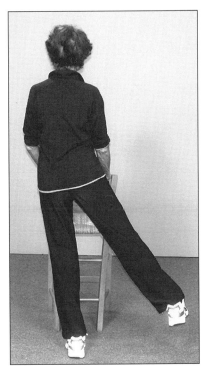

Figure 8.21 Lateral leg lifts.

■ STANDING FORWARD LUNGE

Muscles Targeted

Quadriceps, muscles in the hips, legs, and ankles.

a. Stand with the feet shoulder-width apart and hold onto a chair. Tuck in the abdomen and chin, and keep the head erect and the eyes directed forward. The knees should be slightly flexed. Inhale.

b. Position one foot slightly behind the other and raise the heel (figure 8.22).

c. Slowly flex the back knee toward the floor while also flexing the forward knee. Exhale as the knees are flexed.

d. Pause, then slowly return to the starting position.

e. Repeat the exercise with the opposite leg.

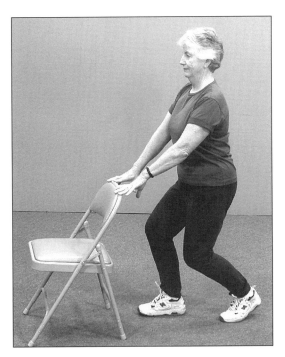

Figure 8.22 Standing forward lunge.

■ SEATED HIP FLEXION

Muscles Targeted
Hip muscles.

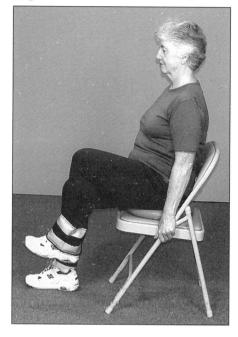

a. Sit with the knees shoulder-width apart.

b. Slowly lift one knee, keeping the upper body erect (figure 8.23).

c. Pause, then slowly lower the leg.

d. Complete 5 to 10 repetitions with the same leg, then repeat the exercise using the other leg.

e. Have participants sit on a Dyna-Disc or balance ball to further challenge balance.

f. This exercise can be performed with or without weights.

Figure 8.23 Seated hip flexion with ankle weights and added balance component.

■ HEEL RAISES

Muscles Targeted
Calf muscles.

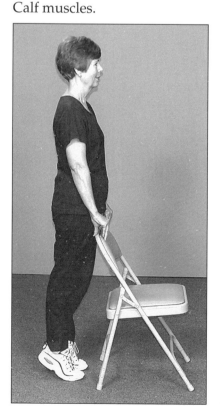

a. Stand tall with the feet flat on the floor and hip-width apart. Hold onto the back of a chair or a wall for additional support. The head should be erect with the eyes directed forward. Inhale.

b. Slowly lift both heels off the floor (figure 8.24). Exhale as the heels lift.

c. Hold the position for 5 to 10 seconds, breathing evenly, then slowly lower the heels to the floor.

d. Repeat the exercise 10 times.

e. Add ankle weights for greater resistance.

Figure 8.24 Heel raises.

■ TOE RAISES

Muscles Targeted

Shin muscles.

   a. Stand tall with the feet flat on the floor and hip-width apart. Hold onto a chair or wall for extra support. Inhale.

   b. Slowly raise the toes off the floor until weight is on the heels only (figure 8.25). Exhale as the toes rise from the floor.

   c. Hold the position for 5 to 10 seconds, breathing evenly, then slowly lower the toes to the floor.

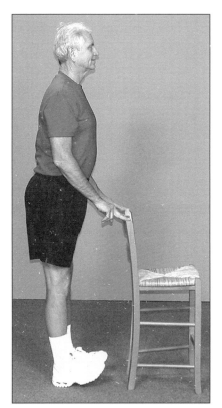

Figure 8.25 Toe raises.

■ FOOT PRESSES

Muscles Targeted

Muscles in the shins, ankles, and feet.

   a. In a seated position, flex the ankle of one foot and place the heel of the other foot on top of the flexed foot (figure 8.26). Inhale.

   b. Slowly push the flexed foot down toward the floor with the heel of the opposite foot. Resist lowering of the flexed foot by continuing to pull the toes of that foot back toward the shin. Exhale.

   c. Complete five repetitions before performing the exercise with the other foot.

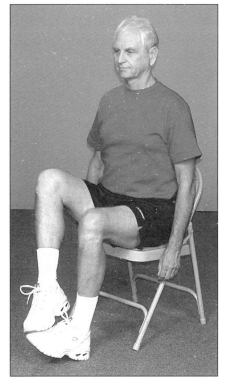

Figure 8.26 Foot presses.

Selected Foot- and Toe-Strengthening Exercises

This final set of exercises is best performed in a seated position with the shoes and socks removed.

■ TOE POINTING AND FLEXION

Muscles Targeted

Plantarflexors and dorsiflexors.

  a. Sit upright toward the front edge of a chair, keeping the trunk erect.
  b. Wrap a resistance band once around the right foot, keeping the left knee flexed and the right knee extended.
  c. Maintaining the tension on the band, slowly point and flex the toes (figure 8.27).
  d. Complete 5 to 10 repetitions before performing the exercise with the opposite leg.

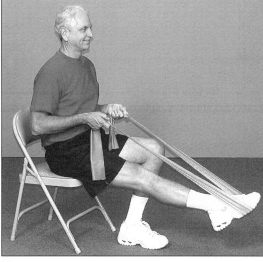
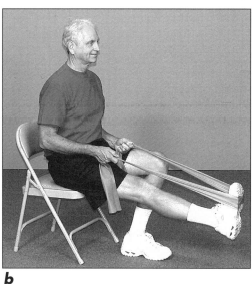

a　　　　　　　　　　　　　　　　　**b**

Figure 8.27　Point *(a)* and flex *(b)* toes.

Muscles Targeted

Muscles of the feet and toes.

  a. In a seated position, slowly raise the heel of one foot and hold for 5 seconds (figure 8.28a).
  b. Continue lifting the heel until the tips of the toes are touching the floor (figure 8.28b).

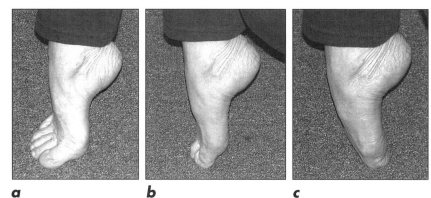

a　　　　　　　　　**b**　　　　　　　　　**c**

Figure 8.28
Toe raise *(a),*
point *(b),* and
curl *(c).*

c. Hold the position for 5 seconds.

d. Gently curl the toes under and hold for 5 seconds (figure 8.28c).

e. Reverse the movement sequence and repeat.

f. This is a good exercise for individuals with hammertoes or toe cramps.

■ TOWEL SCRUNCHES

Muscles Targeted

Muscles of the ankles, feet, and toes.

a. Place a small towel on the floor and pull it toward you, using only the toes (figure 8.29).

b. Increase the resistance by putting a weight on the end of the towel.

c. Relax and repeat the exercise three times before repeating it with the opposite foot.

d. This is a good exercise for individuals with hammertoes, toe cramps, or pain in balls of the feet.

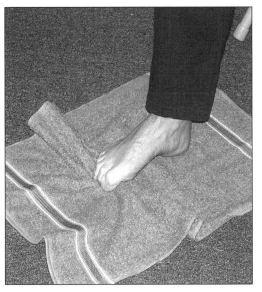

Figure 8.29 Towel scrunches.

■ MARBLE PICK-UP

Muscles Targeted

Muscles of the feet and toes.

a. Place 10 marbles on the floor. Use the toes to pick up one marble at a time and place it in a small bowl (figure 8.30).

b. Continue until all marbles have been retrieved.

c. This is a good exercise for individuals with hammertoes, toe cramps, or pain in the balls of the feet.

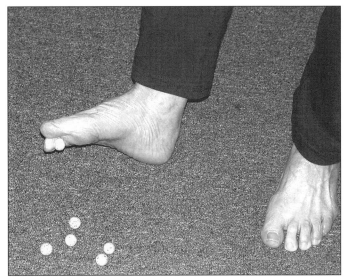

Figure 8.30 Marble pick-up.

Table 8.2   Lower Body Strength and Endurance Exercises at a Glance

Exercise	Muscles targeted	Position	Accessories
1. Wall squats	Front of thighs, hips, back, abdominals	Standing	Small balance ball
2. Sit-to-standing squats	Front of thighs, hips, back, abdominals	Seated	Chair
3. Dyna-Disc thigh squeezes	Front of thighs, adductors, back, abdominals	Seated	Chair, Dyna-Disc
4. Standing leg curls	Back of thighs, calves	Standing	Ankle weights, chair
5. Seated leg extensions	Abdominals, hips, and legs	Seated	Ankle weights
6. Standing flexion and extension	Hips and legs	Standing	Ankle weights, chair
7. Lateral leg lifts	Hip abductors/adductors, legs	Standing	Ankle weights, chair
8. Standing forward lunge	Front of thighs, hips, legs, ankles	Standing	Hand weights
9. Seated hip flexion	Hip muscles	Seated	Ankle weights
10. Heel raises	Calves, feet, toes	Standing	Ankle weights, chair
11. Toe raises	Shins	Standing	Chair
12. Foot presses	Shins, ankles, feet	Seated	Chair
13. Toe pointing and flexion	Ankle muscles	Seated	Ankle weights
14. Toe raise, point, and curl	Feet and toes	Seated	Chair
15. Towel scrunches	Feet and toes	Seated/standing	Towel, weighted object, chair
16. Marble pick-up	Feet and toes	Seated	Marbles

Note: Many of the above strength and endurance exercises can be performed with an added balance component: seated—Dyna-Disc or stability ball (with or without holder); standing—foam balance pad, rocker board.

Summary

Maintaining adequate levels of muscle strength and endurance is important for balance and mobility. Despite the age-related declines observed in absolute muscle strength and power, much can be done to offset the losses by having your clients engage in many different strength and endurance activities of increasing difficulty. As performance improves, the amount of resistance and the number of repetitions performed per set are increased. Finally, many of the strength and endurance activities introduced in this chapter can be performed in a balance environment to further increase the challenge associated with the activity and also simulate the types of challenges that may be encountered in performance of daily activities.

TEST YOUR UNDERSTANDING

1. Men and women over the age of 60 lose muscle mass
   a. more slowly than younger adults
   b. at a rate of 0.5% to 1.0% per decade
   c. at a rate of 0.5% to 1.0% per year
   d. more quickly than muscle power
   e. at a rate of 2% per year

2. Strength exercises should be introduced into the class
   a. during the warm-up and before any flexibility exercises are performed
   b. during the cool-down when the muscles are warm
   c. after the dynamic flexibility component of the warm-up has been completed
   d. when a sufficient amount of postural stability has been achieved
   e. when class participants have reached a level of fatigue that will facilitate better attention to the strength and endurance activities

3. The level of resistance should be increased once class participants are able to
   a. complete three sets of 15 repetitions at a given weight
   b. complete one set of 15 repetitions at a given weight
   c. perform the activity in both seated and standing positions
   d. complete 10 repetitions successfully
   e. perform the activity using correct form

4. Which of the following strength activities would be most appropriate if the goal is to improve the older adult's lateral stability during gait?
   a. wall squats
   b. standing leg curls
   c. standing flexion and extension
   d. lateral leg lifts with ankle weights
   e. heel raises

5. Which of the following activities would be most suited to improving core stability as well as strength in a given muscle group?
   a. standing biceps curls
   b. ball lifts while seated on a balance ball
   c. forward lunge
   d. heel raises while seated on a balance ball
   e. leg extensions while seated on a chair with a backrest and a Dyna-Disc under the buttocks

6. During which phase of a strength activity should you encourage the participant to exhale?
   a. during the action phase of the activity
   b. before the start of the movement
   c. after the movement has been completed

d. before, during, and after the movement

e. at any time during the activity

7. It is most appropriate to adjust the knee angle while performing the wall squat if

a. the client has weak hamstring muscles

b. the client is very tall

c. the client has weak quadriceps muscles

d. the client is experiencing pain in the knees when performing the task

e. both c and d

8. Which additional muscle group is recruited when a client performs a sit-to-standing squat while holding a Dyna-Disc between the thighs?

a. hamstring muscles

b. hip adductor muscles

c. hip abductor muscles

d. quadriceps

e. rectus femoris

9. Which one of the following exercises would you select to improve quadriceps strength with the goal of improving walking?

a. forward lunge

b. standing leg curls with ankle weights

c. standing flexion and extension

d. standing lateral leg lifts

10. Which of the exercises below specifically targets the dorsiflexor and plantarflexor muscles of the feet?

a. towel scrunches

b. marble pick-up

c. point and flex toes

d. heel raises

PRACTICAL PROBLEMS

1. Develop a set of progressive strength and endurance activities for either Jane or Bill after a review of their baseline test results. List the muscle groups you think should be prioritized during this component of the program and provide a rationale for their selection.

2. Describe five strength and endurance activities you would add to the repertoire of activities already provided.

3. Describe how you would manipulate the performance of a given strength activity to emphasize muscle power as opposed to muscle strength.

9

Flexibility Training

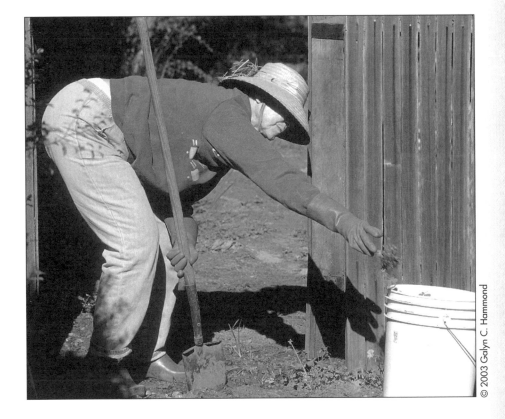

© 2003 Galyn C. Hammond

Objectives

After completing this chapter, you will be able to

- understand the contribution of joint and muscle flexibility to the multiple dimensions of balance and mobility,
- describe the age-associated changes in joint and muscle flexibility,
- develop a set of exercise progressions designed to improve upper and lower body joint and muscle flexibility, and
- incorporate flexibility exercises into a balance environment.

Similar to strength, joint range of motion (ROM) and muscle flexibility gradually decline with age. Specific losses of joint range of motion and muscle strength have been directly linked to the progression of various disabilities among older adults and a declining ability to perform basic and instrumental activities of daily living (Jette, Branch, & Berlin, 1990). More recently, Morey and colleagues (Morey, Pieper, & Cornoni-Huntley, 1998) have also shown that loss of flexibility in shoulder rotation and cervical and spinal rotation is directly related to functional limitations and increased susceptibility to falls among older adults in their 70s. Although declines in joint range of motion and muscle flexibility are inevitable, the rate at which the decline occurs is joint specific (Bell & Hoshizaki, 1981). For example, the loss of flexibility is more evident in the lower as opposed to upper extremity joints. The reduced flexibility observed in the lower body joints, in particular, has important implications for dynamic balance and functional mobility.

> The rate at which joint range of motion and muscle flexibility decline is joint specific.

The aging process results in increased stiffness in all joints of the body and the surrounding muscle tissues. Tendons, ligaments, joint capsules, fascia, and slow-twitch muscle fibers are all affected. Of particular importance is the significant loss of ROM at the ankle joint, especially among older women. Women between the ages of 55 and 85 lose as much as 50% of their ankle ROM, whereas men lose approximately 35% of their ankle ROM (Bandy & Sanders, 2001). Reductions in ankle range of motion, in particular, are likely to place the older adult at heightened risk for falling, especially while walking. Special attention should therefore be given to improving ankle flexibility during this component of the balance and mobility training program.

Age-related changes in muscle structure also lead to increased muscle stiffness and reduced tensile strength. The increase in muscle collagen (known to be very resistant to stretch) with age and the degeneration of elastin fibers (which are less resistant to stretch) contribute to this increased muscle stiffness (Holland, Tanaka, Shigematsu, & Nakagaichi, 2002). As a result, ballistic stretching routines should be avoided at all costs because of the likelihood of injuring older adult muscle. It is also recommended that older adults perform their stretching activities more slowly and maintain a given stretch for a longer duration (i.e., 30 to 60 seconds) once the internal temperature of the body and muscle tissue is sufficiently warm (Asp, 2000). Remember that the most effective stretching program will be one that is not only based on the individual needs of your older adult participants, but is performed regularly. Thus, you should encourage your participants to incorporate a stretching routine into their daily lives. Flexibility exercises should also be assigned as homework once correct form has been taught during class. Incorporating stretching activities into your classes will also be beneficial for older adult clients who are experiencing reduced ROM as a result of musculoskeletal or neuromuscular diseases (e.g., arthritis, Parkinson's disease, multiple sclerosis) A gentle stretching routine has also been shown to be beneficial for older adults who are experiencing chronic pain.

> Ballistic stretching routines should be avoided at all costs due to the likelihood of injury to older adult muscle tissue.

Be sure to review selected test results obtained during the preprogram assessment to determine which areas of the body are less flexible and therefore in need of additional attention. The results of the sit-and-reach and scratch test items, which test lower and upper body flexibility, respectively, on the Senior Fitness Test (Rikli & Jones, 2001) will be particularly helpful to you in deciding how to proceed with the flexibility component of your program. You should also note the level of joint flexibility demonstrated at the hip, knee, and ankle joints during performance of the 50-foot walk test. In addition to reviewing their test results, also review each client's medical history to determine whether you need to modify or delete certain exercises due to predisposing medical conditions or client concerns (e.g., frozen shoulder, osteoporosis).

When incorporating flexibility activities into your balance and mobility training program, consider the following guidelines, some of which have been established by the American College of Sports Medicine (1998):

- Avoid ballistic (bouncing) stretching exercises.
- Incorporate more multijoint, dynamic stretches during the warm-up phase of the class. The continuous contraction of muscles helps warm the muscle tissue and prepare it for subsequent exercise.
- Introduce movements and joint actions that mimic those to be performed later in the class, and progressively increase the range of motion with each repetition.
- Flexibility exercises should be performed two (for maintenance) to seven (to increase range) days per week based on individual needs.
- During static stretches, the stretched position should be maintained for 5 to 40 seconds (depending on which muscle or muscles are stretched). A hold time of 60 seconds may be preferable for certain muscle groups (e.g., hamstrings).
- The stretch should be repeated one to five times (depending on which muscle or muscle groups are being stretched).
- Gradually increase the range through which the muscle is stretched as tolerance increases.
- Have clients perform selected flexibility exercises while seated on a Dyna-Disc™ or balance ball to increase the balance challenge in later classes.
- Be systematic in your approach to performing flexibility exercises (e.g., top to toe, lower body during warm-up and upper body during cool-down).

Selected Neck and Upper Body Flexibility Exercises

■ SEATED CHIN-TO-CHEST

Muscles Targeted

Muscles in the back of the neck.

    a. Sit tall with the lower back pressed firmly against the backrest of a chair. Keep the shoulders relaxed and the chin tucked in so that the ears are directly above the shoulders (figure 9.1). The eyes should be focused on a target directly in front and at eye level. Inhale.

    b. Slowly tuck the chin toward the chest while exhaling.

    c. Hold the position for 5 to 10 seconds while breathing evenly.

    d. Inhale and raise the head back to the starting position, one vertebra at a time.

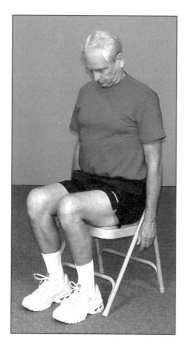

Added balance challenge: Perform the exercise while seated on a Dyna-Disc or balance ball.

Figure 9.1 Seated chin-to-chest.

■ NECK ROTATIONS

Muscles Targeted

Muscles in the back and sides of the neck.

a. Sit tall with the lower back pressed firmly against the backrest of a chair. Keep the shoulders relaxed and the chin tucked in and gently resting on the chest. The eyes should be focused on a target directly in front and at eye level. Inhale.

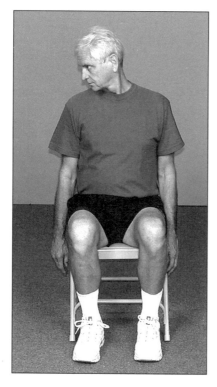

b. With the head in a comfortable position and the chin gently tucked in, slowly turn the chin up toward the right shoulder, then back across the chest and up toward the left shoulder (figure 9.2). Exhale during the rotation.

c. Keep the chin in contact with the chest throughout the rotation.

d. Repeat the exercise three to five times.

Added balance challenge: Perform the exercise while seated on a Dyna-Disc or balance ball or while standing behind a chair.

Figure 9.2 Seated neck rotations.

■ ASSISTED NECK SIDE STRETCH

Muscles Targeted

Muscles in the sides of the neck.

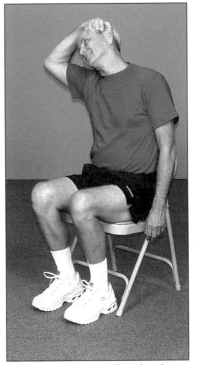

Figure 9.3 Assisted neck side stretch.

a. Sit tall with the lower back pressed firmly against the backrest of a chair. Keep the shoulders relaxed and the head erect, with the eyes focused on a target directly in front and at eye level. Inhale.

b. Slowly bend the head so the right earlobe moves toward the right shoulder. Bend the head as far down as is comfortable while reaching the left hand down toward the floor.

c. Reach the right hand up and over the head until it is resting on the left side of the head (figure 9.3). Use the weight of the hand to increase the stretch to the right side. Exhale as the head bends toward the shoulder.

d. Hold the position for 5 to 10 seconds, breathing evenly.

e. Inhale as the head moves back to the starting position. Repeat the stretch to the left side.

f. Perform the exercise three times to each side.

■ ASSISTED NECK FLEXION

Muscles Targeted

Muscles in the back of the neck, upper back, and shoulders.

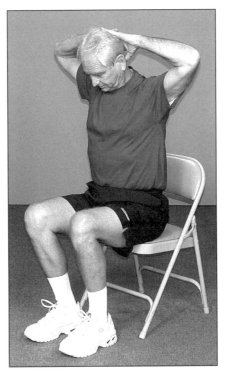

Figure 9.4 Assisted neck flexion.

a. Sit tall with the lower back pressed firmly against the backrest of a chair. Keep the shoulders relaxed and the head erect, with the eyes focused on a target directly in front and at eye level.

b. Position the fingers behind the head (figure 9.4). Inhale.

c. Gently move the chin toward the chest as the shoulders remain level, allowing the weight of the hands to increase the amount of stretch. Exhale during this phase of the stretch.

d. Do not allow the upper back or spine to lean forward during the stretch. The action must be isolated to the neck.

e. Hold the stretch for 5 to 10 seconds, breathing evenly.

f. Inhale as the head returns to the starting position.

g. Repeat the exercise 3 to 5 times.

■ TURTLE

Muscles Targeted

Muscles in the front and back of the neck.

a. This exercise can be performed while seated or standing.

b. Place the thumb side of the hands next to the ears, palms facing forward. Inhale.

c. Gently bring the head backward and past the thumbs (figure 9.5). Be sure to keep the chin level during the movement. Have participants imagine that they are sliding the chin along a tray.

d. Without pausing, move the head forward until it has passed the thumbs again.

e. Repeat 5 to 10 times in the forward and backward directions, breathing evenly throughout the exercise.

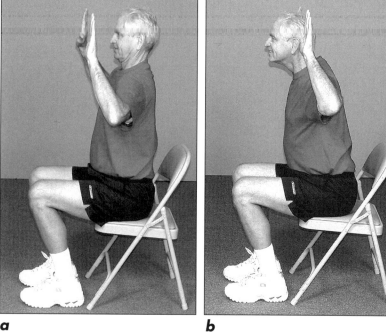

a   *b*

Figure 9.5 Turtle exercise: backward **(a)** and forward **(b)** movements.

■ SHOULDER ROLLS

Muscles Targeted

Muscles in the shoulders, upper back, and chest.

a. This exercise can be performed in a seated or standing position. Inhale before beginning the action.

b. Roll the shoulders up toward the ears and then backward and down as the shoulder blades are squeezed together (figure 9.6). Exhale during the downward phase of the movement.

c. Inhale as the shoulders move back up toward the ears for the start of the second repetition.

d. Repeat five times and then reverse the direction of the shoulder movement for an additional five repetitions.

Added balance challenge: Perform the exercise while seated on a Dyna-Disc or balance ball or while standing on a foam or moving surface (i.e., rocker board).

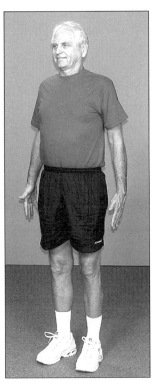

Figure 9.6 Shoulder rolls.

■ ARM CIRCLES

Muscles Targeted

Muscles in the upper back and chest.

a. This exercise can be performed in a seated or standing position.

b. Raise both arms out to the sides at shoulder height with palms facing upwards (figure 9.7). Inhale.

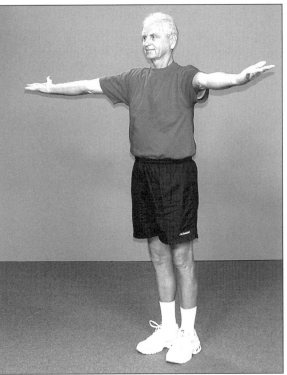

c. Slowly circle both arms backward and in a progressively larger arc with each repetition. Circle the arms backward 10 times, exhaling for two circles and then inhaling for the next two circles, and so on.

d. Pause momentarily, then reverse the direction, circling the arms forward 10 times while using the same breathing pattern.

Added balance challenge: Perform the exercise while seated on a Dyna-Disc or balance ball or while standing on a foam square.

Figure 9.7 Arm circles.

■ FINGER WALK

Muscles Targeted

Muscles in the chest and shoulders.

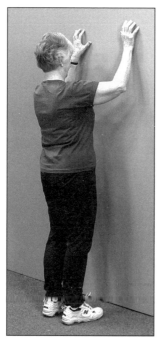

a. Stand tall and facing a wall such that the toes are almost touching. Keep the head erect and the eyes directed forward throughout the exercise.

b. Place the hands at waist level with the palms facing the wall and the fingertips in contact with wall. Inhale.

c. Walk both arms up the wall, leading with the fingertips, until the arms are as far above the head as is comfortable (figure 9.8). Exhale as the fingers are walked up the wall.

d. Inhale and walk the fingers back down the wall without pausing at the top.

e. Repeat the finger-walking exercise 10 times.

Figure 9.8   Finger walking.

■ FULL-BODY STRETCHES

Muscles Targeted

Muscles in the fingers, arms, shoulders, back, and abdomen.

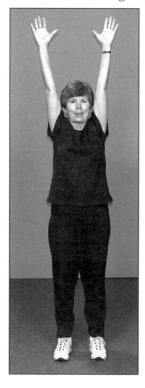

a. Stand tall with the feet shoulder-width apart. The abdomen and chin should be tucked in, with the head erect and the eyes directed forward. The shoulders should be relaxed. Inhale.

b. Slowly extend the arms up over the head to a comfortable height (figure 9.9). Exhale as the arms are lifted; inhale when the arms reach the highest point.

c. Stretch the right arm farther toward the ceiling than the left. Exhale during the upward stretch.

d. Pause and inhale, then stretch the left arm farther toward the ceiling than the right.

e. Repeat the exercise five times with each arm.

Figure 9.9   Full-body stretches.

■ CHEST STRETCHES

Muscles Targeted

Muscles in the front of the shoulders and upper chest.

a. This exercise can be performed while standing or while sitting sideways on a chair with no armrests.

b. Clasp the hands behind the back while maintaining a straight back (do not arch the back) (figure 9.10). Inhale.

c. Exhale as the arms are slowly raised up the back as far as is comfortable.

d. Hold the stretch for 15 to 30 seconds, breathing evenly throughout the hold.

e. Repeat the stretch twice.

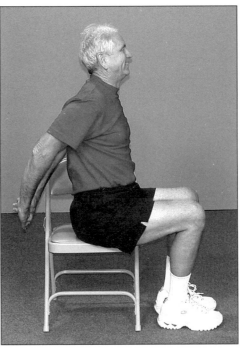

Figure 9.10 Chest stretches.

■ LATERAL SHOULDER STRETCHES

Muscles Targeted

Muscles in the shoulders.

a. This exercise can be performed while seated or standing.

b. Reach one arm across the front of the body and as close to shoulder height as is comfortable. Do not allow the shoulders to lift as the arm reaches across the body.

c. Reach the opposite arm under the outstretched arm and grasp it above the elbow (figure 9.11).

d. Slowly pull the elbow toward the body and slightly in the direction of the outstretched arm to increase the stretch. Exhale during the stretch.

e. Tension should be felt across the shoulders and back.

f. Hold the stretch for 15 to 30 seconds, then repeat the stretch to the opposite side.

g. Repeat the stretch twice to each side.

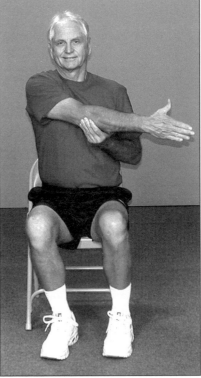

Figure 9.11 Lateral shoulder stretches.

■ WRIST CIRCLES

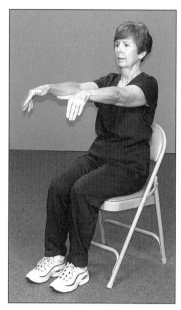

Muscles Targeted

Muscles in the wrists and hands.

    a. Sit tall with the lower back pressed firmly against the backrest of a chair.

    b. Extend and raise arms to shoulder height (figure 9.12).

    c. Begin slowly circling both wrists in a clockwise direction 5 to 10 times, then reverse the direction and repeat the exercise 5 to 10 times.

Figure 9.12 Wrist circles.

■ PALM-UP AND PALM-DOWN WRIST AND FINGER EXTENSIONS

Muscles Targeted

Muscles in the wrists, hands, and forearms.

    a. Sit tall with the lower back pressed firmly against the backrest of a chair. The shoulders should be relaxed, with the head erect and the eyes directed forward.

    b. Extend and raise one arm to shoulder height and flex the wrist so the palm is pointing up toward the ceiling (figure 9.13a). Inhale.

    c. With the other hand, gently press the back of the hand toward the body. Exhale as the hand is stretched.

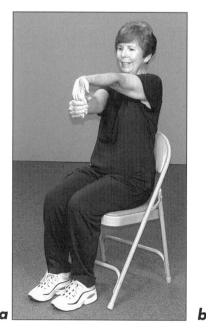
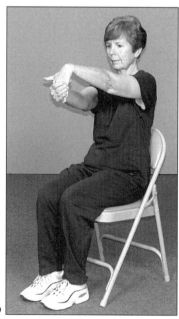

a   b

Figure 9.13 Palm-up *(a)* and palm-down *(b)* wrist and finger extensions.

d. Hold the position for 5 to 15 seconds, breathing evenly throughout the hold.

e. Repeat the exercise with the other hand.

f. Repeat this exercise with the palms facing down (extend and raise each arm to shoulder height with the palm facing down and the fingertips pointing up toward the ceiling) (figure 9.13b).

■ THUMB-TO-FINGER TOUCHES

Muscles Targeted

Muscles in the thumb and fingers.

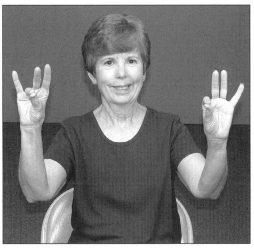

a. Sit tall with the lower back pressed firmly against the backrest of a chair. The shoulders should be relaxed, with the head erect and the eyes directed forward.

b. Open the palms of one or both hands and extend and spread the fingers.

c. Exaggerating each move, touch the tip of the thumb to each finger in sequential order (i.e., thumb to index finger, middle finger, ring finger, little finger) (figure 9.14).

Figure 9.14 Thumb-to-finger touches.

d. Return the thumb and finger to the original starting position before proceeding to the next finger.

e. Repeat the entire finger-touching sequence five times with each hand.

■ SEATED TRUNK TWIST

Muscles Targeted

Muscles on the side of the trunk.

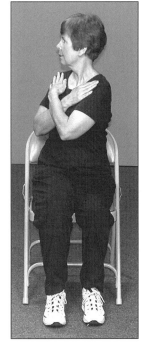

a. Sit tall with the lower back pressed firmly against the backrest of a chair. The shoulders should be relaxed, with the head erect and the eyes directed forward.

b. Fold the arms across the chest. Inhale.

c. Gently rotate the trunk to one side as far as is comfortable (figure 9.15). Exhale during the twisting motion. Hold the end position for 5 to 10 seconds, breathing evenly throughout the hold.

d. Slowly rotate the trunk as far to the opposite side as is comfortable. Exhale during the twisting motion.

e. Keep the hips facing forward throughout the exercise.

f. Repeat the exercise five times to each side.

Added balance challenge: Perform the exercise while seated on a Dyna-Disc or balance ball.

Figure 9.15 Seated trunk twist.

■ STANDING SIDE STRETCH

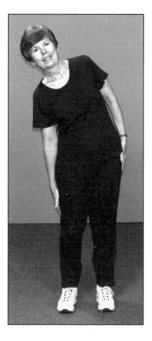

Muscles Targeted

Muscles on the side of the trunk.

a. Stand tall with the feet hip-width apart and the knees slightly bent. The abdomen and chin should be tucked in, the head erect, and the eyes directed forward. The arms should be hanging loosely at the sides. Inhale.

b. Gradually slide the right arm down toward the knee as far as is comfortable (figure 9.16). Keep the head aligned with the trunk during the downward stretch. Exhale as the arm slides down the leg.

c. Slowly return to the starting position, pause momentarily, and then repeat the exercise to the left side.

d. Repeat the exercise three to five times to each side.

Figure 9.16 Standing side stretch.

■ BOWING TO THE GODS

Muscles Targeted

Muscles in the shoulders, upper back, and arms.

a. Holding onto the top of a chair, step backward until the back and arms are extended (figure 9.17). Position the feet shoulder-width apart. Inhale.

b. Gradually tuck the head between the arms and push downward until tension is felt in the shoulders and upper back. Exhale during the stretch.

c. Hold the end position for 10 to 15 seconds, breathing evenly throughout the hold.

d. Relax and walk the feet back toward the chair and roll up slowly.

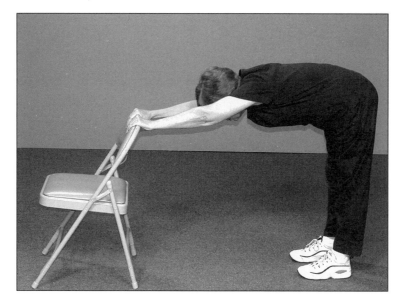

Figure 9.17 Bowing to the gods.

Selected Lower Body Flexibility Exercises

■ HIP ABDUCTOR STRETCH

Muscles Targeted

Hip abductor muscles and muscles in the thighs, sides of the trunk, and upper arms.

a. Stand tall and face sideways to a wall. Keep the abdomen and chin tucked in, the head erect, and the eyes directed forward.

b. Raise the arm closest to the wall above the head and rest it against the wall (figure 9.18). The opposite arm should also be extended and resting against the body. Inhale.

c. Cross the foot closest to the wall behind the ankle of the opposite foot. The knee of the opposite leg should be slightly bent.

d. Slowly lean into the wall, keeping the leg closest to the wall extended during the lean.

e. The stretch should be felt on the outside of the thigh closest to the wall. Exhale during the lean.

f. Hold the stretch for 15 to 30 seconds, breathing evenly throughout the hold. Uncross the leg and turn to face the opposite side. Repeat the stretch.

g. Repeat the exercise three to five times on each side.

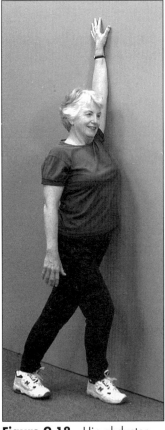

Figure 9.18 Hip abductor stretch.

■ FORWARD LUNGE

Muscles Targeted

Muscles in the front of the thigh.

a. Stand tall with the feet parallel and hip-width apart. Step forward (i.e., lunge) as far as feels comfortable and stable with one foot and bend the knee so that it is aligned with the ankle joint. Use a chair if needed (figure 9.19).

b. Lower the knee of the back leg slowly to the floor. Inhale.

c. Straighten the back leg and slowly lean forward, maintaining a straight back throughout the stretch.

d. Hold the position for 15 to 30 seconds before returning to the starting position. Repeat the stretch with the opposite leg.

e. Repeat the exercise three times on each side.

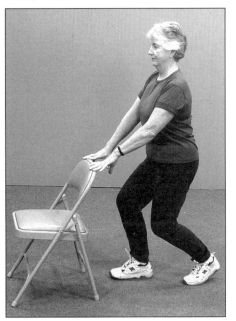

Figure 9.19 Forward lunge.

■ HAMSTRINGS STRETCH

Muscles Targeted

Muscles in the back of the thighs (hamstrings).

  a. This exercise can be performed in a seated or standing position (figure 9.20). If performed in a standing position, the back of a chair positioned against a wall can be used for added support.

  b. Stand tall with the abdomen and chin tucked in, the head erect, and the eyes directed forward. The feet should be parallel and positioned hip-width apart.

  c. Extend the left leg forward, maintaining a slight bend in the knee, and place the heel on the floor with the toes pointing up toward the ceiling.

  d. Bend the right knee, place the hands on the thigh of the extended leg (or on the back of the chair), and slowly lean forward from the hips. Keep the back straight during the forward lean.

  e. Continue leaning forward until gentle tension is felt in the back of the extended leg.

  f. Hold the position for 15 to 30 seconds and repeat with the opposite leg forward.

  g. Be sure to keep your back straight rather than rounded.

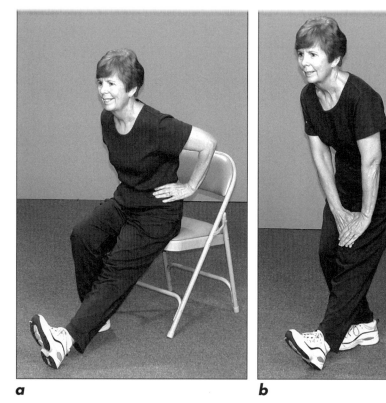

a   *b*

Figure 9.20
Hamstrings stretch in seated *(a)* and standing *(b)* positions.

■ STANDING CALF STRETCH

Muscles Targeted

Muscles in the back of the lower leg.

  a. Stand tall at approximately arm's length from a chair or wall (figure 9.21). Place both hands on the wall with the palms at shoulder height, or on the back of the chair. Position one leg forward with the knee bent and aligned with the ankle of the same leg. The heel should be in contact with the floor.

b. Extend the other leg as far behind the body as possible, with the heel in contact with the floor. Inhale.

c. Lean slowly into the chair, increasing the angle of knee flexion of the front leg. Keep the heel of the back foot in contact with the floor throughout the forward lean.

d. Hold the stretch for 15 to 30 seconds, breathing evenly throughout the hold.

e. Relax and return the front leg to the starting position before repeating the exercise on the other side.

f. Repeat the exercise three times on each side.

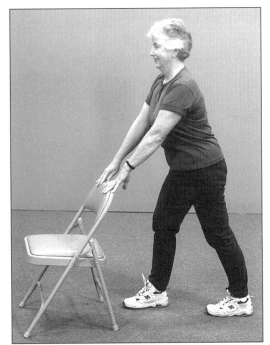

Figure 9.21 Standing calf stretch.

■ ANKLE CIRCLES

Muscles Targeted

Muscles of the ankle and foot.

a. Sit tall with the lower back pressed firmly against the back of a chair. The head should be erect, with the eyes directed forward.

b. Raise one leg off the floor and begin slowly circling the ankle in a clockwise direction (figure 9.22). Make five increasingly larger circles with the ankle before reversing the direction for the same number of circles.

c. Lower the leg to the floor and repeat the exercise with the opposite leg raised off the floor.

d. Repeat the exercise three times on each side.

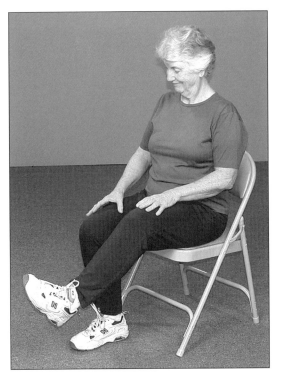

Figure 9.22 Ankle circles.

■ GOLF BALL ROLL

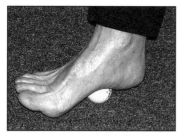

Figure 9.23 Golf ball roll.

Muscles Targeted

Muscles of the foot, particularly the arch.

a. Sit tall with the lower back pressed firmly against the backrest of a chair.

b. Place a golf ball under the ball of the right foot and begin rolling it forward and back for a period of 2 minutes (figure 9.23). Breathe evenly throughout the exercise.

c. Repeat with the other foot for the same amount of time.

d. This is a good exercise for individuals with plantar fasciitis (heel pain), arch strain, or toe cramps.

Table 9.1 Flexibility Exercises at a Glance

Exercise	Muscles targeted	Type of stretch
Seated chin-to-chest	Back of neck	Static
Neck rotations	Back and side of neck	Dynamic
Assisted neck side stretch	Side of neck	Static
Assisted neck flexion	Back of neck, upper back, shoulders	Static
Turtle	Back and front of neck, upper back	Dynamic
Shoulder rolls	Shoulders, upper back, chest	Dynamic
Arm circles	Upper back, chest	Dynamic
Finger walk	Chest, shoulders	Dynamic
Full-body stretches	Fingers, arms, shoulders, back, abdomen	Dynamic
Chest stretches	Front of shoulders, upper chest	Static
Lateral shoulder stretches	Shoulders	Static
Wrist circles	Wrists, hands	Dynamic
Palm-down wrist/finger extensions	Wrists, hands, forearms	Static
Palm-up wrist/finger extensions	Wrists, hands, forearms	Static
Thumb-to-finger touches	Thumbs, fingers	Dynamic
Trunk twist	Side of torso	Static
Standing side stretch	Side of torso	Dynamic
Bowing to the gods	Shoulders, upper back, arms	Static
Hip abductor stretch	Hips, thighs, side of torso, upper arms	Static
Forward lunge	Thigh	Static
Hamstrings stretch	Back of thighs	Static
Standing calf stretch	Back of lower legs	Static
Ankle circles	Ankle, foot	Dynamic
Golf ball roll	Feet	Dynamic

Note: Dynamic stretches are best suited to the warm-up section of the class, whereas static stretches should be incorporated into the cool-down component.

Summary

Each of the exercises presented in this chapter is designed to improve the range of motion in joints and muscles that are required for balance and mobility. Despite the age-related declines in flexibility that occur, much can be done to improve your client's overall level of flexibility. Whereas the dynamic stretching activities presented in this chapter are appropriate for the warm-up component of the class, the static stretching activities will be better suited to the cool-down phase when the internal temperature of the body and muscles is at its warmest. Correct form should be emphasized during the performance of each flexibility exercise, as well as the need to avoid stretching to the point of discomfort or pain. The regular inclusion of flexibility exercises in each class session, combined with daily home exercise, will help your older adult clients improve their overall level of flexibility so they can continue to perform the essential activities of daily living as well as other recreational activities.

TEST YOUR UNDERSTANDING

1. Age-associated declines in flexibility are more evident in
    a. upper body joints and muscles
    b. lower body joints and muscles
    c. muscles in the cervical region
    d. the shoulders

2. Increased muscle stiffness with age is the result of
    a. an increase in muscle collagen and elastin fibers
    b. reduced muscle mass
    c. reduced muscle collagen and an increase in elastin fibers
    d. degeneration of elastin fibers and an increase in muscle collagen
    e. no known reason

3. How much does ankle range of motion decline in women between 55 and 85 years of age?
    a. 10%
    b. 35%
    c. 50%
    d. 65%
    e. 75%

4. Which of the following preprogram assessments will be helpful in deciding what type of flexibility exercises to use to improve range of motion in the upper body?
    a. Fullerton Advanced Balance Scale
    b. Multidirectional Reach Test
    c. scratch test
    d. sit-and-reach test
    e. M-CTSIB

5. Which types of flexibility exercises are best suited for inclusion in the warm-up component of a class?
   a. static stretches
   b. ballistic stretches
   c. dynamic stretches
   d. a combination of static and dynamic stretches
   e. a combination of ballistic and dynamic stretches

6. Which of the following flexibility exercises targets muscles in the side of the neck?
   a. seated chin-to-chest
   b. neck rotations
   c. assisted neck flexion
   d. assisted neck side stretch
   e. turtle

7. Which of the following flexibility exercises is most appropriate for improving stride length during gait?
   a. bowing to the gods
   b. hip abductor stretch
   c. forward lunge
   d. ankle circles
   e. golf ball roll

8. The flexibility exercise called bowing to the gods is specifically designed to improve flexibility in which of the following muscle groups?
   a. upper back and arms
   b. hamstrings
   c. quadriceps and calf muscles
   d. chest and shoulder muscles
   e. hip and ankle muscles

9. Which of the following exercises is specifically designed to increase range of motion in the ankles and feet?
   a. calf stretch
   b. ankle circles
   c. bowing to the gods
   d. forward lunge
   e. golf ball roll

10. How often should flexibility exercises be performed if the goal is to maintain the gains made in range of motion?
    a. three to five times per week
    b. twice a week
    c. every day
    d. twice a day
    e. once per week

PRACTICAL PROBLEMS

1. Develop a list of the flexibility exercises you would select for Jane and Bill based on the results of their sit-and-reach and back scratch tests performed during the Senior Fitness Test. Identify the flexibility exercises you would select that specifically target the key joints and muscles required for good functional mobility.

2. Design a home exercise program for Jane or Bill that targets the joints and muscles most in need of improved range of motion. List the order of exercises, how long each stretch position should be held, and the number of repetitions to be performed.

PART III

Implementing the FallProof Program

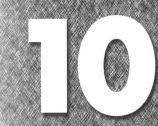

Setting the Stage for Learning

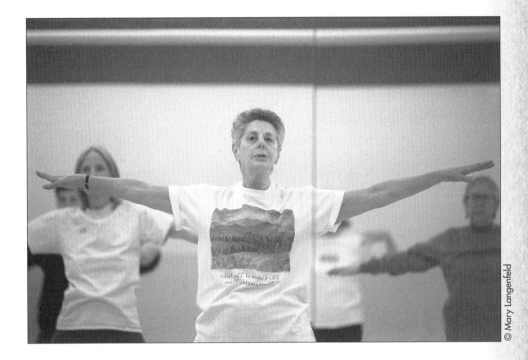

Objectives

After completing this chapter, you will be able to

- identify and apply basic motor learning principles for optimal participant learning and retention,
- understand when and how to apply basic motor learning principles based on each participant's stage of learning,
- design tasks and practice environments that progress participants from a more conscious to less conscious control of balance, and
- understand what type of feedback to present at each stage of learning and how often it should be presented for optimal learning and transfer.

Now that you are familiar with each of the major skill components that make up the FallProof™ program, I want to introduce three motor learning principles that should guide you as you implement each of the exercise components associated with this program. The judicious application of each of the motor learning principles described in this chapter will set the stage for optimal learning and transfer. Although many more principles of motor learning are relevant to effective implementation of the FallProof program, any discussion of them is beyond the scope of this book. Several excellent textbooks on motor learning can be consulted if you wish to learn more about this area of study (Magill, 2001; Rose, 1997; Schmidt & Wrisberg, 2000). The three topics discussed in this chapter include how best to introduce new skills to your participants, how to organize the practice environment effectively, and how to provide feedback to your clients in a meaningful way.

Understanding the Stages of Learning

Several motor learning models have been developed that attempt to describe the cognitive and behavioral changes occurring in the learner at each hypothetical stage of learning (Fitts & Posner, 1967; Vereikjen, 1991; Gentile, 1972). Although each stages-of-learning model provides a unique perspective of the learning process, the model presented in this chapter is one specifically designed to help the practitioner better understand not only what the learner is attempting to do in each of the learning stages described, but also how the practitioner can manipulate the practice environment to facilitate that learning (Gentile, 1972, 1987, 2000). Gentile's model describes two stages of learning. The primary focus of the learner during the first stage is to develop an "understanding of the goal of the movement," whereas in the second stage, the learner's focus shifts to determining how best to "adapt the movement pattern acquired in the first learning stage to the specific demands of the environment in which the skill will ultimately be performed." Let's consider each learning stage in more detail.

> According to Gentile, the learner's major focus during the first stage of learning is to develop an understanding of the goal of the movement, whereas in the second stage, the focus shifts to one of determining how best to adapt the acquired movement pattern to the demands of the performance environment.

regulatory conditions—Characteristics of the performance environment that directly influence how a skill is performed.

nonregulatory conditions—Characteristics of the performance environment that do not or should not influence how a skill is performed.

Getting the idea of the movement is the first task that confronts learners after seeing a new motor skill modeled or hearing it described for the first time. To do that, they must begin to explore how the various parts of the movement pattern must be coordinated to achieve the goal. As a result of trial-and-error practice, learners begin to acquire the basic movement pattern by discriminating between those performance characteristics that determine how the movement is to be performed and others that are present but do not influence how the skill is to be performed. Gentile describes those characteristics of the performance environment that directly influence how a skill is to be performed as the **regulatory conditions,** whereas those characteristics of the performance environment that do not or should not influence how a skill is performed are called the **nonregulatory conditions.**

For example, an older adult who is attempting to reach for an object while standing on a half-foam roller must learn how to coordinate the movements of the body and the arms to retrieve the object successfully while standing on a surface that is narrower than the length of the feet. The regulatory features associated with this task

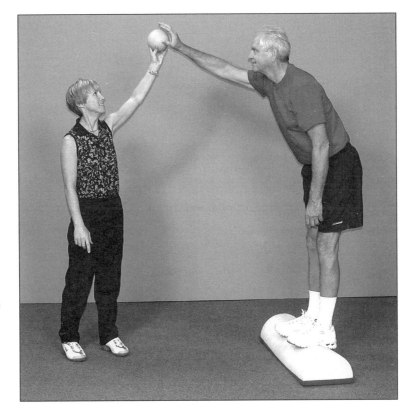

Figure 10.1 The regulatory conditions associated with this task include the size and shape of the object, the distance and height of its position relative to the body, and the width and compliance of the support surface.

include such things as the size and shape of the object, the distance and height it is positioned at relative to the body, and the width and compliance of the raised surface on which the individual is standing (figure 10.1). Conversely, the nonregulatory conditions might include such things as the color of the object to be retrieved, the color of the clothing worn by the person holding the object, or, if the task were taking place in a group setting, the position or movements of other people in the room.

As practice continues, the learner begins to develop a movement pattern that leads to successful completion of the task on most attempts but with a great deal of effort still being expended. At a cognitive level, the learner clearly understands the idea of the movement now despite being unable to perform the task in a consistent and efficient manner on all practice attempts. In the second stage of learning, the learner's goal shifts to one of adapting the acquired movement pattern to the specific demands of the environment in which the task is to be performed. Depending on the type of motor skill being learned, the goal may be one of either **"fixating" or "diversifying" the movement pattern.** For example, if the skill to be learned is to be performed in a closed or unchanging environment, then the learner's goal will be to fine-tune the movement pattern so it is performed with the highest degree of consistency and efficiency.

Conversely, if the type of performance environment in which the skill is ultimately to be performed is open, or frequently changing in its presentation, then the goal is one of learning how to modify the movement pattern to meet a constantly changing set of temporal or spatial conditions. Consider the reaching example just described. We could actually design the environment to be more open or closed depending on how we structure the task demands. For example, if the object was placed on a shelf at the same distance and height from the learner, and the surface on which the learner was standing remained unchanged in terms of its surface characteristics or

fixating the movement pattern—The goal of practice is to perform the same movement pattern as consistently as possible on each subsequent practice attempt.

diversifying the movement pattern—The goal of practice is to vary how the movement pattern is performed on subsequent practice attempts so that the movement pattern becomes more flexible.

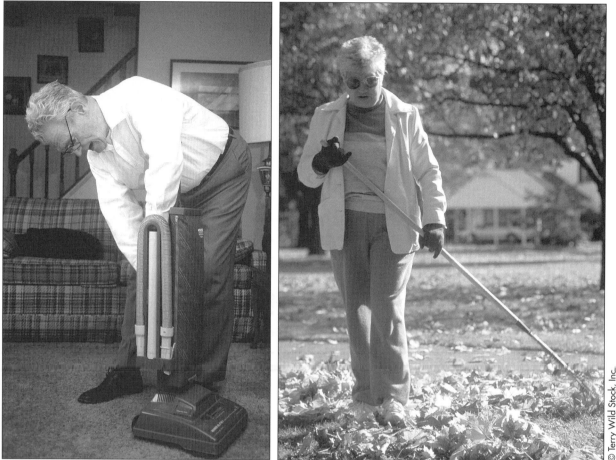

Figure 10.2 Most daily activities require that older adults learn how to diversify the movement pattern.

height from the ground, then the goal for the learner would be to fixate the skill. On the other hand, if the spatial location of the object and its distance from the body were changed on each subsequent trial or the characteristics of the surface on which the learner was standing were frequently interchanged (e.g., half-foam roller, rocker board, Dyna-Disc™), then the goal for the learner would be to diversify the movement pattern to meet the changing task demands and environmental constraints.

Given that in real-life circumstances, the older adult is required to reach for objects of different weights and shapes that are often located at different heights in cupboards, washing machines, wardrobes, or on the floor while standing on different surfaces (e.g., tiled floor, step stool, carpet), the skill of reaching while maintaining upright balance is probably most conducive to being diversified (figure 10.2). In fact, instructors must constantly vary the practice environment by manipulating the regulatory conditions directly associated with the task. For example, in each of the chapters describing the program components, the regulatory conditions associated with many of the balance activities were constantly being manipulated as the level of difficulty increased. These regulatory conditions related to the actual task demands (e.g., weight or shape of objects being retrieved, timing of task, distance of reach) or the constraints imposed by the environment in which the task was performed (e.g., surface type, lighting, visual flow).

As an instructor, you must understand that your participants will often be at different stages in the learning process as they acquire, or in some cases reacquire, the skills necessary to improve their overall balance and mobility. I am sure those of you who are already teaching balance and mobility classes can readily identify some participants in your class who are in the first stage of learning a particular balance skill while others have already moved into the second stage. What is most helpful about Gentile's stages-of-learning model is that it not only describes the learning process from the learner's perspective, but it also provides the instructor with insight into how to shape the learning environment or alter the task demands in each of the learning stages. These ideas are summarized in the box below.

Practical Implications of Gentile's Stages-of-Learning Model for Instruction

Stage 1: Getting the idea of the movement to be learned

Learner's goal: Develop a basic movement pattern that will accomplish the goal of the task. Performance is characterized by inconsistency and lack of efficiency.

Instructor's goal: Provide ample opportunity for the learner to practice and explore different ways of performing the skill. Do not alter the regulatory conditions until some level of performance consistency is achieved (e.g., three out of six practice attempts are successful).

Stage 2: Diversification or fixation of the movement pattern

Learner's goal: If the skill to be learned will be performed in a closed or unchanging environment, the goal is to fine-tune the movement pattern so that it can be performed with a high level of consistency and little cognitive or physical effort.

If the skill to be learned will be performed in an open and frequently changing environment, the goal is to learn how to modify the movement pattern to meet the changing demands of the performance environment.

Instructor's goals (skills to be performed in closed or unchanging environments): Manipulate the nonregulatory conditions while holding the regulatory conditions relatively constant. Certain parameters of the task (e.g., weight or shape of objects) can be manipulated as long as the timing features of the movement pattern required remain relatively the same.

Instructor's goals (skills to be performed in open or changing environments): Manipulate the regulatory conditions (task demands or environmental constraints) so that the movement pattern must be altered on subsequent practice attempts. Begin by varying only the parameters of the task (e.g., weight, shape, height and distance of object from body) and then progress to varying the actual pattern of coordination (e.g., one-handed versus two-handed reach). Characteristics of the surface on which the learner is standing (e.g., foam of different densities and height, rocker board, Dyna-Disc) or environmental conditions (e.g., lighting, amount of visual flow, complexity of visual scene) can also be varied.

Manipulate the nonregulatory conditions (e.g., alter the proximity of other learners practicing similar tasks, play music) as practice progresses so the learner is forced to focus attention on the task being performed despite external distractions.

(Rose 1997).

Introducing the Skill to Be Learned

When instructors decide to introduce a new motor skill to a class of learners, they invariably begin with a brief verbal description of the skill followed by one or more visual demonstrations of the correct movement pattern. Instructors prefer this mode of instruction because they believe it will convey the greatest amount of information in its most meaningful form. Although the use of visual demonstration has been well supported in the motor learning literature, motor learning researchers have recently engaged in a debate as to whether visual demonstrations are always the most effective method of introducing different types of skills. They have also begun addressing such issues as who should actually demonstrate the skill, when and how often a demonstration should be given, and what it should be supplemented with to promote optimal learning (McCullagh & Meyer, 1997; Pollock & Lee, 1992; Weir & Leavitt, 1990).

First, demonstrations appear to be most effective when a new pattern of coordination is to be learned (figure 10.3). Conversely, when the goal is to fine-tune an already-learned skill, other techniques such as verbal cueing may prove more effective (Magill, 2003). Although it is customary to have someone who is highly skilled demonstrate a new motor skill, recent studies have shown that observing initially unskilled performers demonstrating skills can also be beneficial to novice performers. Two probable advantages are associated with the use of this type of model. First, the observer is less likely to try to imitate the action of the unskilled performer, but instead will engage in more problem-solving activities. Second, it is easier to observe the underlying strategy being used to accomplish the goal of the skill when it is demonstrated by someone who is less skilled, particularly when the demonstration is supplemented with corrective feedback delivered by the instructor. The observer can then watch how the strategy is altered on subsequent practice trials. Perhaps the most interesting outcome observed by researchers who have investigated the learning benefits associated with the use of initially unskilled models is that the observers of other novices perform the skill at a significantly higher level than the person who first demonstrated it, once they begin practicing (McCullagh & Meyer, 1997; Pollock & Lee, 1992; Weir & Leavitt, 1990).

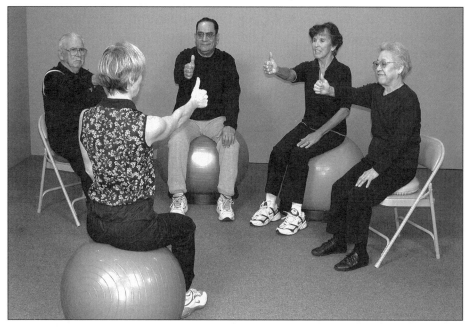

Figure 10.3 Visual demonstrations appear to be most effective when learning new motor skills.

Demonstrations appear to be most effective when a new pattern of coordination is to be learned.

Practical Implications

At a practical level, a balance and mobility class provides many opportunities to incorporate demonstrations by unskilled models. They can be done in small groups, with one member serving as the learning model while several other participants watch the person demonstrate the skill, receive corrective feedback from the instructor, then subsequently attempt the skill again. Although this technique is not always appropriate for teaching young learners, I have found it to be extremely effective when teaching older adults. An alternative strategy is to develop performance checklists that simply describe the key elements of movement skills. Form 10.1 is an example of a performance checklist.

Having your older adult learners work as partners, with one serving as the teacher while the other attempts to perform the skill, is an effective way to use these checklists. The job of the "teacher" is to look for errors in performance by comparing the learner's movements to those described on the checklist. As soon as an error is noticed, the "teacher" provides corrective feedback and then watches how the learner uses it to improve their performance on the next practice attempt. This teaching technique not only provides a valuable learning experience for both "teacher" and learner by fostering a better understanding of the skill to be performed but also makes it easier to manage a large class.

Form 10.1

Multidirectional Weight Shifts in a Seated Position Performance Checklist

BODY ALIGNMENT

_____ Performer is sitting tall and eyes are focused on a target at eye level.

_____ Shoulders are level.

_____ Feet are no more than hip-width apart and pointed forward.

_____ Hands are positioned on ball or chair, on thighs, or folded across chest.

WEIGHT SHIFT

_____ Movement is initiated without hesitation in the correct direction following the cue to move.

_____ Good body alignment is maintained as the hips are moved in the cued direction.

_____ Shoulders remain level and relaxed when weight shifts are performed to either the right or left side.

_____ Feet remain in place during the weight shift.

_____ Eyes are fixed on a target at eye level during each weight shift.

_____ Performer returns to a centered position after each weight shift.

From *FallProof!* by Debra J. Rose, 2003, Champaign, IL: Human Kinetics

implicit learning—
Improvements in the performance of a skill that occur subconsciously—the learner is unaware of how improvements were achieved. Implicit teaching techniques foster self- or guided discovery of a movement solution through manipulation of task and environmental demands.

Even though visual demonstrations have been shown to be highly effective in learning how to perform a new pattern of coordination, an alternative strategy you can employ as an instructor is to allow the participant to learn the desired movement by a process of self- or guided discovery. This is a particularly valuable teaching technique to use in the FallProof program because many of the skills you would like your participants to acquire are not amenable to demonstration or explicit verbal instructions. They are best learned **implicitly.**

A good example of using an implicit approach to teach a new movement technique associated with the FallProof program is attempting to help older adults learn to transition from one type of postural strategy to another (i.e., ankle to hip strategy) to control postural sway. Rather than telling or showing them how and when to switch from an ankle to a hip strategy, the task demands can be manipulated in such a way that the transition becomes inevitable. For example, if you ask an older adult to stand between two chairs and sway in a forward and backward direction to the slow beat of a metronome, you will generally observe a pattern of movement that is largely controlled by the ankle joint as the upper and lower body move in the same direction, or **in phase.**

in-phase movement—
The upper and lower body move in the same direction.

As you increase the speed of the metronome or the distance through which the sway occurs, however, you will observe a relatively spontaneous shift in the movement pattern from one characterized by an in-phase movement to one that is now **out of phase** as use of the larger hip muscles becomes necessary for controlling the sway. In contrast to the in-phase movement that characterized the ankle strategy, the upper body now moves in a direction opposite to the lower body (figure 10.4). Voila! The learner has discovered the hip strategy and not a word has been spoken.

out-of-phase movement—The upper body moves in a direction opposite to the lower body.

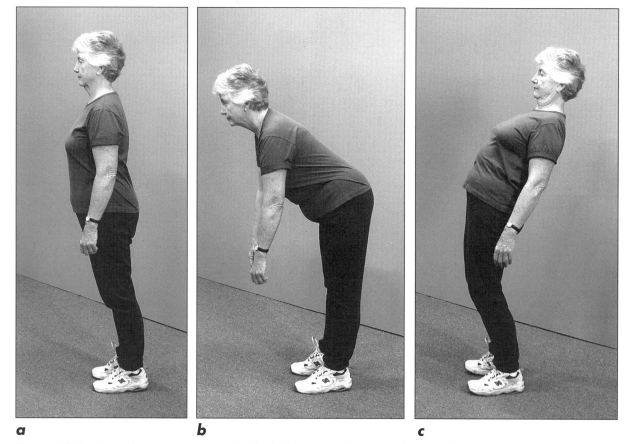

a **b** **c**

Figure 10.4 An ankle strategy requires that the body move in-phase **(a)** whereas a hip strategy results in a forward **(b)** or backward **(c)** out-of-phase body movement.

Just as the use of unskilled models to demonstrate new skills minimizes an observer's tendency to mimic the action when they begin practicing, verbally posing a movement problem to be solved to a group of learners or manipulating the task demands or environmental constraints in such a way that the learner is guided to the solution fosters greater problem solving and a range of solutions that better reflect the individual's unique capabilities. Although according to the old adage, "a picture is worth a thousand words," there are many ways to introduce a new skill to a learner, particularly one who is older and wiser. Certainly, **explicit** teaching techniques, whether in the form of verbal instructions or visual demonstrations, are those most often used to introduce a new skill, but there are many opportunities to use more implicit teaching techniques, particularly when teaching several different balance and mobility activities. These may be invoked by simply having the learner discover a given pattern of coordination by manipulating either the demands of the task or the environment in which it is being performed. At other times, it is sufficient to pose a movement problem to be solved while manipulating either the task demands or the environment in such a way that the solution emerges without the learner ever being consciously aware of how it was achieved.

explicit learning— Improvements in performance of a skill of which the learner is consciously aware. Explicit teaching techniques include verbal instructions and visual demonstrations.

Practicing the Skill

Once participants have acquired a good understanding of how the particular movement pattern is to be performed, begin varying the practice environment so that it better prepares them for performing the skill in a variety of environments and in response to different task demands. As you learned in chapter 4, the challenge associated with performing a particular task can be manipulated by altering the task demands or the environmental constraints. Manipulating either or both of these variables will result in a more varied practice environment that has been shown to benefit learning not only of the skills being practiced, but also of skills learned at a later time.

> Manipulating either the task demands or the environmental constraints will result in a more varied practice environment.

In deciding how best to vary the practice environment, an instructor needs to consider such things as the learner's current level of skill, the characteristics of the skill to be learned, and the type of environment in which the skill will ultimately be performed. As discussed earlier, skills that need to be performed in the same way every time or in an environment that does not change should be fixated, whereas skills that will be performed differently on consecutive attempts and in changing environments should be diversified. Although varying the practice environment is the best way to help learners diversify a skill, it can be argued that it is still valuable to vary the practice environment even when the learner's goal is to fixate a movement skill. Simply by manipulating the regulatory and nonregulatory conditions described in Gentile's two-stage learning model, the practice environment can be varied appreciably. Although both the regulatory and nonregulatory conditions should be manipulated in the case of skills that need to be diversified, manipulating only the nonregulatory conditions is appropriate when the goal is to fixate a skill.

> Varying the practice environment is still valuable even when the learner's goal is to fixate the skill.

contextual interference—A practice method that involves practicing multiple variations of a single skill or multiple skills in a single practice session. Used to increase the variability of a practice session.

blocked practice schedule—The same skill or skill variation is practiced for a given number of practice trials before a new skill or variation is introduced.

random practice schedule—A new variation or skill is practiced on each subsequent practice trial.

In addition to varying the regulatory and nonregulatory conditions associated with a movement skill, an instructor can vary the practice environment by manipulating how variations of one skill or different skills are practiced. For example, learners can practice variations of a single skill or multiple skills simply by varying the type of practice schedule used. This technique increases the level of **contextual interference** or variety introduced into a practice setting and has been shown to be an effective method of improving both the learning and transfer of motor skills among novice and skilled performers alike (Hall, Domingues & Cavazos, 1994; Magill & Hall, 1990; Shea & Morgan, 1979; Wrisberg & Lui, 1991).

The level of contextual variety can be further manipulated by varying the practice environment according to a blocked or random practice schedule. In the case of a **blocked practice schedule,** a particular skill is practiced for a given number of repetitions before a new variation of the same skill or a different movement skill is practiced. Conversely, in a **random practice schedule,** the learner performs a skill or a variation of a skill only once before practicing a different skill or skill variation on the next repetition. The practice order is randomized so that the learner does not know what skill will be practiced on the subsequent trial. Although the latter type of practice schedule is believed to require much greater cognitive effort on the part of learners and results in more errors during practice, it has been shown to significantly benefit skill learning.

Perhaps the best way to progressively increase the level of cognitive effort required of learners is by having them practice different variations of a single skill first according to a blocked schedule and then according to a random schedule. The difficulty of the practice environment can then be further increased by having the participant follow the same practice schedule progression (blocked to random) while practicing two or three different skills in the same practice session. One skill that is particularly well suited to variable practice techniques is that of obstacle negotiation. During the course of a day, the older adult is likely to encounter curbs, stairs, and other types of obstacles that vary in terms of height, width, and surface characteristics. In the center-of-gravity control component of the program, for example, a section is devoted to performing a variety of stepping movements on benches. These movements progress from alternating toe touches to step-up/step-downs on the same and then opposite sides of the bench to step swing-through movement sequences.

A good starting point in varying the practice of these different skills is to vary only the height of the bench on which the participant is performing. For example, a participant might begin practicing toe touches on a bench that is 2 inches high for a set number of repetitions before moving to a bench that is 4 inches high and then to one that is 6 inches in height to practice the same skill (figure 10.5). Practicing the same skill for a set number of repetitions before moving to the next bench height is an example of varying the practice according to a blocked schedule. Conversely, you could have the participant perform only one toe touch with each foot before moving to a different-height bench. Not allowing multiple repetitions of a skill at the same bench height results in a more random practice schedule. The latter practice schedule is considered more cognitively challenging for learners because they must continually change how they perform the skill when a new bench height is encountered. The belief is that a skill is better learned when practiced in this way because the movement must be repeatedly reconstructed and modified to accommodate the bench height changing between practice trials. This is not the case in a blocked practice schedule because participants are able to practice the same skill variation multiple times before moving to a new bench height. They can therefore use the same action

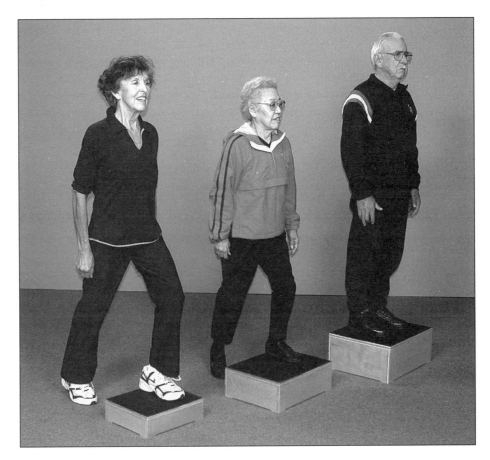

Figure 10.5 Class participants performing stepping sequences on different-height benches.

plan from the previous repetition with little or no modification. Thus, less cognitive effort is expended in this easier practice situation.

A random practice schedule is considered to be more cognitively effortful for learners.

To further increase the level of cognitive effort required of the learner, you can increase the number of different movement skills being practiced on different bench heights within the same practice session. For example, you might have participants practice toe touches, step-up/step-downs, and step swing-through movement sequences according to either a blocked or random practice schedule. Participants would practice one of the three movement skills for a set number of trials before practicing the next movement sequence (i.e., blocked practice schedule) on the same bench height or practice each movement sequence only once before switching to a different movement skill according to a randomly presented order (i.e., random practice schedule).

The final practice variation would be to vary not only the type of movement sequence being performed, but also the height, width, and surface characteristics of the bench. An advantage of this practice technique is that the level of practice difficulty can easily be matched to the capabilities of the learner. For participants who are in the early stages of learning, or perhaps lacking in confidence, the practice can still be varied, but only one skill is practiced for a given number of repetitions before the height of the bench is altered. At the same time, more skilled participants can be practicing different movement sequences in a random order on the same or different bench heights after one or more repetitions.

Previous research has demonstrated that varying the practice environment not only leads to better learning of movement skills, but it also improve a learner's ability to transfer what has been learned in one environment to a different performance environment and from one skill to another (Goode & Magill, 1986; Magill & Hall, 1990). I have also found that introducing practice variability results in a more enjoyable practice environment for the participants, albeit a more cognitively challenging one.

Identifying and Correcting Errors in Performance

One of the most effective ways to help learners identify and correct errors in their own performance is to supplement the feedback they derive from their own internal sensory systems with information provided by the instructor. This externally provided feedback is often referred to as **augmented feedback** in the motor learning literature. The information can be provided in different forms (i.e., verbal, visual, auditory) and either during or after a given performance. It is used to provide learners with information about the outcome of their performance, often referred to as knowledge of results (KR), as well as about the quality of the performance itself. This second type of augmented feedback is called knowledge of performance (KP).

During the first stage of learning, as participants struggle to understand the goal of the movement and how best to achieve that goal, they will derive the greatest learning benefit from receiving a more prescriptive type of feedback that describes not only what they are doing incorrectly, but also what they need to do to correct their errors on subsequent practice attempts **(knowledge of performance).** Once the learner enters the second stage of learning described by Gentile and has a better understanding of how to perform the movement pattern necessary to achieve the goal, the type of feedback provided should shift from being prescriptive to descriptive in nature **(knowledge of results).** That is, the information provided should simply describe the nature of the error (if the learner has not already identified it), not how to correct it.

Previous research on this topic also suggests that a period of time should elapse between the completion of the movement attempt and the delivery of feedback. Moreover, learners should be encouraged to estimate the accuracy of their own performance during the delay between completion of the movement attempt and the delivery of feedback from the instructor (Lui & Wrisberg, 1997; Swinnen, 1990). To further encourage learners to engage in error estimation, the instructor might also consider delivering the augmented feedback in the form of a question rather than a statement of fact. By posing one or more questions to the learner about the accuracy of the previous performance, the instructor encourages the learner to identify not only what went wrong on the previous practice attempt but also what could be done differently to correct the problem on the next attempt. This process nurtures the problem-solving abilities of the learner and over time will result in a more independent learner.

> A period of time should elapse between learners completing a practice attempt and feedback being provided. Learners should also be encouraged to estimate the accuracy of their performance before feedback is provided.

Which of the two types of augmented feedback, KR or KP, is likely to be most meaningful to a learner? For example, should the feedback provided only focus on

augmented feedback—Information provided to a learner from an external source.

knowledge of performance—Information provided to a learner about the quality of the movement.

knowledge of results—Information provided to a learner about the outcome of a movement pattern.

the outcome of a particular skill performance (KR) and whether it was consistent with the intended goal, or should it focus more on the characteristics of the movement that led to the observed outcome (KP)? According to Magill (2003), both types of augmented feedback are beneficial to learners, but for different reasons. He argues that KR is beneficial for skill learning because (a) it can be used by learners to confirm their own assessment of the internal sensory feedback they received about the skill, even though it may be redundant; (b) learners may not be able to determine the actual outcome of their performance based on the intrinsic sensory feedback alone; (c) KR often motivates learners to continue practicing a skill; and (d) by limiting the feedback provided to KR, learners are encouraged to discover how to achieve the desired outcome through self-discovery. Similarly, he also believes that providing KP can be very beneficial to learners, particularly when the skill being learned must be performed in a particular way (i.e., gymnastics maneuver, diving skill). Providing KP to a learner also becomes important when

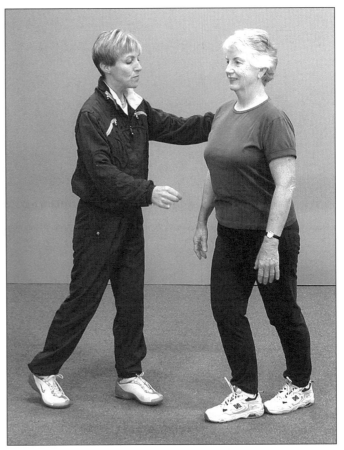

Figure 10.6 Providing knowledge of performance is important when teaching skills that require complex coordination.

certain movement components of a skill that require complex coordination need to be corrected (figure 10.6).

Irrespective of what type of augmented feedback you provide during the learning of a new motor skill, the thing to remember is that more is not better. In fact, research has shown that providing too much feedback to learners actually hinders learning. One reason for this finding is that learners become overly dependent on external feedback if it is provided too often. Conversely, learners who receive feedback less often will be forced to rely on the internal sensory feedback they receive as they perform the skill for making the necessary corrections on subsequent practice attempts. This will help them better recall what needs to be done when the external feedback is no longer available. As an instructor, you need to remember that you will not be there to correct errors that your program participants make during their everyday activities, so you must provide them with the skills needed to become proficient not only at detecting the errors they are making but also at correcting them. Developing these error detection and correction skills is what is most likely to improve their ability to perform daily activities that require good balance and mobility as well as reduce their risk for falling.

More is not better: Learners become overly dependent on augmented feedback when it is provided too often.

Important Guidelines to Follow When Providing Augmented Feedback

- The augmented feedback must direct the learner's attention to the "pivotal error" or component of the skill that, when corrected, will result in an appreciable improvement in performance.

- Augmented feedback should not only provide the learner with information about the elements of a skill that are being performed incorrectly, but it should also inform the learner as to what components of the skill are being performed correctly. This second type of feedback serves to motivate the learner.

- Providing too much feedback too often is detrimental to learning. Although learners need more feedback during the early stages of learning, the frequency should be reduced as their error-detection abilities improve.

- Provide sufficient time for learners to evaluate the accuracy and quality of their own performance before providing feedback after a practice attempt.

- Intersperse error-correcting feedback statements with other feedback statements that are intended to reinforce what the learner is already doing correctly (i.e., "You are clearing the obstacle much better with your rear foot now") or motivate the learner to continue practicing the skill (i.e., "Good effort on that last practice attempt").

Summary

Applying each of the motor learning principles described in this chapter will significantly enhance the quality of the program you create and the outcomes achieved by your participants. When you apply each of these principles, however, will be influenced by such factors as the participants' current stage of learning, their previous motor skill experience, and their particular style of learning. Whereas the principles underlying the presentation of a new motor skill will be applied during the first stage of motor learning, the application of other principles will be deferred to the second stage (i.e., variability of practice) when the learner better understands the goal of the movement they are attempting to learn.

How much augmented feedback is provided to learners will also be influenced by the stage of learning. Although providing more augmented feedback during the early stages of learning will be beneficial to the learner, the frequency with which augmented feedback is provided should be reduced as the learner moves into the second stage. The nature of the feedback provided should also change from information that helps learners detect *and* correct their errors to a form of feedback that only helps them identify the error, if they have not already identified it for themselves.

Always remember that your goal as an instructor is to provide your older adult learners with the skills and strategies needed to accomplish a variety of daily tasks that often vary in the demands they impose and that must be performed across a variety of sensory environments. Given that you cannot always be there to guide them through each of these tasks, you need to structure your class sessions in a manner that is designed to foster their problem-solving abilities. Although the learning environment you create as a result will require much more cognitive effort on the part of your learners, it will lead to optimal learning and the ability to transfer what they have learned in the classroom into their daily lives.

TEST YOUR UNDERSTANDING

1. According to Gentile (1972), during the first stage of motor learning, the learner's primary goal is to
   a. fixate the movement pattern being learned
   b. understand the goal of the movement pattern
   c. diversify the movement pattern so it becomes more flexible
   d. learn how to perform the skill correctly
   e. learn how to identify errors in performance

2. A higher level of cognitive effort is introduced into a practice setting when a learner practices
   a. the same pattern of coordination according to a blocked practice schedule
   b. multiple patterns of coordination in a defined order during a practice session
   c. multiple patterns of coordination in a random order during a practice session
   d. one pattern of coordination for a given time period before practicing a second pattern of coordination
   e. multiple movement skills in a game setting

3. One advantage of using initially unskilled models to demonstrate a new movement pattern to learners is that
   a. they make it much more difficult to learn a motor skill
   b. they prevent learners from imitating the movement to be learned
   c. learners are able to devote all of their attention to the critical components of the skill being modeled
   d. the instructor does not need to be able to perform the skill to teach it
   e. it results in a less difficult learning environment

4. The term *augmented feedback* is defined as
   a. information provided to a learner from an external source either during or following the completion of a movement
   b. outcome information provided to a learner from an external source
   c. process information provided to a learner from an external source
   d. information provided to a learner from an external source at any time before, during, or after the completion of a movement
   e. external information provided to a learner about internal physiological events

5. Information provided to a learner that emphasizes the quality of the form used to perform a skill is called
   a. knowledge of form
   b. augmented sensory feedback
   c. knowledge of results
   d. knowledge of performance
   e. biofeedback

6. Feedback should be provided to a learner
   a. immediately after completion of each practice attempt
   b. immediately after completion of at least five practice attempts

c. following a short temporal delay after a practice attempt

d. only during the performance of the skill

e. following a short temporal delay and preferably in the form of a question

7. Presenting a skilled model is more effective when

   a. the learner is able to correctly reproduce the skill being presented

   b. the skill involves learning a new pattern of coordination

   c. the model also performs the skill incorrectly on some occasions

   d. the learner is attempting to rescale an already familiar movement pattern

   e. the learner is not confident in their ability to perform the skill

8. The regulatory conditions associated with a learning environment include

   a. all the irrelevant aspects associated with the performance of a skill

   b. all the errors that occur during the performance of a skill

   c. both the relevant and irrelevant aspects associated with performance of the skill

   d. the trajectory of the ball and the spatial orientation of the glove in the case of attempting to catch a fly ball in baseball or softball

   e. all those factors that determine whether or not the learner is motivated to learn a particular motor skill

9. According to Gentile (1972), during the second stage of learning,

   a. the primary goal for the learner is to develop a consistent movement pattern

   b. the regulatory conditions associated with the skill to be learned should be manipulated

   c. the primary goal for the learner is to match the movement pattern to the environment in which it is ultimately performed

   d. the nonregulatory conditions associated with the skill to be learned should be manipulated

   e. the learner should begin to vary the type of movement pattern being used to perform the skill

10. Augmented feedback that is prescriptive in nature should be provided

   a. during all stages of learning

   b. only during the early stages of learning

   c. during the later stages of learning

   d. only to older adult learners

   e. after every practice attempt during the early stages of learning

PRACTICAL PROBLEMS

1. Based on your knowledge of Jane and Bill and their entering skill levels, how would you apply each of the following motor learning principles?

   a. Introducing the skill to be learned

   b. Practicing the skill

   c. Identifying and correcting errors in performance

2. Design a performance checklist for two balance exercises that program participants could use during a class session.

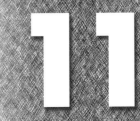

Program Planning and Class Management Techniques

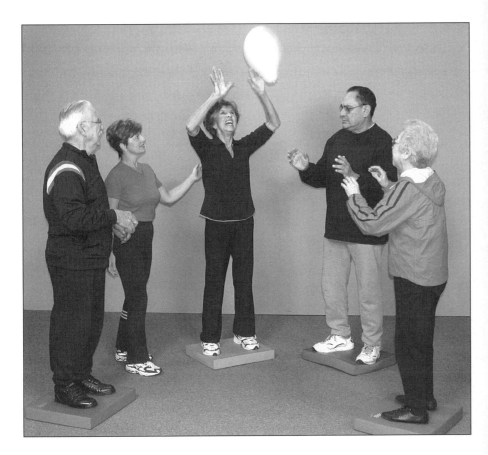

Objectives

After completing this chapter, you will be able to

- effectively plan and implement group-based lessons,
- effectively manage participants in group-based programs to ensure optimal activity levels and safety, and
- communicate effectively with participants.

The focus of this final chapter is to review some of the essential program planning and class management techniques needed to ensure your success as a FallProof™ instructor. Some readers may have many years of experience working with older adults in a group setting, whereas the experience of others may be limited to working one-to-one as a clinician or personal trainer. Although many of the leadership and communication skills are similar, you will find that preparing for and managing group classes requires a different approach from the one you use when instructing individuals. In the sections to follow, I will discuss the various activities you will need to perform (a) following the completion of your assessment and before the program begins, (b) before the start of each class session, (c) during each class session, (d) between class sessions, and finally (e) after each follow-up assessment.

Following the Initial Assessment

As you complete each assessment associated with the FallProof program, you will need to begin identifying and listing the types of balance and mobility problems observed. The test interpretation tables provided in chapter 3 will greatly assist you with this task as well as provide you with ideas as to the type of exercises that will address each of the problems identified. The next step in this process will be to separate the problems you believe to be temporary or amenable to change with targeted exercise progressions from those that you know to be more permanent. For example, if lower body muscle weakness, which we know to be a temporary problem in most cases, is common among the group tested, then you can begin to develop a set of progressive strength exercises to address the problem.

Although there is nothing you can do as an instructor to change the more permanent balance problems an individual is experiencing, you may be able to select several exercises that will help the participant better compensate for the permanent loss. For example, selecting exercises that focus on improving a participant's use of ground cues for balance control will do much to offset permanent changes in the visual system that are associated with such eye diseases as age-related macular degeneration and glaucoma. Categorizing each of the observed balance and mobility problems in this way will not only assist you in deciding where your instructional focus should be during the early stages of the program, but will also help you select the appropriate program components and exercise progressions for each identified balance or mobility problem.

> Following the initial assessment, it will be important to make a list of all temporary problems and a second list of all the permanent balance and mobility problems identified.

During your program planning, you will also need to remember that because multiple systems within the body contribute to good balance and mobility, not all of your program participants will begin at the same starting point in each program component. Although some older adults in your class may be experiencing problems that are sensory in origin, others may be experiencing greater decline in the motor system. Some adults will also tend to move through the exercise progressions more quickly than others because their balance problem is a temporary one (e.g., muscle weakness, reduced range of motion) and therefore easier to resolve. You will also find that your clients' previous motor skill experience and level of current physical activity will influence how quickly they progress during the program. You will therefore need to individualize your lesson plans by selecting a range of exercise progressions

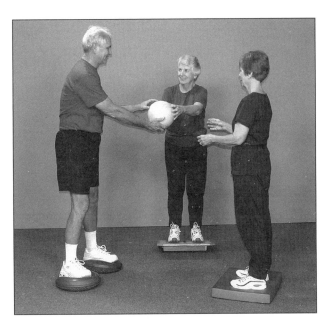

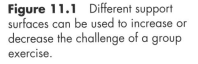

Figure 11.1 Different support surfaces can be used to increase or decrease the challenge of a group exercise.

that can be presented to the same group. This will require a careful review of each participant's test results followed by thoughtful lesson planning.

> The client's previous level of motor skill experience and current level of physical activity will also influence how quickly they progress during the program.

The programming triad that was presented in chapter 1 should guide the process of individualizing the exercises presented within a group setting. By simply manipulating the demands associated with a given exercise or the environment in which it is performed, you can increase or decrease the challenge associated with any exercise presented in the FallProof program (figure 11.1). In fact, this core ingredient of the program is what makes it possible to cater to a broad continuum of functional levels—from the very healthy to the very frail—within the same classroom.

Before Each Class Session

To be a successful instructor and achieve the program outcomes you desire, you will need to spend an adequate amount of time selecting the set of exercises you intend to present during the class. When preparing the early classes in a program, you will not need to select as many exercises as you would for later classes because it will take more time to determine where in the exercise progression each participant should begin. More practice time will also need to be allotted to each exercise so the participants can become familiar with it.

Planning the Lesson

Once you have selected the exercises you plan to use, you need to develop a lesson plan using a format similar to the one presented in form 11.1. The lesson plan should include a warm-up of no less than 10 minutes, a skills section lasting approximately 40 minutes, and a 10-minute cool-down. In addition to listing the exercises to be presented during the skills portion of the class, you should determine which activities you plan to present to the entire class and which activities you will have participants practice in small groups. Your lesson plan should also list all the equipment you plan

Form 11.1

Sample Lesson Plan

Module	Focus	Time	DESCRIPTION OF Activity	VERBAL Cues	Equipment
Warm-Up					
Skill Section: Activity 1					
Skill Section: Activity 2					
Skill Section: Activity 3					
Skill Section: Activity 4					
Culminating Activity					
Cool-Down					

Instructor: _____

Date: _____

 From *FallProof!* by Debra J. Rose, 2003, Champaign, IL: Human Kinetics.

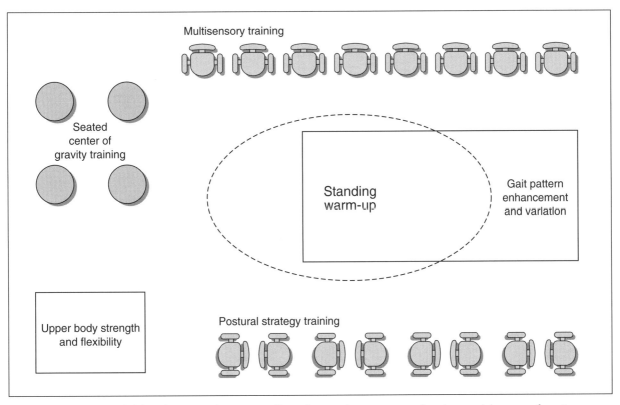

Figure 11.2 It is helpful to diagram where you will conduct each component of a class and the type of equipment you plan to use.

to use during each section of the class. Some instructors also find it helpful to include a column that lists the verbal cues associated with each exercise.

As a further time-saving practice, you or your program assistants should retrieve the equipment you plan to use during a particular class from its storage area and place it in different areas of the room in preparation for the activities you have included in your lesson plan. (An example of a possible classroom setup is provided in figure 11.2.) For example, if you are planning to have participants work on seated balance activities, you should have the necessary number of chairs, Dyna-Discs™, balance balls, and ball holders available to accommodate the different ability levels of your participants.

As a standard practice, you should also develop a master list that indicates whether a participant generally performs the seated balance activities on a Dyna-Disc, ball with ball holder, or ball alone. The size of the ball that each participant uses should also be recorded. This list will be particularly helpful in the early stages of the program so that your assistants can get the equipment ready and it can be assigned to participants efficiently. Even though the type of surface a client will be seated on is likely to change as their skill improves, it will still be helpful to maintain this type of master list, particularly if you teach multiple classes. Similarly, if you are planning to practice standing activities on altered surfaces, it will be helpful to have chairs arranged in another section of the room with the surface(s) to be used already positioned beneath or behind the chairs. In this way, participants can move easily between stations and start the next set of activities immediately. This preclass preparation will save you valuable time during the class and will also facilitate group transitions between exercise stations. I will talk more about group transition skills later in this chapter.

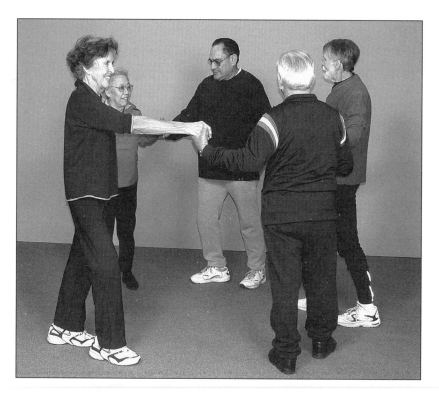

Figure 11.3 Using circle formations during a warm-up allows the instructor to observe all participants easily and increases the safety and confidence of the clients by having them hold hands.

Warm-Up

The warm-up section of a balance and mobility class tends to be a little shorter in duration than in a more traditional fitness class. Although its primary purpose is still to elevate the heart rate and prepare the muscles and joints for activity, this can usually be accomplished within a 10-minute time frame. Because the clients you are likely to be serving in this program will tend to be more deconditioned as a result of their balance and mobility problems, the warm-up should adequately prepare them for the balance activities to follow but should not lead to undue fatigue that will affect the quality of their physical performance as well as diminish their ability to focus their attention.

> The warm-up should adequately prepare clients for the balance activities to follow but should not lead to undue fatigue.

Many of the activities described in the center-of-gravity control, gait pattern enhancement and variation, and strength and flexibility components of the program are well suited to this section of the class (figure 11.3). Fun warm-up activities include starts and stops to music, seated balance ball activities, and progressive aerobic exercise sequences combining upper and lower body coordination. Do not be concerned about developing a new warm-up for every class because older adults often enjoy performing the same set of activities on a regular basis. Repeating the same set of warm-up activities often will also allow participants to focus more on actually performing the activity than on thinking about what they have to do. Simply adding one or two new movements to a repeating aerobic sequence or adding arm or leg movements to a balance ball movement sequence can create sufficient variety. Progressively adding new movements also challenges the working memory skills of your program participants.

Skills Section

The skills section of the class is where you introduce the various balance exercises you have selected based on the results of your initial assessment. During the 40 minutes that have been planned for this section, you will be able to present three or four program components. Depending on the size of your class and the availability of equipment, you may choose to present certain activities to the class as a whole or divide the class into smaller groups according to a station format. Although teaching the activity to the whole class allows you to monitor the progress of your participants more directly, it requires greater attention to creating a safe practice environment, particularly if the exercise being practiced is one of the more challenging progressions. How well you match the demands of the exercise to be performed to the capabilities of each participant will significantly affect the level of safety achieved. For example, teaching seated center-of-gravity activities to a larger group can be easily and safely accomplished by making sure that the more unstable participants are seated on Dyna-Discs on chairs with a back and armrests while the more stable participants are seated on balance balls with or without a ball holder for added stability.

> How well you match the demands of the exercise to be performed to the capabilities of each participant will significantly affect the level of safety achieved.

Allowing for adequate space between participants or placing a chair next to a participant seated on a balance ball will also enhance the safety of the activity. Similarly, positioning the group close to a wall with chairs placed directly in front of each participant will maximize safety when they are practicing a particular set of progressions while standing on altered surfaces (e.g., half-foam roller, foam pad, rocker board). The level of safety can also be increased by again matching the difficulty of the support surface to the participant's abilities. Finally, the challenge of the exercise can be easily manipulated just by altering the height and width of the half-foam rollers, the height and density of the foam pads, or the degree of tilt associated with any rocker boards used during the exercises.

Creating exercise stations can also be an effective means of implementing the skills section of a class. Organizing the class into smaller groups provides the opportunity for individualizing the program a little more by allowing participants to work at a specific exercise station or for a longer time period at a station that addresses their particular balance problems. The use of multiple exercise stations also allows you to better distribute your available equipment. While one group is working on seated balance activities requiring Dyna-Discs, balance balls, and ball holders, a second group could be practicing standing transfer activities using a set of different-height benches, and a third group could be engaged in strength or flexibility exercises using resistance bands, hand weights, or no equipment at all.

In your planning, allocate an appropriate length of time for practice at each station (i.e., 8-10 minutes at each of four stations) before having each group transition to a new station. Be sure to organize the exercise station so that the activities designed for the next station logically follow from those assigned at the previous one (i.e., seated to standing) and vary in terms of their balance challenge or aerobic intensity. As the program progresses, the activities planned for each station also will need to increase in difficulty.

Cool-Down

Just as the warm-up is used to create a clear beginning to a class, the cool-down brings closure to a class. The activities planned for this section should be designed to lower both the heart rate and anxiety level of the participants. Remember that a large number of the activities you present in the skills section of the class will be unfamiliar or anxiety inducing because they often push participants beyond a certain comfort level and increase their fear of falling on occasion. Relaxation exercises, in particular, should be incorporated regularly into this section of the class. These can take the form of gentle stretching activities performed in a comfortable seated position, rhythmic breathing to music, inspirational readings, self- or partner massage, and postural awareness activities. Planning cool-down activities that involve class participants lying on mats on the floor will also provide you with an excellent opportunity to review the floor-to-standing transition strategies described at the end of the center-of-gravity chapter following completion of the cool-down. I recommend that you not precede this activity with relaxation exercises, however, because for many older adults, getting up from the floor is anything but relaxing.

> The activities presented during the cool-down should be designed to lower both the heart rate and anxiety level of participants.

In addition to lowering the heart rate and anxiety level of your participants, the cool-down provides an opportunity to review what has taken place during the class, solicit feedback from class participants, recognize the efforts of individual participants and the class as a whole, and assign homework to be done before the next class. Your goal in this section is to prepare your participants to leave the class and transition back into their daily lives in a relaxed and satisfied state. If you have planned your lessons carefully, they will leave each class with a sense of accomplishment as well as an eagerness to attend the next class.

Before beginning any relaxation exercises you may have planned for the cool-down section, first create a conducive atmosphere by dimming the lighting in the room, closing any doors to outside noise, and playing soft instrumental music. Lower the volume of your voice and speak more slowly so that it has a calming effect on your participants as you present each exercise, read an inspirational poem, or verbally guide your participants through a series of visual images (e.g., floating down a river, stepping onto a cloud). Avoid ending the cool-down abruptly. Allow the participants to take additional time as needed before you increase the room lighting or open the doors to the outside world. Be mindful that any abrupt movements or a change in voice volume can quickly reverse the relaxed state you have helped your participants achieve.

During Each Class Session

By taking the time to develop a clear lesson plan before the start of each class, you have already done much to ensure that each session will be a successful one. Going into a class with a clear idea of what you plan to do will minimize the time wasted in transitioning between activities and maximize the amount of time each participant is engaged in activity. By knowing the order of activities in each section of the class, you will not only teach with a greater level of confidence, but you will also be perceived by your class participants as a well-organized and knowledgeable instructor.

Begin your class promptly with the warm-up so that you set the tone for the entire session. Be positive in your presentation style and provide clear verbal instructions before starting each new exercise in the warm-up or moving on to a new movement in your aerobic sequence. Ensure that all participants are positioned so that they can see what you are doing and hear what you are saying. Encourage participants with particularly poor vision or impaired hearing to stand closer to you during the warm-up. If you use music during your warm-up, which many older adults enjoy, remember to choose music that is age-appropriate, has a moderate tempo (i.e., approximately 100 to 120 beats per minute) and strong beat, and is played at a volume that allows for verbal instructions to be heard.

> Be sure that all participants are positioned so that they can see what you are doing and hear what you are saying.

Where you position yourself relative to your class members when leading the warm-up, introducing a new exercise, monitoring group activities, or making skill corrections is particularly important when working in group settings. In general, when leading the warm-up or introducing a new exercise or balance skill, position yourself where all students can see you clearly. For example, if you choose to incorporate seated activities into your warm-up, have your class sit on the appropriate surface in a semicircle, with you seated directly in front of them. Be sure to position individuals with hearing or visual impairments on the edges of the semicircle (figure 11.4). When leading standing warm-up exercises, organize your class into staggered rows, with the shorter people toward the front. Position yourself in front of the class and facing the group. Although it is often more difficult for older adults to mirror your movements when you are facing them, it is more important that you be able to watch closely to ensure that they are being monitored by any program assistants or holding onto a chair if extra support is needed. You can minimize any confusion that might arise by verbalizing and pointing in the direction you want them to go just before changing the movement sequence.

If you have planned to set up several exercise stations during the skills section of the class, the two major difficulties you are likely to encounter as an instructor are (a) where to position yourself in the room so you can monitor the activities of each group and (b) how to move efficiently between the groups so you can provide additional instruction and corrective feedback. Certainly, if you have additional program assistants to help you during each class, this problem is easier to resolve. How many assistants you will require will depend greatly on the functional level of the participants in the class. If clients are only moderately impaired, you may only need a ratio of one assistant to every four to six participants, whereas if participants are more severely impaired, as is likely to be the case in programs operating in residential care facilities, the ratio may need to be as high as one assistant for every two to three clients. Knowing how many assistants are available for each class lesson will also guide you in determining your class size. Although it is not always possible to set a class maximum, particularly if you are employed by a community college district or other state-funded organization, it may be possible to divide the class into two smaller groups and shorten the lesson to 30 minutes to better ensure the safety of your clients while providing a sufficient level of challenge that will lead to observable improvements in balance and mobility.

A program assistant can be given a list of appropriate activities to present and then assigned to lead a small group. Alternatively, you might appoint a participant in each group to lead the activities. If you have established your groups in planning the

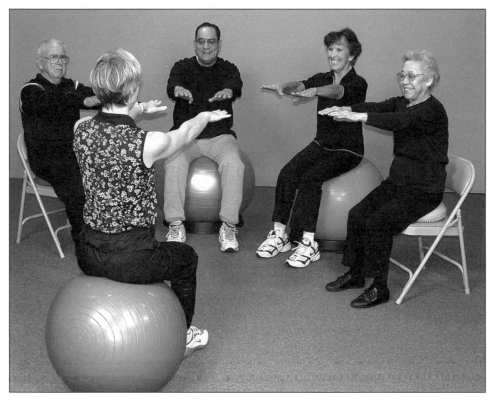

Figure 11.4 Position class participants with hearing or visual problems on the edges of a semicircle so they are closer to you.

class, you can identify an appropriate participant who is at a higher level of function and possesses good leadership skills. However you decide to organize the activities within each group, remember to position yourself on the perimeter of the group you are instructing so you can easily view each of the other groups in the room. In addition, be sure to assess which group activities require expert instruction or involve the greatest level of challenge to participants and lead those yourself. As mentioned earlier, taking the time to plan your lesson and prepare your classroom in advance will result in smooth transitions between activities and exercise stations.

> It is important to position yourself on the perimeter of the group you are instructing so you can easily view other groups in the room.

Between Class Sessions

As soon as possible after each class, take time to evaluate what went well and what did not in each section. If you determine that there are problems associated with the set of exercises you selected, make any changes to the lesson plan you think are appropriate to resolve them. You also need to evaluate how effectively you matched the difficulty of the exercise progression to each participant's individual capabilities. Remember that your goal is to maximize the challenge associated with each activity as well as minimize the risk to participants. You also want them to experience some level of success when performing the various exercises. Being successful, at least part of the time, raises each participant's balance-related self-confidence. Carefully review the exercise progressions in the appropriate chapter and decide how to adjust the difficulty level if you plan to present the same set of exercises in the next class.

Being successful, at least a good proportion of the time, is important for raising each participant's balance-related self-confidence.

In addition to evaluating how effectively you selected and progressed the exercises, another way to evaluate your class management skills is to estimate how much time your participants were actually engaged in exercising during the hour they spent in class. For example, how much time elapsed between the completion of one set of exercises and the start of the next set? How long did it take to get the exercises started at each station or to move the groups between stations? Did all members of a group appear to be actively engaged in the exercise for the allotted time? Although you need to provide sufficient rest for your participants between activities to avoid undue fatigue, this can often be accomplished simply by sequencing the activities effectively. For example, following a more vigorous set of gait pattern activities with a set of seated head-eye coordination exercises will allow time for your participants to rest the muscles of their legs while still engaging in other balance activities. You can also make use of the time participants spend waiting to move through an obstacle course or perform an activity that requires individualized attention by having them complete a set of exercises they can safely perform unsupervised. Good "waiting" exercises could include upper body strength and flexibility exercises that can be performed in a seated position with or without a partner.

An important way to evaluate your class management skills is to estimate how much time your class participants were actually engaged in exercise during the time they spent in class.

As the program progresses, you should maintain a log of the exercise components and progressions you present in each class session. This log will help you remember (1) to select exercises from each of the five program components so that each dimension of balance is addressed on a regular basis, and (2) which level(s) in the exercise progression of each component your class has reached at any point during the program. These two elements of the program will be particularly important for you to monitor if you teach multiple classes a week. An example of a program log is presented in form 11.2.

After Each Follow-Up Assessment

Regularly assessing the performance of your class participants is essential for several reasons. In addition to providing your participants with information about their individual progress, it will assist you in evaluating your own effectiveness as an instructor. From a programming perspective, the collective results of each individual test, once compared to previous test outcomes, can also be used to identify which dimensions of balance are beginning to show improvement and which might require more attention in the coming weeks. Regular follow-up assessments are also an effective way of motivating your participants to continue attending the program because of the improvement they have made in one or more areas of balance. Because you are continually increasing the difficulty of most exercises, it is often hard for a participant to see the positive changes resulting from each class. Thus, these tests become a means of objectively demonstrating those positive changes.

Regularly assessing the performance of your class participants is essential.

Sample Program Exercise Log

Lesson Plan Checklist   FallProof™ Program   Date: _____

WARM-UP ACTIVITIES

_____ Stop and start with music

_____ Seated warm-up activities

_____ Standing warm-up activities

_____ Dynamic flexibility exercises

CENTER-OF-GRAVITY CONTROL TRAINING

I.   Seated balance activities

_____ L1:   Seated balance

_____ L2:   With voluntary arm movements

_____ L3:   With voluntary trunk movements

_____ L4:   With voluntary leg movements

_____ L5:   While resisting perturbations

_____ L6:   With dynamic weight shifts

_____ L7:   With dynamic weight shifts against gravity

CULMINATING ACTIVITIES

_____ Seated bunny hop

_____ "Pass the potato, please"

_____ "Hot potato!"

_____ Balloon volleyball

_____ "Shift around the clock"

_____ Seated soccer

II: Standing balance activities

_____ L1:   Checking standing posture

_____ L2:   Quasi-static standing with altered base of support (BOS)

_____   With added cognitive task

_____   With added manual task (upper body)

_____   With added manual task (lower body)

_____ L3:   Multidirectional weight shifts

_____ L4:   Weight transfers with head and body movements

_____ L5:   Dynamic weight transfers through space

_____ L6:   Kicking stationary objects

_____ L7:   Weight shifts and transfers against gravity

CULMINATING ACTIVITIES

____ "Pass the potato, please"

____ "Hot potato!"

____ Balloon volleyball

____ "Shift around the clock"

____ Fast feet

____ Line passing

____ Creek crossing

____ Rock hopping

____ Circle soccer

FLOOR-TO-STANDING TRANSFERS

____ L1: Floor-to-standing transfer progressions

MULTISENSORY TRAINING

I: Multisensory training

Somatosensory focus

____ Seated exercises

____ Standing exercises

____ Moving exercises

Visual focus

____ Seated exercises

____ Standing exercises

____ Moving exercises

Vestibular focus

____ Seated exercises

____ Standing exercises

____ Moving exercises

II: Eye-head coordination exercises

____ L1: Eye movements with stationary head

____ Smooth-pursuit eye movements

____ Saccadic eye movements

____ L2: Combination head and eye movements (seated)

____ L3: Head and eye movements while weight shifting (standing)

____ L4: Head and eye movements while walking

(continued)

CULMINATING ACTIVITY

_____   "Walk the gauntlet"

POSTURAL STRATEGY TRAINING

I: Ankle, hip, and step

_____   L1:   Voluntary postural strategies—ankle, hip, step

_____   L2:   Involuntary postural strategies—ankle, hip, step

GAIT PATTERN TRAINING

I: Variation and enhancement

_____   L1:   Walking with directional changes and abrupt starts and stops

_____   L2:   Walking with altered base of support

_____   L3:   Gait pattern variations—braiding and tandem walking

_____   L4:   Gait pattern enhancement/variation obstacle course

STRENGTH TRAINING

_____   Upper body

_____   weights   _____   bands

_____   Lower body

_____   weights   _____   bands

FLEXIBILITY TRAINING

_____   Upper body

_____   Lower body

From *FallProof!* by Debra J. Rose, 2003, Champaign, IL: Human Kinetics.

All of the tests that make up the FallProof assessment have been selected based on their reliability, their validity, and their ability to detect changes in performance over time. As long as you conduct each test using the same care you exercised during the initial assessment, you are sure to see positive and meaningful changes in one or more of the dimensions of balance and mobility you are reevaluating. Because you probably have not conducted the tests within the previous two months (the recommended minimum time between follow-up assessments), you will need to review the test instructions for each test so you can readminister them reliably. You should also review the participant's file just before conducting each follow-up test to see whether certain tests were modified during the initial assessment. For example, some older adults may have needed to use an assistive device while performing mobility tests such as the 8-foot up-and-go and the 50-foot walk or may have required additional support while performing other tests (e.g., used hands to rise from the chair during the chair stand). To ensure that your follow-up test results are valid, participants should perform each test in exactly the same way as on the previous assessment. Certainly, if time permits, you could also allow them to perform the test without the assistive device or additional support, but that should not occur during the first readministration of the test.

To ensure that your follow-up test results are valid, participants should perform each test in exactly the same way or using the same assistive device they did on the previous assessment.

Once you have completed the reevaluation of each participant, share the results with them in a timely fashion (figure 11.5). This can be done via a short interview or by giving them a report card that indicates the actual changes (if any) in test scores, what the changes mean in terms they can understand, and any areas that may require more attention during and between future class sessions. A sample report card is provided in form 11.3.

The amount of change in performance you observe between tests is likely to vary among the participants in your class due to differences in their initial functional level and the type of balance and mobility problems they are experiencing (e.g., temporary versus permanent). Thus, class participants should be actively discouraged from comparing their test scores to others in the class and should focus only on their own individual improvements. In

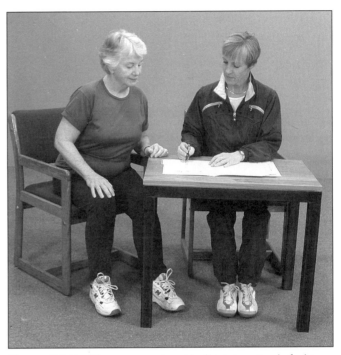

Figure 11.5 Share test results with clients in a timely fashion.

this regard, you should show participants how the changes you are seeing in their balance and mobility are likely to influence their performance of daily activities. It is often a good idea to ask participants whether they think the program has positively influenced their performance of daily tasks, and in what ways, before sharing the test results with them. Also spend time reviewing each participant's program goals and how they feel about their progress toward meeting those goals. This conversation will not only help form a personal connection between you and each of your clients, but it will also provide you with information for selecting the next set of progressive exercises for them.

Communicating With Class Participants

Although it is beyond the scope of this instructor guide to discuss the many techniques associated with good leadership, I would like to discuss one particularly important area. This area relates to how you communicate with your program participants, both verbally and nonverbally. I am sure you would agree that good communication skills are essential to the success of any program in which you are trying to motivate individuals to change their behavior. In the FallProof program, in particular, how well you deliver feedback to your class participants relative to their performance will often determine how well they perform on subsequent practice attempts.

How well you deliver feedback to your class participants relative to their performance will often determine how well they perform on subsequent practice attempts.

FallProof Program Report Card

Name: _____ Center: _____

Balance test	Baseline score	Rating	Additional comments
Fullerton Advanced Balance (FAB) Scale	/40		
M-CTSIB (30 second trials)	Condition 1 __ sec Condition 2 __ sec Condition 3 __ sec Condition 4 __ sec		
8-foot up-and-go (circle best trial)	Trial 1 Trial 2		
"Walkie-talkie" test * (circle one)	Positive Negative		
50-foot walk (preferred speed) (fast speed)	ft/sec ft/sec		
Multidirectional reach test (measured in inches reached)	FWD: BWD: RLAT: LLAT:		
Arm curl (left/right) (circle one)	in 30 sec		
30-second chair stand	in 30 sec		
Sit-and-reach test	in.		
Scratch test	in.		
2-minute step	steps		
Balance Efficacy Scale	/100		

*"Walkie-talkie": Positive = participant had to stop in order to respond to question; Negative = participant able to continue walking while talking.

Note: M-CTSIB=Modified Clinical Test of Sensory Interaction in Balance; FWD=forward; BWD=backward; RLAT=lateral reach right; LLAT=lateral reach left.

From *FallProof!* by Debra J. Rose, 2003, Champaign, IL: Human Kinetics.

Among the many leadership skills that are desirable if you are going to be an effective and successful instructor of older adults is the ability to express a genuine professional interest in and concern for each individual who attends your classes. This is conveyed not only by what you say to individual clients before, during, and after each class but also by what you do not say but nevertheless convey through body language. Tailor your communication to the individual personalities within your class. Whereas some class participants will need lots of reassuring and motivating words during a class, others will prefer less positive reinforcement and more corrective feedback on their performance. When in doubt, ask your class participants if they feel they are receiving sufficient and meaningful feedback.

Addressing class participants in a respectful manner is essential for effective communication. Substitute slang terms such as "you guys" with more appropriate ones such as "ladies and gentlemen" or "class" when addressing the group as a whole. Also take the time to learn the names of your participants as soon as possible. A good way to do this during the early classes is to provide participants with name tags to help you and other class members learn each other's names. Knowing the names of each of your class participants will not only facilitate good communication, but will also make them feel just that little bit more special.

As important as it is to communicate effectively, it is equally important to listen. Never interrupt class participants when they are speaking, and always maintain good eye contact. If you need to end a conversation in order to start the class or change activities, indicate your need to curtail the conversation but also let the participant know that you would be happy to continue the conversation at the end of class or before the next class.

If possible, allow time after class to talk with participants and answer any questions. This is also a good time to provide positive feedback to participants so that they leave the class feeling successful and optimistic about their progress. In addition, be sure to thank each of them for coming to class and tell them how much you are looking forward to seeing them the next time. For participants with more severe balance problems, a change in performance will not come quickly; so you need to provide these participants with feedback that acknowledges their efforts and motivates them to attend regularly.

> Allow time after class to talk with participants and answer any questions.

Take the time to evaluate your communication skills periodically. Consider videotaping yourself instructing a class so you can evaluate your communication skills in that setting. During your review, focus on what you are saying, when and how often you are saying it, and the tone you are using. In addition, consider soliciting feedback from class members at various points during the program, particularly those who often appear to have difficulty understanding what you are asking them to do. It is helpful to know if they have any areas of concern or confusion about any of the exercise progressions you have been teaching and whether they understand how the various types of activities relate to their daily lives. Because some activities are included in the instructor guide that may not seem immediately meaningful to your class participants, you must explain how an activity might be related to certain daily activities, how it might influence how well a certain task is ultimately performed, or how it may help them cope with different sensory environments.

> It will be important to explain how the balance activities presented in class relate to the performance of certain daily activities.

Summary

The success of the program described in this instructor guide will be determined not only by how well you plan each class session, but also by how effectively you present the content you have selected for that class. Good organization skills are essential if you are going to be an effective FallProof instructor. Just as it will take time to learn how to interpret the results of the comprehensive assessment you conduct before the start of each program and then match the appropriate exercise progressions to the capabilities of your participants, developing your class organization skills will also require time and effort on your part. Individualizing the content of a program used in a group setting is not an easy task, but it is a necessary skill to master if you are going to optimize the progress of each participant in your program. Programming for older adults with balance and mobility disorders can also be challenging because many of them will have developed elaborate ways of compensating for their problems over the years that are often inappropriate or difficult to change. Careful planning, good communication skills, and patience will be the keys to your success as a FallProof program instructor. I have no doubt that this program's success over the years is due not only to the quality of the exercise progressions developed, but also to the many effective instructors I have watched deliver it.

TEST YOUR UNDERSTANDING

1. After completion of the preprogram assessment, the first task is to
   a. begin selecting appropriate exercises based on the results obtained
   b. identify and list the types of balance and mobility problems observed
   c. determine which clients should use a Dyna-Disc as opposed to a balance ball during the seated center of gravity balance activities
   d. develop a list of the balance problems observed that are permanent and a list of the impairments that are more temporary in nature
   e. assign certain exercises for homework

2. Which of the following will *not* determine the starting point for each participant in the program?
   a. previous motor skill experience
   b. current level of physical activity
   c. type of impairments identified during the initial assessment
   d. age and gender of the participant
   e. level of balance-related self-confidence

3. It is suggested that each class include the following components:
   a. 10-minute warm-up, 40-minute skills section, and 10-minute cool-down
   b. 15-minute warm-up, 35-minute skills section, and 10-minute cool-down
   c. 20-minute warm-up, 40-minute skills section, and no cool-down
   d. a warm-up, skills section, and cool-down of any length the instructor chooses
   e. 40-minute skills section and 20-minute cool-down

4. The major advantage of presenting certain activities to the whole class is that
   a. the social atmosphere of the class is enhanced
   b. you do not have to repeat your verbal instructions to multiple groups
   c. you are able to monitor each client's progress more directly
   d. the class participants do not have to move between groups so their risk for falling is decreased
   e. transition time between groups is eliminated

5. The primary reason for incorporating small-group station activities into a class is so the instructor can
   a. take a well-earned rest from teaching the class
   b. individualize the program a little more for each participant
   c. group participants according to ability
   d. use more of the space available
   e. better distribute his or her attention among the groups

6. The primary reason for including a cool-down at the end of each class is to
   a. elevate the heart rate following the skills section
   b. solicit feedback from participants about the class
   c. assign homework to be completed before the next class
   d. lower the heart rate and anxiety level of class participants
   e. recognize the efforts of individual participants

7. When working with class participants who have very low balance-related self-confidence,
   a. make sure that the exercises performed are easy enough that the participant will always be successful
   b. always provide close supervision and additional manual support
   c. have them perform all exercises in a seated position so their risk for falling is decreased
   d. present challenging balance activities that will help them forget they have a confidence problem
   e. select exercises that will challenge their balance abilities but also ensure that they are successful on a large percentage of practice attempts

8. The best way to evaluate your class management skills is to
   a. determine how quickly class participants move from one activity to the next
   b. ask the participants for feedback during the cool-down
   c. estimate the amount of time the class participants spent exercising during the time allocated for the class
   d. check whether your class ends at the designated time
   e. determine how long it requires you or your assistants to get all the necessary equipment needed for the class

9. Which of the following is *not* a good reason for conducting regular balance and mobility assessments?
   a. to identify which dimensions of balance are beginning to show improvement in each client
   b. to identify which dimensions of balance still need improving in each client
   c. to evaluate your effectiveness as an instructor
   d. to practice your test administration skills
   e. to motivate participants to continue attending classes

10. The following are all examples of effective communication skills *except*
    a. addressing class participants in a respectful manner

b. taking the time to point out each individual class member's errors during the cool-down

c. knowing the names of class participants

d. not interrupting when a client is speaking

e. allowing time to talk with clients individually after class

PRACTICAL PROBLEMS

1. Develop a complete lesson plan (using the proposed lesson plan format presented in form 11.1) for a class of 20 participants. Indicate whether the lesson plan is one that will be presented early or later in the program.

2. Videotape yourself leading an activity class for a group of older adults. Review the tape with the goal of evaluating the following:

a. Classroom management skills (i.e., record time participants were engaged in activity, efficiency of classroom setup)

b. Communication skills

c. Positioning during class and quality of verbal cuing and feedback provided to participants

Be sure to make a list of all the things you felt you did well in addition to a list of the things you feel need improvement.

Balance Kit Inventory

☐ Lightweight balls (6)

- 3 small
- 3 large

☐ Swiss balls (5)

- 1 55-cm ball
- 2 65-cm balls
- 1 75-cm ball
- 1 80-cm ball

☐ Medicine balls (3)

- 1 1-kg ball
- 1 2-kg ball
- 1 3-kg ball

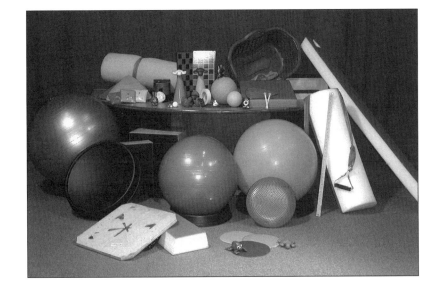

☐ Dyna-Discs (3)

☐ Stacking cones, small (set of 30)

☐ Stacking cones, large (set of 10)

☐ 8-inch stacking cones

☐ Rocker board (2)

☐ Wobble board (1)

☐ Nested benches (2 sets of 2-, 4-, 6-, and 8-inch benches)

☐ Naugahyde wedge (1 large, 12 × 24 × 28 inches)

☐ Naugahyde wedge, (1 small, 10 × 24 × 28 inches

☐ Egg crate pad

☐ Foam squares (4)

☐ 2 medium-density squares

☐ 2 firm-density squares

☐ Airex mats (2)

☐ Half foam roll (2 mats, 6 × 36 inches)

☐ Half foam roll (2 mats, 12 × 36 x .5 inches)

☐ Spot sets

☐ Theraband

☐ Air inflator or compressor

☐ Laundry basket

☐ Masking tape (2 rolls)

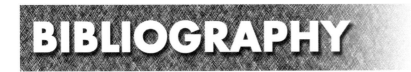

BIBLIOGRAPHY

Akima, H., Kano, Y., Enomoto, Y., Ishizu, M., Okada, M., Oishi, Y., Katsuta, S., & Kuno, S. Y. (2001). Muscle function in 164 men and women aged 20-84 yr. *Medicine and Science in Sports and Exercise*, 33: 220-226.

Alexander, N. (1994). Postural control in older adults. *Journal of the American Geriatrics Society*, 42: 93-108.

Allison, L., & Rose, D.J. (1998). The relationship between postural control system impairments and disabilities in older adults. *Physical Therapy*, 78 (5): S69-70.

Aloia, J.F., McGowan, D.M., Vaswani, A.N., Ross, P., Cohn, S.H. (1991). Relationship of menopause to skeletal and muscle mass. *American Journal of Clinical Nutrition* 53: 1378-1383.

American College of Sports Medicine. (1998). Position stand on exercise and physical activity for older adults. *Medicine and Science in Sports and Exercise*, 30: 992-1008.

American College of Sports Medicine (2002). Progression models in resistance training for healthy adults. *Medicine and Science in Sports and Exercise*, 34: 364-380.

American Heart Association (2002). *Heart facts 2002: All Americans.* Dallas, TX.

Arroyo, J.F., Herrmann, F., Saber, H., et al. (1994). Fast evaluation test for mobility, balance, and fear: A new strategy for the screening of elderly fallers. *Arthritis Rheumatology*, 37: S416. Abstract.

Asp, K. (2000). The role of stretching exercises: From warm-ups to cool-downs. *IDEA Fitness Edge*, November-December: 7-10.

Bandy, W.D., & Sanders, B. (2001). *Therapeutic exercise.* Baltimore: Lippincott Williams & Wilkins.

Barry, A.J., Steinmetz, J.R., Page, H.F., & Rodahl, K. (1967). The effects of physical conditioning on older individuals: II. Motor performance and cognitive function. *Journal of Gerontology*, 21: 192-199.

Basmajian, J.V., & De Luca, C.J. (1985). *Muscles alive: Their functions revealed by electromyography*, (5th ed.). Baltimore: Williams & Wilkins.

Bassett, C., McClamrock, E., & Schmelzer, M.A. (1982). A 10-week exercise program for senior citizens. *Geriatric Nursing*, 3: 103-105.

Bell, R., & Hoshizaki, T. (1981). Relationships of age and sex with joint range of motion of seventeen joint actions in humans. *Canadian Journal of Applied Sport Sciences*, 6: 202-206.

Berg, K.O., Maki, B.E., Williams, J.I., et al. (1992). Clinical and laboratory measures of postural balance in an elderly population. *Archives of Physical Medicine and Rehabilitation*, 73: 1073-1080.

Berg, K., Wood-Dauphinee, S., & Williams, J.I. (1995). The balance scale: Reliability assessment with elderly residents and patients with acute stroke. *Scandinavian Journal of Rehabilitation Medicine*, 27: 27-36.

Berg, K., Wood-Dauphinee, S.L., Williams, J.I., & Gayton, D. (1989). Measuring balance in the elderly: Preliminary development of an instrument. *Physiotherapy Canada*, 41: 304-311.

Berg, K.O., Wood-Dauphinee, S.L., Williams, J.I., & Maki, B. (1992). Measuring balance in the elderly: Validation of an instrument. *Canadian Journal of Public Health*, 2: S7-S11.

Bernstein, N. (1967). *The coordination and regulation of movement.* London: Pergamon.

Berthoz, A., & Pozzo, T. (1994). Head and body coordination during locomotion and complex movements. In S.P. Swinnen, H. Heuer, J. Massion, & P. Casaer (Eds.), *Interlimb coordination: Neural, dynamical and cognitive constraints* (pp. 147-165). San Diego: Academic Press.

Binder, E.F., Brown, M.B., & Birge, S.J. (1991). Effects of moderate intensity exercise program at reducing risk factors for falls in frail older adults. *Journal of the American Geriatric Society*, 39: A50.

Bogle Thorbahn, L.D., & Newton, R.A. (1996). Use of the Berg Balance Test to predict falls in elderly persons. *Physical Therapy*, 76 (6): 576-583.

Bohannon, R.W. Comfortable and maximum walking speed of adults aged 20-79 years: Reference values and determinants. *Age and Ageing*, 26: 15-19.

Bohannon, R.W., & Leary, K.M. (1995). Standing balance and function over the course of acute rehabilitation. *Archives of Physical Medicine and Rehabilitation*, 76: 994-996.

Brandt, K.D., & Slemenda, C.W. (1993). Osteoarthritis epidemiology, pathology, and pathogenesis. In H.R. Schumacher Jr. (Ed.), *Primer on the rheumatic disease.* (10th ed., pp184-187). Atlanta: Arthritis Foundation.

Brauer, S.G., Woollacott, M., & Shumway-Cook, A. (2002). The influence of a concurrent cognitive task on the compensatory stepping response to a perturbation in balance-impaired and healthy elders. *Gait and Posture*, 15: 83-93.

Brill, P.A., Matthews, M., Mason, J., Davis, D., et al. (1998). Improving functional performance through a group-based free weight strength training program in residents of two assisted living communities. *Physical and Occupational Therapy in Geriatrics*, 15(3): 57-69.

Brown, L.A., Shumway-Cook, A., & Woollacott, M.H. (1999). Attentional demands and postural recovery: The effects of aging. *Journal of Gerontology*, 54A: M165-171.

Buchner D.M., Cress M.E., de Lateur B.J., Esselman P.C., Margherita A.J., Price R., & Wagner E.H. (1997). The effect of strength and endurance training on gait, balance, fall risk, and health services use in community-living older adults. *Journal of Gerontology*, 52: M218-M224.

Campbell, A., Borrie, M.J., & Spears, G.F. (1989). Risk factors for falls in a community-based prospective study of people 70 years and older. *Journal of Gerontology*, 44: 112-117.

Center for Successful Aging (2003). *Training and operations manual* Fullerton, CA:.California State University, Fullerton.

Chandler, J.M. (1996). Invited commentary. *Physical Therapy*, 76: 584-585.

Chandler, J.M., & Hadley, E.C. (1996). Exercise to improve physiologic and functional performance in old age. *Clinics in Geriatric Medicine*, 12: 761-784.

Chen, H-C., Ashton-Miller, J.A., Alexander, N.B., & Schultz, A.B. (1991). Stepping over obstacles: Gait patterns of healthy young and old adults. *Journal of Gerontology*, 46: M196-203.

Chiodo, L.K., Gerety, M.B., Mulrow, C.D., Rhodes, M.C., & Tuley, M.R. (1992). The impact of physical therapy on nursing home patient outcomes. *Physical Therapy*, 72: 168-173.

Chong, R.K.Y., Horak, F.B., Frank, J., & Kaye, J. (1999). Sensory organization for balance: Specific deficits in Alzheimer's but not in Parkinson's disease. *Journal of Gerontology: Medical Sciences*, 54A(3): M122-M128.

Clark, S., & Rose, D.J. (2001). Evaluation of dynamic balance among community-dwelling older adult fallers: A generalizability study of the limits of stability. *Archives of Physical Medicine and Rehabilitation*, 82: 468-474.

Clark, S., Rose, D.J., & Fujimoto, K. (1997). Generalizability of the limits of stability test in the evaluation of dynamic balance among older adults. *Archives of Physical Medicine and Rehabilitation*, 78: 1078-1084.

Close, J., Ellis, M., Hooper, R., Glucksman, E., Jackson, S., & Swift, C. (1999). Prevention of falls in the elderly trial (PROFET): A randomized controlled trial. *The Lancet*, 353: 93-97.

Crilly, R.G., Willems, D.A., Trenholm, K.J., Hayes, K.C., & Delaquerriere-Richardson, L.F.O. (1989). Effect of exercise on postural sway in the elderly. *Gerontology*, 35: 137-143.

Cutson, T.M. (1994). Falls in the elderly. *American Family Physician.* 49: 149-157.

Danneskiold-Samsoe, B., Lyngberg, K., Risum, T., & Telling, M. (1987). The effect of water exercise therapy given to patients with rheumatoid arthritis. *Scandinavian Journal of Rehabilitation Medicine*, 19: 31-35.

Daschle et al., 1999. Unpublished Masters Project. Pacific University, Pacific Grove, OR.

Day, L., Fildes, B., Gordon, I., Fitzharris, M., Flamer, H., & Lord, S. (2002). Randomised factorial trial of falls prevention among older people living in their homes. *British Medical Journal,* 325: 128-133.

Deyle, G.D., Henderson, N.E., Matekel R.L., Ryder, M.G., Garber, M.B., & Allison, S.C. (2000). Effectiveness of manual physical therapy and exercise in osteoarthritis of the knee. *Annals of Internal Medicine,* 132: 129-133.

Diener, H.C., & Nutt, J.G. (1997). Vestibular and cerebellar disorders of equilibrium and gait. In J.C. Masdeu, L. Sudarsky, & L. Wolfson (Eds.), *Gait disorders of aging. Falls and therapeutic strategies* (pp. 261-272). Philadelphia: Lippincott-Raven.

Di Fabio, R.P., & Seay, R. (1997). Use of the "Fast Evaluation of Mobility, Balance and Fear" in elderly community dwellers: Validity and reliability. *Physical Therapy,* 77: 904-917.

Di Pietro, L. (1996). The epidemiology of physical activity and physical function in older people. *Medicine and Science in Sports and Exercise,* 28: 596-600.

Duncan, P.W., Studenski, S.A., Chandler, J., & Prescott, B. (1992). Functional reach: Predictive validity in a sample of elderly male veterans. *Journal of Gerontology: Medical Sciences,* 47: M93-M97.

Duncan, P.W., Weiner, D.K., Chandler, J., & Studenski, S.A. (1990). Functional reach: A new clinical measure of balance? *Journal of Gerontology: Medical Sciences,* 45: M192-M197.

Eisenberg, D.M., Kessler, R.C., Foster, C., Norlock, F.E., Calkins, D.R., & Delbanco, T.L. (1993). Unconventional medicine in the United States: Prevalence, costs, and patterns of use. *New England Journal of Medicine,* 328: 246-252.

Eisenberg, D.M., Davis, R.B., Ettner, S.L., Appel, S., Wilkey, S., Van Rompay, M., & Kessler, R.C. (1998). Trends in alternative medicine use in the United States, 1990-1997. Results of a follow-up national survey. *Journal of the American Medical Association,* 280: 1569-1575.

Elble, R.J. (1997). Changes in gait with normal aging. In J.C. Masdeu, L. Sudarsky, & L. Wolfson (Eds.), *Gait disorders of aging. Falls and therapeutic strategies* (pp. 93-106). Philadelphia: Lippincott-Raven.

Elble, R.J., Thomas, S.S., Higgins, C., & Colliver, J. (1991). Stride-dependent changes in gait of older people. *Journal of Neurology,* 238: 1-5.

El-Kashlan, H.K., Shepard, N.T., Asher, A.M., Smith-Wheelock, M., & Telian, S.A. (1998). Evaluation of clinical measures of equilibrium. *The Laryngoscope,* 108, March: 311-319.

Engardt, M., Knutsson, E., Jonsson, M., & Sternhag, M. (1995). Dynamic muscle strength training in stroke patients: Effects on knee extension torque, electromyographic activity, and motor function. *Archives of Physical Medicine and Rehabilitation,* 76: 419-425.

Erim, Z., Beg, M.F., Burke, D.T., & De Luca, C.J. (1999). Effects of aging on motor-unit control properties. *Journal of Neurophysiology,* 82: 2081-2091.

Ettinger, W.H., Burns, R., & Messier, S.P. (1999). A randomized trial comparing aerobic exercise and resistance exercise with a health education program in older adults with knee osteoarthritis. The Fitness Arthritis and Seniors Trial (FAST). *Journal of the American Medical Association,* 277: 1361-1369.

Fiatarone, M.A., Marks, E.C., Ryan, N., Meredith, C.N., Lipsitz, L.A., & Evans, W.J. (1990). High-intensity strength training in nonagenarians. *Journal of the American Medical Association,* 263(22): 3029-3034.

Fitts, P.M. & Posner, M.I. (1967). *Human performance.* Belmont, CA: Brooks/Cole.

Foldvari, M., Clark, M., Laviolette, L.A., Bernstein, M.A., Kaliton, D., Castaneda, C., Pu, C. T., Hausdorff, J.M., Fielding, R.A., Fiatarone-Singh, M.A. (2000). Association of muscle power with functional status in community-dwelling elderly women. *Journal of Gerontology,* 55A: M192-M199.

Ford-Smith, C.D., Wyman, J.F., Elswick, Jr., R.K., Fernandez, T., & Newton, R.A. (1995). Test-retest reliability of the sensory organization test in noninstitutionalized older adults. *Archives of Physical Medicine and Rehabilitation,* 76: 77-81.

Gardner, M.M., Robertson, M.C., & Campbell, A.J. (2000). Exercise in preventing falls and fall related injuries in older people: A review of randomised controlled trials. *British Journal of Sports Medicine,* 34: 7-17.

Gentile, A.M. (1972). A working model of skill acquisition with application to teaching. *Quest,* Monograph XVII: 3-23.

Gentile, A.M. (1987). Skill acquisition: Action, movement, and neuromotor processes. In J.H. Carr, R.B. Shephard, J. Gordon, A.M. Gentile, & J.M. Held (Eds.), *Movement science. Foundations for physical therapy in rehabilitation* (pp. 93-154). Rockville, MD: Aspen.

Gentile, A.M. (2000). Skill acquisition: Action, movement, and neuromotor processes. In J.H. Carr, & R.B. Shephard (Eds.), *Movement science. Foundations for physical therapy in rehabilitation* (2nd ed., pp. 111-187). Rockville, MD: Aspen.

279

Gibson, J.J. (1966). *The senses considered as perceptual systems.* Boston: Houghton Mifflin.

Gillespie, L.D., Gillespie, W.J., Robertson, M.C., Lamb S.E., Cumming, R.G., & Rowe, B.H. (2002). Interventions for preventing falls in elderly people (Cochrane Review). In: *The Cochrane Library*, Issue 3. Oxford: Update Software.

Goode, S.L., & Magill, R.A. (1986). The contextual interference effect in learning three badminton serves. *Research Quarterly for Exercise and Sport*, 57: 308-314.

Grisso, J.A., Capezuti, E., & Schwartz, A. (1996). Falls as risk factors for fractures. In R. Marcus, D. Feldman, & J. Kelsey (Eds.), *Osteoporosis.* New York: Academic Press.

Gunter, K.B., White, K.W., Hayes, W.C., & Snow, C.M. (2000). Functional mobility discriminates nonfallers from one-time and frequent fallers. *Journal of Gerontology: Medical Sciences*, 11: M672-M676.

Gutman, G.M., Herbert, C.P., & Brown, S.R. (1977). Feldenkrais versus conventional exercises for the elderly. *Journal of Gerontology*, 32: 562-572.

Hall, K.G., Domingues, D.A., & Cavazos, R. (1994). Contextual interference effects with skilled baseball players. *Perceptual and Motor Skills*, 78: 835-841.

Hamid, M.A., Hughes, G.B., & Kinney, S.E. (1991). Specificity and sensitivity of dynamic posturography: A retrospective analysis. *Acta Otolaryngology* (Stoch.), Suppl. 481: 596-600.

Harada, N., Chiu, V., Damron-Rodriguez, J., Fowler, E., Siu, A., & Reuben, D.B. (1995). Screening for balance and mobility impairment in elderly individuals living in residential care facilities. *Physical Therapy*, 75: 462-469.

Harada, N., Chiu, V., Fowler, E., Lee, M., & Reuben, D.B. (1995). Physical therapy to improve functioning of older people in residential care facilities. *Physical Therapy*, 75: 830-838.

Herdman, S.J. (1999). *Vestibular rehabilitation* (2nd ed.). Philadelphia: F.A. Davis.

Hill, K.D., Schwarz, J.A., Kalogeropoulos, A.J., & Gibson, S.J. (1996). Modified Falls Efficacy Scale. *Archives of Physical Medicine and Rehabilitation*, 77: 1025-1029.

Holland, G.J., Tanaka, K., Shigematsu, R., & Nakagaichi, M. (2002). Flexibility and physical functions of older adults: A review. *Journal of Aging and Physical Activity*, 10: 169-206.

Horak, F.B. (1994). Components of postural dyscontrol in the elderly: A review. *Neurobiology of Aging*, 10: 727-738.

Horak, F.B., & Nashner, L.M. (1986). Central programming of postural movements: Adaptations to altered support surface configurations. *Journal of Neurophysiology*, 55: 1369-1381.

Hoyert, D.L., Kochanek, K.D., & Murphy, S.L. (1999). Deaths: Final data for 1997. *National Vital Statistics Reports*, 47: 19. Hyattsville, MD: National Center for Health Statistics.

Hu, M.H., & Woollacott, M. (1994a). Multisensory training of standing balance in older adults: I. Postural stability and one-leg stance balance. *Journal of Gerontology*, 49: M52-M61.

Hu, M.H., & Woollacott, M. (1994b). Multisensory training of standing balance in older adults: II. Kinetic and electromyographic postural responses. *Journal of Gerontology*, 49: M62-M71.

Jette, A.M., Branch, L.G., & Berlin, J. (1990). Musculoskeletal impairments and physical disablement among the elderly. *Journal of Gerontology*, 45: M203-M208.

Kisner, C., & Colby, L.A. (1990). *Therapeutic exercise foundations and techniques* (2nd ed.). Philadelphia: Davis.

Kugler, P.N., & Turvey, M.T. (1987). *Information, natural law and the self-assembly of rhythmic movement.* Hillsdale, NJ: Erlbaum.

Landers, K. A., G. R. Hunter, C. J. Wetzstein, M. M. Bamman, & R. L. Wiensier (2001). The interrelationship among muscle mass, strength, and the ability to perform physical tasks of daily living in younger and older women. *Journal of Gerontology*, 56A: B443-B448.

Leape, L.L. (2000). Preventable medical injuries in older patients. *Archives of Internal Medicine*, 160: 2717-2728.

Lee, D.N. (1978). The functions of vision. In H. Pick & E. Salzman (Eds.), *Modes of perceiving and processing information* (pp. 159-170). Hillsdale, NJ: Erlbaum.

Leipzig, R.M., Cumming, R.G., & Tinetti, M.E. (1999a). Drugs and falls: A systematic review and meta-analysis: I. Psychotropic drugs. *Journal of American Geriatric Society*, 47: 30-39.

Leipzig, R.M., Cumming, R.G., & Tinetti M.E. (1999b). Drugs and falls: A systematic review and meta-analysis II. Cardiac and analgesic drugs. *Journal of American Geriatric Society*, 47: 40-50.

Lichtenstein, M.J., Shields, S.L., Shiavi, R.G. & Burger, M.C. (1989). Exercise and balance in aged women: A pilot controlled clinical trial. *Archives of Physical Medicine and Rehabilitation*, 70: 138-143.

Lindle, R.S, Metter, E.J., Lynch, N.A., Fleg, J.L., Fozard, J.L., Tobin, J., Roy, T.A., & Hurley, B.F., (1997). Age and gender comparisons of muscle strength in 654 women and men aged 20-93 yr. *Journal of Applied Physiology*, 83: 1581-1587.

Lipsitz, L.A., Jonsson, P.V., Kelley, M.M., & Koestner, J.S. (1991). Causes and correlates of recurrent falls in ambulatory frail elderly. *Journal of Gerontology*, 46: M114-M122.

Liston, R.A.L., & Brouwer, B.J. (1996). Reliability and validity of measures obtained from stroke patients using the balance master. *Archives of Physical Medicine and Rehabilitation*, 77: 425-430.

Lui, J., & Wrisberg, C.A. (1997). The effect of knowledge of results delay and the subjective estimation of movement form on the acquisition and retention of a motor skill. *Research Quarterly for Exercise and Sport*, 68: 145-151.

Lundin-Olsson, L., Nyberg, L., & Gustafson, Y. (1997). "Stops walking when talking" as a predictor of falls in elderly people. *Lancet*, 349: 617.

Magill, R.A. (2001). *Motor learning. Concepts and applications.* (6th ed.). Boston: McGraw Hill.

Magill, R.A., & Hall, K.G. (1990). A review of the contextual interference effect in motor skill acquisition. *Human Movement Science*, 9: 241-289.

Mann, G.C., Whitney, S.L., Refern, M.S., Borello-France, D.F., & Furman, J.M. (1996). Functional reach and single leg stance in patients with peripheral vestibular disorders. *Journal of Vestibular Research*, 6: 343-353.

McCartney, N., Hicks, A.L., Martin, J., & Webber, C.E. (1995). Long-term resistance training in the elderly: Effects on dynamic strength, exercise capacity, muscle, and bone. *Journal of Gerontology: Biological Sciences*, 50A(2): B97-B104.

McCullagh, P., & Meyer, K.N. (1997). Learning versus correct models: Influence of model type on the learning of a free-weight squat lift. *Research Quarterly for Exercise and Sport*, 68: 56-61.

McMurdo, M.E.T., & Burnett, L. (1992). Randomized controlled trial of exercise in the elderly. *Gerontology*, 38: 292-298.

Means, K.M., Rodell, D.E., O'Sullivan, P., & Cranford, L.A. (1996). Rehabilitation of elderly fallers: Pilot study of a low to moderate intensity exercise program. *Archives of Physical Medicine and Rehabilitation*, 77: 1030-1036.

Medell, J.L., & Alexander, N.B. (2000). A clinical measure of maximal and rapid stepping in older women. *Journal of Gerontology: Medical Sciences*, 55A(8): M429-M433.

Miller, E.W., Black, K., Eble, T., & Welch, A. (1998). The influence of height and age on functional reach. *Neurology Report*, 22(5): 161. Abstract.

Mills, R.M. (1994). The effect of low-intensity aerobic exercise on muscle strength, flexibility and balance among sedentary elderly persons. *Nursing Research*, 43: 207-211.

Minor, M.A., Hewett, J.E., Anderson, S.K., & Ray, D.A. (1989). Efficacy of physical conditioning exercise in patients with rheumatoid arthritis and osteoarthritis. *Arthritis Rheumatology*, 32: 1396-1405.

Moore, S., & Woollacott, M.H. (1993). The use of biofeedback devices to improve postural stability. *Physical Therapy Practice*, 2(2): 1-19.

Morey, M.C., Pieper, C.F., & Cornoni-Huntley, J.C. (1991). Physical fitness and functional limitations in community dwelling older adults. *Medicine and Science in Sports and Exercise*, 30: 715-723.

Morrison, R.S., Chassin, M.R., & Siu, A.L. (1998). The medical consultant's role in caring for patients with hip fracture. *Annals of Internal Medicine*, 128: 1010-1020.

Mulrow, C.D., Gerety, M.B., Kanten, D., Cornell, J.E., DeNino, L.A., Chiodo, L., et al. (1994). A randomized trial of physical rehabilitation for very frail nursing home residents. *Journal of the American Medical Association*, 271: 519-523.

Myers, A.M., Fletcher, A.H., & Sherk, W. (1998). Discriminative and evaluative properties of the Activities-specific Balance Confidence (ABC) Scale. *Journal of Gerontology: Medical Sciences*, 53A(4): M287-M294.

Myers, A.M., Powell, L.E., Maki, B.E., Holliday, P.J., Brawley, L.R., & Sherk, W. (1996). Psychological indicators of balance confidence: Relationship to actual and perceived abilities. *Journal of Gerontology: Medical Sciences*, 51A(1): M37-M43.

Nagi, S.Z. (1991). Disability concepts revisited: Implication for prevention. In A.M. Pope & A.R. Tarlov (Eds.), *Disability in America: Toward a national agenda for prevention* (pp. 309-327). Washington, DC: National Academy Press.

Nashner, L.M. (1990). Sensory, neuromuscular, and biomechanical contributions to human balance. In P.W. Duncan (Ed.), *Balance: Proceedings of the APTA Forum*. Virginia: American Physical Therapy Association.

Nashner, L., & McCollum, G. (1985). The organization of human postural movements: A formal basis and experimental synthesis. *Behavioral and Brain Sciences*, 9: 135-172.

National Institutes of Health (1994). *Total hip replacement: NIH Consensus Statement, 12*: 1-31. Bethesda, MD: U.S. Dept. of Health and Human Services.

Nevitt, M.C. (1997). Falls in the elderly: Risk factors and prevention. In J.C. Masdeu, L. Sudarsky, & L. Wolfson (Eds.), *Gait disorders of aging. Falls and therapeutic strategies* (pp. 13-36). Philadelphia: Lippincott-Raven.

Nevitt, M.C., Cummings, S.R., Kidd, S., & Black, D. (1989). Risk factors for recurrent nonsyncopal falls: A prospective study. *Journal of the American Medical Association*, 261: 2663-2668.

Newell, K.M. (1986). Constraints on the development of coordination. In M.G. Wade & H.T.A. Whiting (Eds.), *Motor development in children: Aspects of coordination and control*, (pp. 341-360). Boston: Martinus Nijhoff.

Newton, R.A. (1997). Balance screening of an inner city older adult population. *Archives of Physical Medicine and Rehabilitation*, 78: 587-591.

Newton, R.A. (2001). Validity of the Multi-Directional Reach Test: A practical measure for limits of stability in older adults. *Journal of Gerontology: Medical Sciences*, 56A(4): M248-M252.

O'Brien, K., Pickles, B., & Culham, E. (1998). Clinical measures of balance in community-dwelling elderly female fallers and non-fallers. *Physiotherapy Canada*, Summer: 212-217, 221.

Overstall, P.W., Exton-Smith, A.N., Imms, F.J., & Johnson, A.C. (1990). Falls in the elderly related to postural imbalance. *British Journal of Medicine*, 1: 261-264.

Patla, A.E. (1997). Understanding the roles of vision in the control of human locomotion. *Gait and Posture*, 5: 54-69.

Patla, A., & Shumway-Cook, A. (1999). Dimensions of mobility: Defining the complexity and difficulty associated with community mobility. *Journal of Aging and Physical Activity*, 7: 7-19.

Perret, E., & Reglis, F. (1970). Age and the perceptual threshold for vibratory stimuli. *European Neurology*, 4: 65-76.

Physicalmind Institute®. 2001. Osteoporosis. Exercise protocols. Santa Fe, NM: Physicalmind Institute.

Podsiadlo, D., & Richardson, S. (1991). The timed "up and go": A test of basic functional mobility for frail elderly persons. *Journal of the American Geriatric Society*, 39: 142-148.

Pollock, B.J., & Lee, T.D. (1992). Effects of the model's skill level on observational learning. *Research Quarterly for Exercise and Sport*, 63: 25-29.

Powell, L.E., & Myers, A.M. (1995). The Activities-specific Balance Confidence (ABC) Scale. *Journal of Gerontology: Medical Sciences*, 50A: M28-M34.

Province, M.A., Hadley, E.C., Hornbrook, M.C., Lipsitz, L.A., Miller, J.P., Mulrow, C.D., et al. (1995). The effects of exercise on falls in elderly patients. A preplanned meta-analysis on the FICSIT trials. *Journal of the American Medical Association*, 273: 1341-1347.

Ray, W.A., & Griffin, M.R. (1990). Prescribed medications and the risk of falling. *Topics in Geriatric Rehabilitation*, 5: 12-20.

Ray, W.A., Taylor, J.A., Meador, K.G., Thapa, P.B., et al. (1997). A randomized trial of a consultation service to reduce falls in nursing homes. *Journal of the American Medical Association*, 278: 557-562.

Reuben, D.B., & Sui, A.L. (1990). An objective measure of physical function of elderly outpatients: The Physical Performance Test. *Journal of the American Geriatric Society*, 38: 1105-1112.

Rhodes et al., 2000.

Riccio, G.E., & Stoffregen, T.A.(1988). An ecological theory of orientation and the vestibular system. *Psychological Review*, 95: 3-14.

Riccio, G.E., Martin, E.J., & Stoffregen, T.A. (1992). The role of balance dynamics in the active perception of orientation. *Journal of Experimental Psychology: Human Perception and Performance*, 18: 624-644.

Riddle, D.L., & Stratford, P.W. (1999). Interpreting validity indexes for diagnostic tests: An illustration using the Berg Balance Test. *Physical Therapy*, 79: 939-948.

Rikli, R.E., & Jones, C.J. (1997). Assessing physical performance in independent older adults: Issues and guidelines. *Journal of Aging and Physical Activity*, 5: 244-261.

Rikli, R.E., & Jones, C.J. (1998). The reliability and validity of a 6-minute walk test as a measure of physical endurance in older adults. *Journal of Aging and Physical Activity*, 6: 363-375.

Rikli, R.E., & Jones, C.J. (1999a). The development and validation of a functional fitness test for community-residing older adults. *Journal of Aging and Physical Activity*, 7: 129-161.

Rikli, R.E., & Jones, C.J. (1999b). Functional fitness normative scores for community-residing adults, ages 60-94. *Journal of Aging and Physical Activity*, 7: 162-181.

Rikli, R.E., Jones, C.J. (2001). *Senior Fitness Test Manual.* Champaign, IL: Human Kinetics.

Robbins, A.S., Rubenstein, L.Z., Josephson, K.R., et al. (1989). Predictors of falls among elderly people. *Archives of Internal Medicine*, 149: 1628-1633.

Rodriquez, A.A., Black, P.O., Kile, K.A., Sherman, J., Stelberg, B., et al. (1996). Gait training efficacy using a home-based practice model in chronic hemiplegia. *Archives of Physical Medicine and Rehabilitation*, 77: 801-805.

Rose, D.J. (1997). A multilevel approach to the study of motor control and learning. Boston, MA: Allyn & Bacon.

Rose, D.J. (2001a). Central nervous system: Motor function. In G.L. Maddox (Ed.), *The Encyclopedia of Aging: A Comprehensive Resource in Gerontology and Geriatrics* (3rd ed., pp. 189-191). New York: Springer.

Rose, D.J. (2001b). Age-related balance changes affect athletic performance. *BioMechanics*, 8:79-85.

Rose, D.J. (2001c). Reducing fall risk in older adults: There is no quick fix! *Gerontologist*, 41 (1): 297.

Rose, D.J. (2002). Promoting functional independence among "at risk" and physically frail older adults: The need for a multidimensional and targeted programming approach. *Journal of Aging and Physical Activity*, 10: 207-225.

Rose, D.J., & Clark, S. (2000). Can the control of bodily orientation be improved in a group of older adults with a history of falls? *Journal of the American Geriatric Society*, 48: 275-282.

Rose, D.J., Jones, C.J., & Lemon, N. (2001). Effectiveness of a fall risk reduction program for older adult women with arthritis. Paper presented at the 1st Joint Conference of The American Society on Aging and The National Council on the Aging, 8-11 March, New Orleans, LA.

Rose, D.J., Jones, C.J., Lemon, N., & Bories, T. (1999). The effect of a community-based balance and mobility training program on functional performance and balance-related self-confidence in older adults with a history of falls. *Journal of Aging and Physical Activity*, 7(3): 265.

Rose, D.J., Jones, C.J., & Lucchese, N. (2002). Predicting the probability of falls in community-residing older adults using the 8 foot up and go: A new measure of functional mobility. *Journal of Aging and Physical Activity*, 10:466-475.

Rubenstein, L.Z., & Josephson, K.R. (1992). Causes and prevention of falls in elderly people. In B. Vellas et al. (Eds.), *Falls, Balance and Gait Disorders in the Elderly*, (pp. 21-38). Paris: Elsevier.

Rubenstein, L.Z., Josephson, K.R., Trueblood, P.R., Loy, S., Harker, J.O., Pietruszka, F.M., & Robbins, A.S. (2001). Effects of a group exercise program on strength, mobility, and falls among fall-prone elderly men. *Journal of Gerontology: Medical Sciences*, 55A: M317-M321.

Schmidt, R.A., & Wrisberg, C.A. (2000). *Motor learning and performance.* Champaign, IL: Human Kinetics.

Seidler, R.D., & Martin, P.E. (1997). The effects of short term balance training on the postural control of older adults. *Gait and Posture*, 6: 224-236.

Shea, J.B., & Morgan, R.L. (1979). Contextual interference effects on the acquisition, retention, and transfer of a motor skill. *Journal of Experimental Psychology: Human Learning and Memory*, 5: 179-187.

Shumway-Cook, A., Baldwin, M., Polissar, N.L., & Gruber, W. (1997). Predicting the probability for falls in community-dwelling older adults. *Physical Therapy*, 77(8): 812-819.

Shumway-Cook, A., Brauer, S., & Woollacott, M. (2000). Predicting the probability for falls in community-dwelling older adults using the timed up and go test. *Physical Therapy*, 80: 896-903.

Shumway-Cook, A., Gruber, W., Baldwin, M., & Liao, S. (1997). The effect of multidimensional exercises on balance, mobility, and fall risk in community-dwelling older adults. *Physical Therapy*, 77(1): 46-56.

Shumway-Cook, A., & Horak, F.B. (1986). Assessing the influence of sensory interaction on balance: Suggestions from the field. *Physical Therapy*, 66: 1548-1550.

Shumway-Cook, A., & Woollacott, M. (2000). Attentional demands and postural control: The effect of sensory context. *Journal of Gerontology*, 55A: M10-M16.

Shumway-Cook, A., & Woollacott, M.H. (2001). *Motor Control. Theory and Practical Applications* (2nd ed.). Philadelphia: Lippincott Williams & Wilkins.

Shumway-Cook, A., Woollacott, M., Baldwin, M., & Kerns, K. (1997). The effects of cognitive demands on postural sway in elderly fallers and non-fallers. *Journal of Gerontology: Medical Sciences*, 52A: M232-M240.

Skelton, D.A., & Dinan, S.M. (1999). Exercise for falls management: Rationale for an exercise programme aimed at reducing postural instability. *Physiotherapy Theory and Practice*, 15: 105-120.

Skelton, D.A., Young, A., Greig, C.A., & Malbut, K.E. (1995). Effects of resistance training on strength, power, and selected functional abilities of women aged 75 and older. *Journal of the American Geriatric Society*, 43: 1081-1087.

Sowden, A., Sheldon, T., Pehl, L., Eastwood, A., Clenny, A-NI, & Long, A. (1996). Preventing falls and subsequent injury in older people. *Effective Health Care*, 2: 1-16.

Spirduso, W. W. (1995). *Physical dimensions of aging*. Champaign, IL: Human Kinetics.

Stelmach G.E., Phillips, J., DiFabio, R.P., & Teasdale, N. (1989). Age, functional postural reflexes, and voluntary sway. *Journal of Gerontology: Biological Sciences*, 44: B100-B106.

Stewart, M.G., Chen, A.Y., Wyatt, R., Favrot, S., Beinart, S., Coker, N.J., & Jenkins, H.A. (1999). Cost-effectiveness of the diagnostic evaluation of vertigo. *The Laryngoscope*, 109, April: 600-605.

Stoffregen, T.A., & Flynn, S.B. (1994). Visual perception of support-surface deformability from human body kinematics. *Ecological Psychology*, 6: 36-63.

Stoffregen, T.A., Riccio, G.E. (1988). Affordances as constraints on the control of stance. *Human Movement Science*, 7: 265-300.

Studenski, S., Duncan, P.W., Chandler, J., Samsa, G., Prescoh, B., et al. (1994). Predicting falls: The role of mobility and nonphysical factors. *Journal of American Geriatric Society*, 42: 297-302.

Swinnen, S.P. (1990). Interpolated activities during the knowledge of results and post knowledge of results interval: Effects of performance and learning. *Journal of Experimental Psychology: Learning, Memory, and Cognition*, 19: 1321-1344.

Thapa, P.B., Gideon, P., Cost, T.W., Milam, A.B., & Ray, W.A. (1998). Antidepressants and the risk of falls among nursing home residents. *New England Journal of Medicine*, 339: 875-882.

Thelen, E., Kelso, J.A.S., & Fogel, A. (1987). Self-organizing systems and infant motor development. *Developmental Reviews*, 7: 39-65.

Thorbahn, L., & Newton, R. (1996). Use of the Berg Balance Test to predict falls in elderly persons. *Physical Therapy*, 76: 576-585.

Tideiksaar, R. (1997). Environmental factors in the prevention of falls. In J.C. Masdeu, L. Sudarsky, & L. Wolfson (Eds.), *Gait disorders of aging. Falls and therapeutic strategies* (pp. 395-414). Philadelphia: Lippincott-Raven.

Tinetti, M.E. (1986). Performance-oriented assessment of mobility problems in elderly patients. *Journal of the American Geriatric Society*, 34: 119-126.

Tinetti, M.E., Baker, D.I., McAvay, G., Clans, E.B., Garrett, P., Gottschalk, M., Koch, M.L., Trainor, K., & Horwitz, R.I. (1994). A multifactorial intervention to reduce the risk of falling among elderly people living in the community. *New England Journal of Medicine*, 331: 821-827.

Tinetti, M.E., Mendes de Leon, C.F., Doucette, J.T., & Baker, D.I. (1994). Fear-of-falling and fall-related efficacy in relationship to functioning among community-living elders. *Journal of Gerontology*, 49: M140-M147.

Tinetti, M.E., Richman, D., & Powell, L. (1990). Falls efficacy as a measure of fear of falling. *Journal of Gerontology: Psychological Sciences*, 45(6): P239-243.

Tinetti, M.E., Speechley, M., & Ginter, S.F. (1988). Risk factors for falls among elderly people living in the community. *New England Journal of Medicine*, 319: 1701-1707.

Tinetti, M.E., Williams, T.F., & Mayewski, R. (1986). Fall risk index for elderly patients based on numbers of chronic disabilities. *American Journal of Medicine*, 80: 429-434.

Urton, M.M. (1991). A community home inspection approach to preventing falls among the elderly. *Public Health Reports*, 106: 192-195.

Van den Ende, C.H.M., Vliet Vlieland, T.P.M., Munneke, M., & Hazes, J.M.W. (1998). Dynamic exercise therapy in rheumatoid arthritis: A systematic review of randomized clinical trials. *British Journal of Rheumatology*, 42: 677-687.

Van Dijk, P.T., Meulenberg, O.G., van de Sande, H.J., & Habbema, J.D. (1993). Falls in dementia patients. *Gerontologist*, 33: 200-204.

VanSwearingen, J.M., Paschal, K.A., Bonino, P., & Yang, J-F. (1996). The modified gait abnormality rating scale for recognizing the risk of recurrent falls in community-dwelling elderly adults. *Physical Therapy*, 76(9): 994-1001.

Vereijken, B. (1991). The dynamics of skill acquisition. Unpublished dissertation, Free University, Netherlands.

Wee, J.Y.M., Bagg, S., & Palepu, A. (1999). The Berg Balance Scale as a predictor of length of stay and discharge destination in an acute stroke rehabilitation setting. *Archives of Physical Medicine and Rehabilitation, 80:448-452.*

Weiner, D.K., Bongiorni, D.R., Studenski, S.A., Duncan, P.W., & Kochersberger, G.G. (1993). Does functional reach improve with rehabilitation? *Archives of Physical Medicine and Rehabilitation*, 74: 796-799.

Weiner, D.K., Duncan, P.W., Chandler, J., & Prescott, B. (1992). Functional reach: A marker of physical frailty. *Journal of the American Geriatric Society*, 40: 203-207.

Weir, P.L., & Leavitt, J.L. (1990). The effects of model's skill level and model's knowledge of results on the acquisition of an aiming task. *Human Movement Science*, 9: 369-383.

Wernick-Robinson, M., Krebs, D.E., & Giorgetti, M.M. (1999). Functional reach: Does it really measure dynamic balance? *Archives of Physical Medicine and Rehabilitation*, 80: 262-268.

WHO Study Group. (1994). Assessment of fracture risk and its application to screening for postmenopausal osteoporosis. *WHO Technical Report Series, no. 843* (pp. 1-129). Geneva, Switzerland: World Health Organization.

Winstein, C.J., & Schmidt, R.A. (1990). Reduced frequency of knowledge of results enhances motor skill learning. *Journal of Experimental Psychology: Learning, Memory, and Cognition*, 16: 677-691.

Winstein, C.J., Gardner, E.R., McNeal, D.R., Barto, P.S., & Nicholson, D.E. (1989). Standing balance training: Effect on balance and locomotion in hemiparetic adults. *Archives of Physical Medicine and Rehabilitation*, 70: 755-762.

Wolf, S.L., Barnhart, H.X., Kutner, N., McNeely, E., Coogler, C., et al. (1996). Reducing frailty and falls in older persons: An investigation of tai chi and computerized balance training. *Journal of the American Geriatric Society*, 44: 489-497.

Wolfson, L. (1997). Balance decrements in older persons: Effects of age and disease. In J.C. Masdeau, L. Sudarsky, & L. Wolfson (Eds.), *Gait disorders of aging. Falls and Therapeutic Strategies*, pp. 79-92. Philadelphia, PA: Lippincott-Raven.

Wolfson, L., Whipple, R., Amerman, P., & Tobin, J.N. (1990). Gait assessment in the elderly: A gait abnormality rating scale and its relation to falls. *Journal of Gerontology*, 45: M12-M19.

Wolfson, L., Whipple, R., Judge, J., Amerman, P., Derby, C., & King, M. (1993). Training balance and strength in the elderly to improve function. *Journal of the American Geriatric Society*, 41: 341-343.

Wolfson, L., Whipple, R., Derby, C., Judge, J., King, M., Amerman, P., Schmidt, L., & Smyers, D. (1996). Balance and strength training in older adults: Intervention gains and T'ai Chi maintenance. *Journal of the American Geriatrics Society*, 44: 498-506.

Wrisberg, C.A., & Lui, Z. (1991). The effect of contextual variety on the practice, retention, and transfer of an applied motor skill. *Research Quarterly for Exercise and Sport*, 62: 406-412.

Yaffe, K., Barnes, D., Nevitt, M., Lui, L.Y. , & Covinski, K. (2001). A prospective study of physical activity and cognitive decline in elderly women: Women who walk. *Archives of Internal Medicine*, 161: 1703-1708.

Yelin, E. & Felts, W. (1990). A summary of the impact of the musculoskeletal conditions in the United States. *Arthritis Rheumatology*, 33: 750-755.

AUTHOR INDEX

A

Akima, H. 194
Alexander, N. 15, 182
Allison, L. 65
Aloia, J.F. 194
American College of Sports Medicine 194, 219
American Heart Association 33-34
Amerman, P. 14, 17, 140
Anderson, S.K 34
Ashton-Miller, J.A. 182
Asp, K. 218

B

Baker, D.I. 42
Baldwin, M. 10, 17
Bamman, M.M. 194
Bandy, W.D. 218
Barnes, D. 16
Basmajian, J.V. 4
Beg, M.F. 15
Bell, R. 218
Berg, K. 55
Berg, K.S. 65, 73-76, 76t
Berlin, J. 218
Berthoz, A. 181
Black, D. 12
Bohannon, R.W. 80t
Bories, T. 17, 82
Borrie, M.J. 40
Branch, L.G. 218
Brandt, K.D. 34
Buchner, D.M. 17

Burke, D.T. 15
Burns, R. 34

C

Campbell, A.J. 30, 40
Capezuti, E. 31f, 31t, 32f, 32t
Cavazos, R. 248
Center for Successful Aging, The 18f-20f, 22f-24f, 51-54, 79, 83-85
Chandler, J. 50, 62
Chen, H.C. 182
Clark, S. 17
Colby, L.A. 35
Colliver, J. 182
Cornoni-Huntley, J.C. 218
Cost, T.W. 40
Covinski, K. 16
Cumming, R.G. 40
Cummings, S.R. 12

D

Danneskiold-Samsoe, B. 34
Daschle 72
Day, L. 30
De Luca, C.J. 4, 15
Derby, C. 14, 17, 140
Deyle, G.D. 34
Di Pietro, L. 50
Diener, H.C. 39
DiFabio, R.P. 15
Domingues, D.A. 248
Doucette, J.T. 42

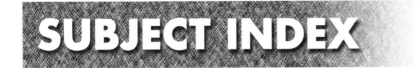

SUBJECT INDEX

Note: The italicized *f* or *t* following a page number denote a figure or table on that page, respectfully. The italicized *ff* or *tt* following a page number denotes multiple figures or tables on that page.

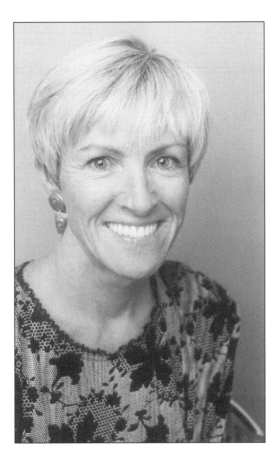

Debra Rose, PhD, is a professor in the division of kinesiology and health promotion and co-director of the Center for Successful Aging at California State University at Fullerton. She is also a professor in the physical therapy department at Chapman University at Orange, California. Her primary research focus is on the enhancement of mobility and the prevention of falls in later years.

Dr. Rose is nationally and internationally recognized for her work in fall risk reduction assessment and programming. Her research in fall risk reduction in the elderly has been published in numerous peer-reviewed publications, including the *Journal of the American Geriatric Society, Archives of Physical Medicine and Rehabilitation, Neurology Report,* and the *Journal of Aging and Physical Activity.* The innovative fall risk reduction program she developed and describes in this manual was recognized by the National Council on Aging as one of seven meritorious programs nationwide that promotes a healthy, active lifestyle. She is a fellow of the Research Consortium of AAPHERD, former executive board member of the North American Society for the Psychology of Sport and Physical Activity, and coeditor of the *Journal of Aging and Physical Activity.*